Systems Approaches to
Developmental Neurobiology

NATO ASI Series

Advanced Science Institutes Series

A series presenting the results of activities sponsored by the NATO Science Committee, which aims at the dissemination of advanced scientific and technological knowledge, with a view to strengthening links between scientific communities.

The series is published by an international board of publishers in conjunction with the NATO Scientific Affairs Division

A	**Life Sciences**	Plenum Publishing Corporation
B	**Physics**	New York and London
C	**Mathematical**	Kluwer Academic Publishers
	and Physical Sciences	Dordrecht, Boston, and London
D	**Behavioral and Social Sciences**	
E	**Applied Sciences**	
F	**Computer and Systems Sciences**	Springer-Verlag
G	**Ecological Sciences**	Berlin, Heidelberg, New York, London,
H	**Cell Biology**	Paris, and Tokyo

Recent Volumes in this Series

Series A: Life Sciences

Systems Approaches to Developmental Neurobiology

Edited by

Pamela A. Raymond

University of Michigan
Ann Arbor, Michigan

Stephen S. Easter, Jr.

University of Michigan
Ann Arbor, Michigan

and

Giorgio M. Innocenti

Institute of Anatomy
Lausanne, Switzerland

Plenum Press
New York and London
Published in cooperation with NATO Scientific Affairs Division

Proceedings of a NATO Advanced Study Institute on
Systems Approaches to Developmental Neurobiology,
held June 1-14, 1989,
in Varenna, Italy

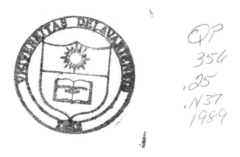

QP
356
.25
.N37
1989

Library of Congress Cataloging-in-Publication Data

NATO Advanced Study Institute on Systems Approaches to Developmental
  Neurobiology (1989 : Varenna, Italy)
    Systems approaches to developmental neurobiology / edited by
  Pamela A. Raymond, Stephen S. Easter, Jr., and Giorgio M. Innicenti.
      p.   cm. -- (NATO ASI series. Series A, Life sciences ; vol.
  192)
    "Proceedings of a NATO Advanced Study Institute on Systems
  Approaches to Developmental Neurobiology, held June 1-14, 1989, in
  Varenna, Italy"--T.p. verso.
    "Published in cooperation with NATO Scientific Affairs Division."
    Includes bibliographical references and index.
    ISBN 0-306-43594-2
    1. Developmental neurophysiology--Congresses.   I. Raymond, Pamela
  A. II. Easter, Stephen S. III. Innocenti, Giorgio M. IV. North
  Atlantic Treaty Organization. Scientific Affairs Division.
  V. Title. VI. Series: NATO ASI series. Series A, Life sciences ;
  v. 192.
  QP356.25.N37 1989
  591.1'8--dc20   90-7333
                                                          CIP

© 1990 Plenum Press, New York
A Division of Plenum Publishing Corporation
233 Spring Street, New York, N.Y. 10013

Printed in the United States of America

PREFACE

It is appropriate at the outset of this book to pose a question that was often asked -- of the organizers before the meeting took place and later among those who participated in the meeting -- "What is meant by 'Systems Approaches' in the study of developmental neurobiology?" The answer, as we originally conceived it, can be succinctly summarized by the word "interactions". That brief epithet was expanded during the general discussion portion of the meeting, where the following definition was offered:

"Systems approaches in developmental neurobiology are unified by attention to the emergent properties of the developing system under investigation and by a focus on the aspects of development of the nervous system that depend on interactions among its various elements, be they molecular, intracellular or multicellular."

As opposed to ignoring complexity or trying to wish it away, those of us who utilize a systems approach embrace the principle that complexity is what makes the nervous system special. We have come to recognize that wherever we look, we find interactions which are to be probed and eventually understood. Even the so-called "simple systems", a term that has been used to describe many invertebrate preparations, are embraced under the above definition, since with further study it is becoming increasing clear that such systems are not as simple as once thought. We also include molecular genetics under the systems rubric. After all, genes regulate other genes which regulate others, and so it goes.

After examining the list of chapter titles and contributors included in this book a cynical observer might conclude that we used the term "Systems Approaches" as a catch-all, a flimsy umbrella, to allow us to invite a rather eclectic group of hand-picked colleagues who might otherwise be difficult to lump together into a single NATO-Advanced Study Institute. The cynic might also note that the term has a refreshing ring to it, a pleasant change from the over-used "Cell and Molecular" descriptor, and he might be aware that this aspect of novelty is not without merit in the competitive world of grantsmanship. We must confess that these crasser considerations did in fact play a role in our initial planning and choice of topic. However, the underlying validity of the scientific premise stated above -- when one is interested in interactions one is by definition using a systems approach -- was clearly substantiated during the course of the meeting. The participants were drawn from fields as disparate as molecular biology, behavior, and computer modeling, and their technical expertise was as varied as their native tongues, but in a surprising number of cases, common ideas and principles emerged. We hope the essence of these communications, the "emergent features" of this scientific interchange, if you will, have been captured in this volume.

The structure of this Advanced Study Institute was by design different from most meetings, and a brief summary of the organization is warranted here so that the reader can appreciate the organization of this book. There were 15 "Lecturers", each of whom was given a two-hour slot in which to deliver a formal presentation. One of the other lecturers was assigned as the "Discussant", whose task was to lead the one-hour discussion period that followed. Selected questions of special interest or obvious significance have been incorporated into the text of each chapter. Each question posed and the Lecturer's response is enclosed by horizontal lines to set it apart from the main body of the discourse. It was our hope that by including these exchanges in the written report, we would convey to the reader a sense of the interactive ambience that pervaded the meeting. Additional opportunities for interaction were provided by poster displays. All participants were encouraged to bring a poster (most did), and these were viewed and discussed during several evening sessions. Abstracts of the posters presented are collected at the end of this volume.

The last half-day session of the meeting was devoted to a general discussion, in which the participants and lecturers broke into smaller subgroups and distributed themselves among four topics that the group as a whole had identified as major, recurring themes. The topics were: evolution and species differences, axon pathfinding, juvenile/adult plasticity, and competition. We then met once more as a body, and each subgroup presented a report of their discussion. Following is a very brief synopsis of what was said.

EVOLUTION AND SPECIES DIFFERENCES

Evolution is development. Evolution is no more than the cumulative ontogeny of many individuals over the epochs. Therefore, both evolution and development address the fundamental origins of life biology. The process of evolution of the nervous system, like all other parts of the organism, involves a concatenated series of slight modifications of what is already there. The theme of evolution ran as an undercurrent through many of the talks, and it was explicitly addressed in one lecture (Marois and Meinertzhagen, 1990, this volume) and in an impromptu chalk-talk by Ghysen. From studies of the phyletic diversity and the ontogenetic history of neural organization has come the growing awareness that the nervous system is built on a simple orthogonal pattern of connectives and commissures (Blagburn and Bacon, Ross and Easter, 1990, this volume) that form a scaffolding upon which more complex networks, such as the mammalian cortex (Kind and Innocenti, Shulz and Frégnac, 1990, this volume), are built by processes that include both addition and deletion. Similarly, morphologically complex synaptic structures, which by inference convey enhanced functional abilities, appear to have evolved from the sequential addition or modification of pre-existing units (LaMantia, Marois and Meinertzhagen, 1990, this volume). Common principles may govern cell determination (Ruiz-Gómez, Jimenez and Campos-Ortega, Braisted and Raymond, Metcalfe and Westerfield, 1990, this volume) and segmentation (Ruiz-Gómez, Metcalfe and Westerfield, 1990, this volume) between vertebrates and invertebrates.

Not all of those present were convinced of the usefulness of studying evolution, however, and this prompted a lively discussion. For one used to designing experiments it is frustrating not to be able to manipulate phylogeny. Nevertheless, the point was made that an awareness of the building-block process of evolution and the links between ontogeny and phylogeny may provide insights that will prove helpful in gaining a better understanding of how the nervous system develops.

AXONAL PATHFINDING

Many of the chapters address this topic, which is *au courant* in developmental neurobiology. The discussion focused on three principles governing axonal outgrowth:

Substrates. These mediate the "stick and let go" of axon growth. Guidance by the substrate can be a facilitatory or an inhibitory phenomenon (Allsopp and Bonhoeffer, 1990, this volume). The question of how axons know which way to grow has not been resolved, but an enthusiastic search for polarity cues continues (Taylor and Gaze, Hankin and Lund, Gaspar and Sotelo, 1990, this volume). The role of chemotactic factors released by the target is another area of hot pursuit (Hankin and Lund, 1990, this volume).

Guidepost cells. These special features of the cellular environment through which an axon grows have been documented in invertebrates, where they appear to play a significant role in directing the growing axon, thereby establishing the basic architecture of axon pathways. Experimental studies in which guidepost cells have been ablated have given contradictory results, so just how important the guidepost cells are remains unclear, as does the issue of whether there are homologues in vertebrates.

Pioneer fibers. These are the first axons that grow out, thereby establishing the future pathways over which later cohorts of axons will travel. The first axons that colonize virgin territory (the pioneers) must be responding to exogenous guidance cues, whereas those that follow have the much easier task of fasciculating with their predecessors. Although the concept of pioneer neurons was first developed in invertebrates (Blagburn and Bacon, 1990, this volume), recent work suggests that it is valid for vertebrates, too (Ross and Easter, Metcalfe and Westerfield, 1990, this volume).

The usual models for studying axonal guidance have all involved axons that travel long distances (e.g. the retinotectal system, Taylor and Gaze, Hankin and Lund, 1990, this volume). What about short distance axons involved in generating the complex organization of the synaptic neuropil? What cues guide growth of those processes? Essentially nothing is known about this important aspect of axonal outgrowth, and it is not clear how it can be addressed experimentally in a meaningful way.

JUVENILE/ADULT PLASTICITY

The issue that consumed the participants in this discussion was the principle of critical periods. What is a "critical period"? The definition may vary from one system to another (Marois and Meinertzhagen, Stanford and Sherman, Shulz and Frégnac, 1990, this volume). With regard to the mammalian visual cortex, where the volume of work on critical periods justifies designating it as the archetype, two types of critical period have been recognized:

1. The developmental period during which the cortex can adapt to the environment.
2. The period during which environmental features are necessary for normal development.

Questions related to evolution were also posed. How did critical periods evolve? They have not been seen in phylogenetically old systems, although perhaps no one has looked carefully enough. What is the purpose of a critical period? If it conveys some advantage, why does it end?

COMPETITION

Here again, there was a struggle to come up with a meaningful and consistent definition. There were many opinions, including:

1. Elements searching to obtain limited resources.
2. An interaction among axonal or dendritic processes to establish a balance in the parcellation of territory and/or an optimal axonal or dendritic size.

Another issue was the question of what the neurons are competing for. Again, several alternatives were suggested, including trophic factors, postsynaptic "space", presynaptic inputs, and economical representation in the target field. Although the term "competition" is heavily used, and the principle has been demonstrated in several different systems, the underlying meaning and mechanisms are proving difficult to pin down. This has not dissuaded many from continuing their efforts, however, and several of the chapters dealt with competitive phenomena (Kind and Innocenti, Stanford and Sherman, Shulz and Frégnac, 1990, this volume).

Finally, a word on authorship of the chapters. Each Lecturer selected in advance a Scribe, whose job was to take notes during the lecture and discussion, then to produce a manuscript. In some cases the Scribe was a colleague and associate of the Lecturer, and the work the Lecturer described was in part attributable to the Scribe. In other instances, the Scribe had not participated in the work, and played the role of a reporter only. Lecturers all had the opportunity to comment on the manuscript produced by the Scribe, and some played a more active role in the actual writing. Therefore, the issue of authorship has been left up to each Lecturer/Scribe team, with the general stipulation that if both are to be authors, the Scribe is first author. In some cases, the Lecturer chose not to be an author. A footnote on the title page of each chapter indicates the authorship for the purpose of citation.

October, 1989

P.A. Raymond
S.S. Easter, Jr.
G.M. Innocenti

CONTENTS

NEURAL DEVELOPMENT IN INSECTS: NEURON BIRTH, PATHFINDING, SYNAPTOGENESIS, COMPETITION [*]

Jonathan M. Blagburn (scribe)

Institute of Neurobiology and Department of Physiology
University of Puerto Rico Medical Sciences Campus
Old San Juan, Puerto Rico, USA

Jonathan P. Bacon (lecturer)

School of Biological Sciences
University of Sussex
Falmer, Brighton, UK

This lecture provides an introduction to the development of the insect nervous system. Insect nervous systems are particularly useful for investigating the cellular and molecular mechanisms which give rise to neuronal specificity, because they are made up of relatively small numbers of neurons, many of which can be reliably identified as individuals. The first sections deal with the development of the CNS, focussing on how the pattern of neuroblasts and their progeny of identified neurons is set up, and the way in which axons fasciculate in the initial orthogonal array of axon tracts. The next section examines genetic studies of synapse formation between identifed neurons. The last, and longest, sections address the development of the sensory neurons of the insect's peripheral nervous system (PNS), and its usefulness as a model system for studying the rules by which sensory axons grow into the CNS, and establish and modify synaptic connections in the CNS.

ESTABLISHMENT OF NEURONAL IDENTITY

The basic pattern of the arthropod CNS consists of a chain of cephalic, thoracic and abdominal ganglia; the three thoracic ganglia contain approximately 2000 neurons each, and the abdominal ganglia, about 500 (Thomas et al., 1984). Many studies have utilized Orthopteroid insects (locusts, grasshoppers, crickets and cockroaches) because their large, individually identifiable neurons permit a detailed cellular analysis of developmental events. The powerful techniques of molecular genetics can more easily be applied to the Dipteran, *Drosophila melanogaster*, allowing a molecular analysis of neuronal development. Despite the fact that Orthoptera and Diptera are not closely related phylogenetically, the pattern of neuroblasts in each segment, and even the stereotyped way in which identified neurons extend their axons and form the basic tracts and commissures of the CNS, appear to have been conserved throughout the 300 million years during which the various groups have diverged (Thomas et al., 1984). The existence of a common developmental plan has recently been corroborated at the molecular level by the finding that homologous genes are expressed in the developing nervous systems of both locust and *Drosophila* (Zinn et al., 1988).

The insect CNS develops from a sheet of neuroectodermal cells running along the ventral surface of the embryo. There are two steps in this process: first, ectoderm cells enlarge into neuroblasts (NBs); second, each NB generates a specific family of neurons. Out of approximately 150 undifferentiated neuroectoderm cells per hemisegment, 25 - 30 enlarge to become NBs, while others form epidermal cells and the less numerous midline precursors, glial precursors, or the neuroblast support cells (Doe et al., 1985). The pattern in which these cells develop is repeated (with minor variations) from segment to segment. The neuronal precursors can be identified not only according to

---

[*] This chapter to be cited as: Blagburn, J. M., and Bacon, J. P., 1990, Neural development in insects: neuron birth, pathfinding, synaptogenesis, competition, in: "Systems Approaches to Developmental Neurobiology," P. A. Raymond, S. S. Easter, Jr., and G. M. Innocenti, eds., Plenum Press, New York.

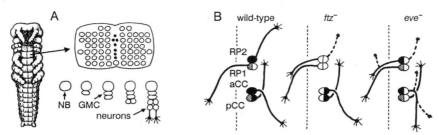

Fig. 1. A. Drawing of a grasshopper embryo (ventral view) at 32% of embryogenesis, showing the metameric arrangement of cephalic, three thoracic, and eleven abdominal segments. A diagrammatic representation of the neuroepithelium of the prothoracic segment, showing the characteristic pattern of neuroblasts (open circles) and midline precursors (filled, small circles). Below is shown the temporal sequence (left to right) of the production of neuroblast progeny (NB, neuroblast; GMC, ganglion mother cell). B. Cartoon of the RP1, RP2, aCC and pCC neurons, in normal embryos, embryos without neural *ftz* expression *(ftz⁻)*, and embryos without functional *eve* protein *(eve⁻)*. The relative strength of gene expression is indicated by the shading of the neuron cell body: the left half represents *ftz* expression and the right half, the presence or absence of functional *eve* protein. Black indicates a high level of expression, hatching a low level. The solid axons represent the most frequent pattern of growth, while broken lines indicate other pathways taken by the axon. The vertical dotted lines indicate the midlines of the embryos. (Based on results in Doe et al., 1988 a, b.)

their position within the array, but also according to the family of identified neurons which they generate. Each neuroblast divides asymmetrically to form a chain of ganglion mother cells (GMCs) which in turn divide once to form families of neurons (Fig. 1A). Midline precursors divide once only, to form two neurons each, while the glial precursors form a family of glial cells which migrate through the segment (Doe and Goodman, 1985).

The identity of a neuroblast appears to be determined by the position in the array in which it enlarges. Prior to this, any one of a cluster of undifferentiated neuroectoderm cells is capable of becoming the NB, but only one of them does so. Cell interactions then prevent neighbouring cells from differentiating into NBs. Laser ablation experiments in grasshoppers have shown that neuroectoderm cells are pluripotent; i.e., cells within a cluster can regulate for a missing NB, and furthermore, if a whole cell cluster is ablated, nearby neuroectoderm cells (that would normally differentiate into other neuroblasts) can differentiate into the missing NB (Doe and Goodman, 1985). Transplantation experiments in *Drosophila* also indicate that interactions take place between neuroectoderm cells during early neurogenesis, and analysis of mutants in which overproduction of neurons occurs has provided an insight into the molecular basis of these interactions (Jimenez and Campos-Ortega, 1990, this volume).

Neuroectodermal cells can regulate for missing near neighbors, but over a longer range, are neuroectoderm cells determined to produce anterior or posterior NBs before they differentiate?

"Determination" is an operational term that depends on transplantation (Slack, 1983). To answer this question, therefore, it would be neccessary to carry out the technically very difficult experiment of removing ectodermal cells from one end of a segment, and transplanting them to the other end, and then determining the identity of the NBs which they produced. It is not known if a neuroectoderm cell from the posterior region of a segment would be capable of forming an anterior NB if transplanted to an anterior position.

The identity of a neuron appears to be determined firstly by its lineage, and secondly by interactions with its sibling. Thus a particular mitotic division of a NB will always produce the same ganglion mother cell. The daughters of that GMC are born equivalent and their respective fates are determined by cell interactions, with one fate preferred and dominant over the other (Kuwada and Goodman, 1985). Recent evidence suggests that one way in which *Drosophila* neurons assume their characteristic fates is via transcription of segmentation genes.

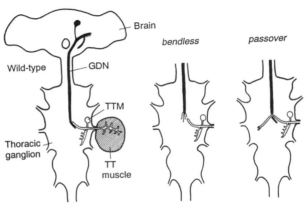

Fig. 2. Cartoons of the *Drosophila* escape system in the wild-type (left), *bendless* (center) and *passover* (right) mutants. The giant descending neuron (GDN) sends an axon from the brain to the thoracic ganglion, where it normally forms an electrical synapse with the tergotrochanteral motoneuron (TTM). The latter innervates the tergotrochanteral (TT) muscle which extends the leg. In the mutants, the GDN - TTM synapse is absent, possibly due to disruption in the system by which the neurons recognize each other. (Based on results in Thomas and Wyman, 1983.)

CONTROL OF NEURONAL FATE BY SEGMENTATION GENES

Segmentation genes are transcribed in the early embryo, and their products delineate progressively finer subdivisions of the embryo. The first to be transcribed are the gap genes (for example, *Krüppel* and *hunchback*), then the pair-rule genes, such as *even-skipped (eve)* and *fushi tarazu (ftz)* which are expressed in alternate parasegments, and finally the segment polarity genes, such as *engrailed (en)* which is expressed in 14 blastoderm stripes, a few cells wide. With segment number and polarity established, the expression of homeotic selector genes, such as *Ultrabithorax (Ubx)*, then determines segment identity (Akam, 1987).

After playing their cardinal role in blastoderm pattern formation, many segmentation genes are again expressed transiently later in development, in the embryonic CNS. However, the pattern of CNS expression is not merely an inheritance of the blastoderm pattern. For example, the *ftz* gene is first expressed in 7 blastoderm stripes, in alternate parasegments, but later is expressed in small, segmentally repeated sets of GMCs, neurons and glial precursor cells (but not neuroblasts). The patterns of *ftz* and *eve* expression have been examined in detail in two pairs of sibling neurons, aCC and pCC, and RP1 and RP2. Both aCC and RP2 express *ftz* strongly, but pCC and RP1 express the gene weakly. The aCC and pCC express *eve* strongly, as does RP2, but *eve* protein is absent from RP1 (Fig. 1B; Doe et al., 1988a).

It is difficult to examine these neurons in embryos homozygous for a *ftz* null allele because segmentation and subsequent development of the nervous system is severely disrupted. Fortunately, the *ftz* gene contains separate control elements for expression of the striped blastoderm pattern and for the later expression in the CNS. This enabled the neurogenic element to be deleted, and transformant mutant lines were made which express *ftz* normally in the blastoderm and so establish a normal segmentation pattern, but do not express *ftz* in the CNS. In such *ftz*⁻ embryos, aCC, pCC and RP1 are all normal (judged by the criterion of axon morphology) but the RP2 axon, instead of extending anteriorly and then laterally to follow the intersegmental nerve, follows the RP1 axon. RP2 sometimes also extends a second axon anteriorly. In the *ftz*⁻ mutants, RP2 also fails to express *eve* (Fig. 1B). In the absence of ftz, RP2 behaves similarly to its sibling, RP1, in terms of axon path and lack of *eve* expression (Doe et al., 1988a).

As with *ftz*, it is not possible to study the CNS of embryos with no *eve* expression because of the disruption of segment formation. The existence of a temperature-sensitive allele of *eve* permitted *eve* function to be disrupted in the CNS after the embryos were raised at a temperature which permitted normal blastoderm pattern formation. RP2 is also abnormal in these *eve*⁻ embryos, even though *ftz* expression is normal. In the absence of functional *eve* protein aCC axon morphology is aberrant whereas the pCC axon is normal (Fig. 1B; Doe et al., 1988b). It seems reasonable to

3

conclude that ftz is required for the activation of eve expression in RP2 (but not in other neurons such as aCC) and that *eve* product is involved in the control of RP2 axon morphology.

AXONAL PATHFINDING

The growth cones of developing neurons navigate their way through the tangle of the developing nervous system by fasciculating selectively with other neurons in a carefully orchestrated temporal sequence (the "labelled pathways hypothesis" (Raper et al., 1983)). In this way, quite complex axon morphologies can be built by sequentially following orthogonally arranged axon tracts that have been laid down earlier by other neurons.

A family of surface glycoproteins has been found in grasshopper and/or *Drosophila* that appear to be involved in selective axonal fasciculation, namely, the proteins fasciclin I, II and III (Bastiani et al., 1987; Patel et al., 1987; Zinn et al., 1988). At least one of these molecules, fasciclin II, is homologous and analogous to the axonal glycoproteins such as N-CAM and L1 which are found in vertebrates (Harrelson and Goodman, 1988). Antibodies to the fasciclins show that they are expressed on different but overlapping subsets of axon bundles; in locust some axons transiently express fasciclin I within the commissures but then express fasciclin II in the longitudinal pathways. In *Drosophila*, fasciclin III is expressed on a subset of axons in the commissures and the intersegmental nerve, and the axon of RP1 stains strongly for the protein while the RP2 axon shows no staining (Patel et al., 1987). A possible explanation for the aberrant pathway choice by the RP2 axon in the absence of functional *eve* protein (see above) is that *eve* may normally suppress the expression of the fasciclin III gene. In its absence, both RP1 and RP2 may express fasciclin III, causing them to fasciculate together.

Deleting the *Drosophila* fasciclin III gene causes some disruption in the developing CNS, including broader (less tightly fasciculated) commissures, and abnormalities in the trajectory of the RP1 axon (Jacobs et al., 1987). Blocking fasciclin II molecules with antibody partially interferes with the ability of an identified grasshopper neuron, MP1, to recognize and selectively fasciculate with a longitudinal axon pathway (Harrelson and Goodman, 1988). The fact that axonal growth is not as drastically affected as when individual pathway neurons are laser-ablated (Raper et al., 1984), suggests that there are several adhesion or recognition molecules which serve to "label" a particular pathway, so that blocking only one of them causes little disruption.

SYNAPTIC RECOGNITION

Having navigated to the appropriate region of the developing CNS, neurons must then recognize their correct synaptic partners. Less is known about this aspect of neuronal specificity, although it is possible that recognition between potential synaptic partners may be a process similar to selective fasciculation of axons. One approach to investigating synaptic recognition mechanisms is to isolate *Drosophila* mutants in which pairs of identified neurons fail to make synaptic connections.

The largest neurons in the *Drosophila* CNS are those which make up the escape system, and these are present also in larger Diptera (Thomas and Wyman, 1983; Bacon and Strausfeld, 1986). The giant descending neuron (GDN, also known as GF) conveys visual and mechanosensory information from the brain to the fused thoracic ganglia, where it forms (among other connections) an electrical synapse with the tergotrochanteral motoneuron (TTM) of the midleg extensor muscle (Fig. 2). Thus the fly is able to jump away rapidly at the approach of a predator. It is relatively simple to assay for the presence of escape system mutants in mutagenized *Drosophila*. Two mutants (*bendless* and *passover*) were isolated because of their inability to escape in response to a visual stimulus. In these animals the latency between GDN and TTM spikes is 2.2 ms, instead of the normal 0.8 ms, suggesting that the electrical synapse between the neurons fails to develop normally.

In the wild type animal the GDN exhibits a characteristic bend at the end of the axon where it contacts the TTM. In *bendless (ben)* mutants, the GDN bend is missing and the axon does not contact the TTM, but instead sometimes forms filopodia-like extensions as though searching for its postsynaptic target (Fig.2). In the *passover (pass)* mutants, the GDN anatomy appears normal but the TTM continues growing on past the ganglion midline, as though failing to recognize and therefore failing to synapse with GDN (Fig. 2). It seems that both these mutations affect the recognition system between the two cells at the time during pupal development when synaptogenesis between these cells would normally occur (Thomas and Wyman, 1983). The *ben* and *pass* genes are currently being cloned.

4

Could the changes in the GDN-TTM synapse in these mutants simply be due to the presence of barriers to growth which prevent the GDN and TTM from reaching each other?

It will be important to eliminate possible explanations for the lack of connectivity, such as the existence of barriers, by studying the development of this synapse in the pupa, or by creating mosaic animals in which a mutant neuron grows into a normal ganglion. It is interesting to note that in these mutants many defects occur throughout the nervous system, implying that the putative recognition molecules which are used in the formation of the escape system are also used in the development of other neuronal circuits.

THE CERCAL SENSORY SYSTEM

The development of the insect peripheral nervous system is physically separate from that of the CNS. Individual epidermal cells undergo two mitotic divisions to produce a clonally-related group of 4 cells which then differentiate into the various components of a sense organ or sensillum. The determination of the positions of these sensilla is dealt with in detail by Ruiz-Gómez (1990, this volume). The 4 cells differentiate into a sensory neuron, a sheath cell which wraps the neuron, a cell which secretes the hair or bristle (trichogen) and a cell which secretes the socket (tormogen). The axons of sensory neurons grow towards the CNS, usually following the pioneer axons which, together with motoneurons, establish the pattern of the peripheral nerves at an early stage when the distances from the periphery to the CNS are short.

The cercal sensory system of Orthopteroid insects, in particular the cricket, *Acheta domesticus*, and the cockroach, *Periplaneta americana*, has become a popular model system for studying questions relating to synapse formation and synaptic plasticity, because both the pre- and postsynaptic cells are identifiable and amenable to anatomical and physiological study. The cerci, conical appendages on the caudal end of the animal, bear long, thin (filiform) hairs, innervated by single sensory neurons which send axons to the terminal abdominal ganglion, where they arborize and form synapses. A filiform hair is free to move in response to air movements, but its elliptical socket imposes on it a single plane of movement. However, the underlying sensory neuron is excited by hair movement in only one direction. In the cricket, there are two major planes of hair movement, and thus 4 main classes of receptor, each of which is sensitive to a different wind direction. These 4 receptor types are segregated according to their circumferential position of the cercus, for example, transversely-mobile hairs (T hairs) are found on the dorsal and ventral aspects of the cercus, while longitudinally-mobile hairs (L hairs) are situated on the medial and lateral aspects. Within these regions are strips of sensilla with different directions of excitation (Bacon and Murphey, 1984). The projections of the sensory neurons within the terminal ganglion were revealed by staining single cells with cobalt chloride, by placing a Co^{++}-filled micropipette over cut hairs. It was found that a kind of "cercotopic" projection of hair afferents exists within a defined region of neuropil of the terminal ganglion, the so-called cercal glomerulus. Each physiological receptor type arborizes in a different region of the glomerulus, thus dividing the neuropil functionally, according to wind direction (Fig. 3A).

Within the terminal ganglion of crickets and cockroaches are a set of interneurons often termed "giant interneurons" (GIs) because of the large diameter and length of their axons. These neurons form dendritic arborizations within the terminal ganglion and some of them receive monosynaptic input from the cercal sensory axons (Shepherd and Murphey, 1986; Blagburn, 1989). The GI axons extend up the nerve cord to the thoracic ganglia where they excite interneurons, and in turn, leg motoneurons, thus triggering the animal's escape response. In crickets, the projection of a GI's dendritic branches within the cercal glomerulus is correlated with the synaptic inputs it receives from the wind afferents, and thus with its directional sensitivity (Bacon and Murphey, 1984).

Cross-species transplantation experiments have shown that the cercal receptor cells are programmed according to the position at which they arise on the cercal circumference. This positional information appears to determine the plane of hair movement, the directionality of the sensory neuron, and also guides formation of synaptic contacts with the correct set of interneurons (Kämper and Murphey, 1987). In some of these transplants cercal axons enter the terminal ganglion via the wrong nerve yet still arborize in the correct region of neuropil, thus ruling out the possibility that they simply follow their neighbors within the cercal nerve to the correct destination. Also, the results of these experiments are inconsistent with the hypothesis that the temporal order in which the axons grow into

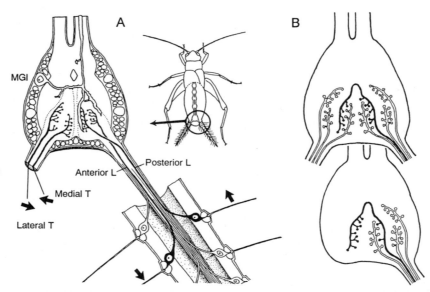

Fig. 3. A. The cricket cercal - to - giant system. A cricket is shown with the abdominal CNS exposed. The main panel is a horizontal section of the terminal abdominal ganglion showing the projections of the four types of afferents as well as one interneuron, MGI. Note that the posterior L afferent is in contact with the MGI, but the anterior L afferent is not. Arrows indicate the major excitatory wind direction of each of the 4 receptor types. B. The axon of the X neuron (shown in black) before (upper) and after (lower) deafferentation. Removal of afferents from the left side of the ganglion results in the redistribution of the arborization of X to the deafferented side. (Based on results in Bacon and Murphey, 1984; Murphey, 1986.)

the terminal ganglion determines their synaptic connectivity. There is no evidence for the existence of gradients of diffusible molecules in this system. Instead, the available experimental evidence supports the idea that the axons are guided by cell surface labels to the appropriate areas.

PLASTICITY OF INSECT SYNAPSES

Despite the apparent "simplicity" of these systems, insect synaptic connections are not entirely genetically hard-wired; they also depend upon interactions between neurons during development. In the cricket, a small number (25 out of 1000) of filiform hair afferents, the "X neurons", cross the midline and synapse with GI dendrites in both cercal glomeruli (Fig. 3B). Counts of the number of putative synaptic boutons showed that normally the arborization of the X neuron is more or less equally distributed on either side of the midline. Unilateral cercotomy removes approximately 90 - 95% of the X neuron's contralateral neighboring axons within the defined region of glomerulus to which the X neuron is restricted, whereas only 5 - 10% of the ipsilateral neighbors are removed. It was found that the X neuron shifted boutons from the afferented to the deafferented side of the ganglion, in which the number of neighboring axons was greatly reduced (Murphey and Lemere, 1984). Quantal analysis of EPSPs in the medial GI supports the idea that the number of X neuron synapses is increased on the deafferented side (Shepherd and Murphey, 1986).

The X neurons responded most effectively to cercotomy when it was carried out at early stages, when the rate of growth of the arborizations is normally at its fastest (Murphey, 1986). It is interesting to note that (1) the X neuron arborization retained its position within the neuropil, and did not sprout into other deafferented regions; and (2) that the total size of the arborization appears to be intrinsically limited. These results demonstrate that interactions between afferent axons regulate the number of synaptic contacts that they can form with postsynaptic cells. It is possible that these axons are competing for a limited resource, such as postsynaptic sites on the target interneurons.

In some respects this is not such a simple system - it is more complex than the vertebrate autonomic ganglion or neuromuscular junction, where the neurons are able to make 4 or 5 times more synapses in the absence of competitors. Do you think the X neurons might not be so constrained in the size of their arborizations, if it were possible to denervate totally, as with the neuromuscular junction?

Even though total denervation of one cercal glomerulus is not possible, because there may be inputs from noncercal sensory afferents or presynaptic interneurons, cercotomy does produce a major reduction in afferentation which should allow the X neurons to expand their arbors if they were capable of doing so. In fact, deafferentation before the X neuron is born sometimes allows it to extend an extra branch into an "incorrect" region of the glomerulus, but even in this case there is no overall increase in the total size of these X neurons (Murphey, 1986). There does in fact seem to be more constraint on the total size of the X neuron arbor than on the arbors of vertebrate motoneurons or preganglionic neurons.

A simpler system, at least in terms of the number of presynaptic axons, is that found in the first instar cockroach (Blagburn and Beadle, 1982). In the newly-hatched nymph there are only two filiform hairs on each cercus, yet the 4 hairs allow the animal to perform its escape response with as great a directional sensitivity as the adult cockroach with its 440 hairs (Dagan and Volman, 1982). The afferents, termed the lateral (L) and medial (M) because of their positions on the cercus, arborize within non-overlapping regions of the cercal glomerulus and synapse onto giant interneurons which are analogous to those in the cricket. The patterns of connections between the filiform afferents and GIs are highly stereotyped from animal to animal. For example, GI3 always receives strong synaptic input from the L afferent, while GI2 receives input only from the M afferent (Blagburn, 1989).

As an alternative to surgical manipulation, mutants can be sought where the normal pattern of sensory projection is altered. In routine studies of the cockroach (Bacon and Blagburn, 1989), first instar animals were discovered which bore one extra filiform hair sensillum on one or both of their cerci, thus representing a dramatic 50% increase in the number of afferents to the cercal glomerulus. The most common mutant phenotype, termed "Space Invader" (SI) had a supernumerary hair in the same circumferential plane as the L hair, but located more proximally. These mutants animals represent approximately 2% of the inbred laboratory colony. By selecting and crossing such animals, F1, F2 and F3 populations have been produced, in which the occurrence is increased to, respectively, 11%, 24% and 36%, thus indicating a genetic basis to the phenomenon. The probabilities of the supernumerary hair arising on the left or the right cercus are equal.

Is the appearance of the supernumerary sensillum dependent on the size of the cercus? If the embryonic cercus were larger, epidermal cells might be released from inhibition by the existing sense organs, and be free to differentiate into extra sensilla.

We considered this, but in fact quantitative measurements of wild-type and SI cerci show that there is no difference in size. The possibility that the SI hair might be a prematurely- differentiating second instar hair was also considered, but in fact the supernumerary sensillum can be identified on second instar cerci.

The SI hair is innervated by its own neuron, called the SIN, which sends its axon to the cercal glomerulus. The SIN axon is similar in appearance to the L afferent, although it is thinner and makes a more sparse arborization, and it arborizes in the same region of glomerulus as the L axon. Hence the name Space Invader - the supernumerary invades the space occupied by the L axon. Electrophysiological recording shows that, like the L axon, the SIN synapses with GI3 and not GI2. The SIN EPSPs are smaller than those from the normal afferent, which is consistent with its more sparse arborization.

There is surprisingly little variation in the position of the supernumerary hair, so it is not possible to use the supernumerary afferent as a "wandering probe" to test the effects of positional information on the CNS arborization. However, in the F3 and now the F4 populations more double SI animals were found, as well as animals with a supernumerary medial hair in addition to the SI hair.

These supernumerary medials seem to behave like the M afferent, so there seem to be distinct lateral and medial territories across the circumference of the cercus.

Recent results indicate that there are interactions, possibly competitive in nature, between SIN and the L axon. Attention has been focussed on the connections made by L and SIN to GI3. In wild-type animals, L produces EPSPs in GI3 with a mean amplitude of 6.3 mV. However, in the presence of SIN in mutant animals, these EPSPs are reduced to a mean of 4.7 mV. The mutant neuron produces EPSPs of mean amplitude 2.5 mV in GI3. Control experiments show synaptic transmission to be otherwise normal in the mutants. This fine tuning of synaptic efficacy is competitive in the sense that the strength of connections is not genetically predetermined but depends on an interaction between the two afferents and their target interneuron.

Why is the SIN always the smaller of the two afferents, and evokes the smallest EPSPs? Is this because it grows in later and thus "loses" the competition? What would happen if the L afferent were ablated?

We have indications that the SIN may be born later, but this does not have to be the reason it is smaller. Transplanting the cercus of a cricket into the contralateral socket will induce supernumerary cerci to grow, and these bear the same identified sensory neurons as in normal cerci. The arborizations of these supernumerary neurons occupy the same neuropilar territory as the normal axons but they are no smaller than normal, even though the "competition" within the cercal glomerulus is much greater (Murphey et al., 1983). We are now performing experiments in which either SIN or the L neuron is ablated, to investigate the morphological and physiological effects on the remaining afferent.

There are no obvious morphological differences in the L afferent arborization in the presence of SIN. Experiments are in progress to determine if there are effects on the branching pattern of the postsynaptic GIs. This mutant first instar cockroach cercal system, with its two identified competing afferents, and one identified postsynaptic cell, may represent an ideal preparation for studying the cellular and molecular mechanisms of competition (Bacon and Blagburn, 1989).

ACKNOWLEDGEMENTS

J.M. Blagburn is supported by NIH grant NS 07464, and J.P. Bacon by the S.E.R.C. (U.K.).

REFERENCES

Akam, M., 1987, The molecular basis for metameric pattern in the *Drosophila* embryo, *Development*, 101: 1.

Bacon, J.P., and Blagburn, J.M., 1989, Mutant cockroach neurons compete with wild-type cells for central targets, in: "Proceedings 17th Göttingen Neurotagung," Georg Thieme Verlag, Stuttgart, p. 41.

Bacon, J.P., and Murphey, R.K., 1984, Receptive fields of cricket giant interneurones are related to their dendritic structure, *J. Physiol.*, 352: 601.

Bacon, J.P., and Strausfeld, N.J., 1986, The Dipteran "Giant fibre" pathway: neurons and signals, *J. Comp. Physiol.*, A158:529.

Bastiani, M.J., Harrelson, A.L., Snow, P.M., and Goodman C.S., 1987, Expression of Fasciclin I and II glycoproteins on subsets of axon pathways during neuronal development in the grasshopper, *Cell*, 48:745.

Blagburn, J.M., 1989, Synaptic specificity in the first instar cockroach: patterns of monosynaptic input from filiform hair afferents to giant interneurones, *J. Comp.Physiol* A, in press.

Blagburn, J.M., and Beadle, D.J., 1982, Morphology of identified cercal afferents and giant interneurones in the hatchling cockroach *Periplaneta americana*, *J. Exp. Biol.*, 97: 421.

Campos-Ortega, J.A., 1988, Cellular interactions during early neurogenesis of *Drosophila melanogaster*, *Trends Neurosci.*, 11: 400.

Dagan, D., and Volman, S., 1982, Sensory basis for directional wind detection in first instar cockroaches, *Periplaneta americana.*, *J. Comp. Physiol.*, A147: 471.

Doe, C.Q., and Goodman, C.S., 1985, Early events in insect neurogenesis. II. The role of cell interactions and cell lineage in the determination of neuronal precursor cells, *Dev. Biol.*, 111: 206.

Doe, C.Q., Hiromi, Y., Gehring, W.J., and Goodman, C.S., 1988a, Expression and function of the segmentation gene *fushi tarazu* during *Drosophila* neurogenesis, *Science*, 239: 170.

Doe, C.Q., Smouse, D., and Goodman, C.S., 1988b, Control of neuronal fate by the *Drosophila* segmentation gene *even-skipped*, *Nature*, 333: 376.

Doe, C.Q., Kuwada, J.Y., and Goodman, C.S., 1985, From epithelium to neuroblasts to neurons: the role of cell interactions and cell lineage during insect neurogenesis, *Phil. Trans. R. Soc. Lond. [Biol.]*, 312: 67.

Harrelson, A.L, and Goodman, C.S., 1988, Growth cone guidance in insects: fasciclin II is a member of the immunoglobulin superfamily, *Science*, 242: 700.

Jacobs, J.R., Patel, N.H., Elkins, T., and Goodman, C.S., 1987, Genetic analysis of fasciclin III in *Drosophila*: deletion of the gene leads to abnormal axon fasciculation, *Soc. Neurosci. Abstr.*, 13: 1222.

Kämper, G., and Murphey, R.K., 1987, Synapse formation by sensory neurons after cross-species transplantation in crickets: the role of positional information, *Dev. Biol.*, 122: 492.

Kuwada, J.Y., and Goodman, C.S., 1985, Neuronal determination during embryonic development of the grasshopper *(Schistocerca americana)* nervous system, *Dev. Biol.*, 110: 114.

Murphey, R.K., 1986, Competition and the dynamics of axon arbor growth in the cricket, *J. Comp. Neurol.*, 251:100.

Murphey, R.K., Johnson, S.E., and Sakaguchi, D.S., 1983, Anatomy and physiology of supernumerary cercal afferents in crickets: implications for pattern formation, *J. Neurosci.*, 3: 312.

Murphey, R.K., and Lemere, C.A., 1984, Competition controls the growth of an identified axonal arborization, *Science*, 224: 1352.

Patel, N.H., Snow, P.M., and Goodman, C.S., 1987, Characterization and cloning of Fasciclin III, a glycoprotein expressed on a subset of neurons and axon pathways in *Drosophila*, *Cell*, 48: 975.

Raper, J.A., Bastiani, M.J., and Goodman, C.S., 1983, Pathfinding by neuronal growth cones in grasshopper embryos. II. Selective fasciculation onto specific axonal pathways, *J. Neurosci.*, 3: 31.

Raper, J.A., Bastiani, M.J., and Goodman, C.S., 1984, Pathfinding by neuronal growth cones in grasshopper embryos. IV. The effects of ablating the A and P axons upon the behavior of the G growth cone, *J. Neurosci.*, 4: 2329.

Shepherd, D., and Murphey, R.K., 1986, Competition regulates the efficacy of an identified synapse in crickets, *J.Neurosci.*, 6: 3152.

Slack, J.M.W., 1983, "From egg to embryo," Cambridge University Press, Cambridge.

Thomas, J.B., Bastiani, M.J., Bate, C.M., and Goodman, C.S., 1984, From grasshopper to *Drosophila*: a common plan for neuronal development, *Nature*, 310: 203.

Thomas, J.B., and Wyman, R.J., 1983, Normal and mutant connectivity between identified neurons in *Drosophila*, *Trends Neurosci.*, 6: 214.

Zinn, K., McAllister, L., and Goodman, C.S., 1988, Sequence analysis and neuronal expression of fasciclin I in grasshopper and *Drosophila*, *Cell*, 53: 577.

DEVELOPMENT OF THE PERIPHERAL NERVOUS SYSTEM IN *DROSOPHILA* [*]

Mar Ruiz-Gómez (scribe), Alain Ghysen (lecturer)

Laboratory of Genetics
Université Libre de Bruxelles
Bruxelles, BELGIUM

INTRODUCTION

The sense organs of insects are epidermal derivatives composed of one or more sensory neurons and a set of support (nonneural) cells (see chapter by Blagburn and Bacon, this volume). The neuron(s) and support cells that form one sense organ are descendants of a single precursor cell, the sensory mother cell (SMC). Before being committed to its developmental fate this cell is indistinguishable from the neighbouring cells which will differentiate as epidermal cells and secrete cuticle. Thus the generation of a specific sense organ is the result of two consecutive events: the determination of precursor cells at specific locations of the epidermis, and the cellular differentiation of their progeny. Dr. Ghysen and colleagues have studied this process in the case of the peripheral nervous system (PNS) of *Drosophila*, where all larval and many adult sensory organs (SO) can be uniquely identified according to position and type. The reproducibility of the patterns, together with the known advantages of *Drosophila* for genetic studies, make the fly PNS an excellent model system to investigate how defined arrays of neurons arise during the development and how position affects cellular behavior.

THE DETERMINATION OF SENSORY NEURONS

The Adult System

Two general models have been developed to explain pattern generation. One of them assumes that cells can interpret positional cues which are distributed along the tissue. The other assumes that local interactions between cells can generate large-scale patterns. A simple form of the positional cues postulated in the first model would be a gradient of concentration of some signal molecule, with a maximal concentration (source) at one edge of the tissue and a minimal concentration (sink) at the other edge, such that any cell could assess its position in the tissue by "reading" the local concentration of the signal. An interesting example of the cell interactions postulated in the second model was proposed by Wigglesworth to explain the regular spacing of bristles in some insects (1940). As soon as an epidermal cell has chosen to become a SMC, this cell would inhibit its neighbors from becoming SMCs (for example by sequestering from the medium a molecule required for this activity). This process of lateral inhibition will generate a pattern of regularly spaced bristles,

---

[*] This chapter to be cited as: Ruiz-Gómez, M., 1990, Development of the peripheral nervous system in *Drosophila*, in: "Systems Approaches to Developmental Neurobiology," P. A. Raymond, S. S. Easter, Jr., and G. M. Innocenti, eds., Plenum Press, New York.

even if the initial decision to become a SMC is taken at random. As divisions occur, the existing bristles will be separated by more and more epidermal cells until some of these cells escape from inhibition and additional bristles are intercalated.

In adult flies, SO are arranged in different patterns depending on the type of SO and the part of the body. Some of these patterns could be accounted for by Wigglesworth's lateral inhibition, for example the regular spacing of bristles on the abdominal segments. However other patterns seem difficult to explain along the same line, most notably the pattern of large bristles on the thorax and head of the fly. Each of these large bristles occupies a fixed, unique position. How can such a precise pattern be generated? To answer this question early investigators looked for mutations that alter the pattern of sensory elements. They found a number of mutations that eliminate specific bristles. Many of these mutations occur in the same location, near the tip of the X chromosome and were named *achaete* (ac) or *scute* (sc) depending on which bristles they removed. All *ac* and *sc* mutations are recessive and correspond to a partial loss-of-function. Another kind of mutation in the same region, the *Hairy-wing* mutations (Hw), have the opposite effect: they increase the number of bristles. These mutations are dominant and correspond to a gain-of-function. García-Bellido (1981) clearly demonstrated that both loss and gain of function mutations affect the same gene. This result strongly supports the idea that this gene is involved in the initial decision of making a bristle at a given place, since the inactivation of the gene (loss-of-function mutations) leads to an absence of bristles, while the overactivity of the gene (gain-of-function mutations) leads to the formation of supernumerary bristles. Genetic and developmental analysis of this locus showed that the mutations define not a single gene but a gene complex called Achaete-Scute Complex (AS-C). This complex contains four genes: *achaete* and *scute* , with loss of function mutations affecting complementary sets of sense organs in the adult fly, lethal of *scute* (l'sc), which is required for the appropriate development of the CNS, and *asense* (ase), which affects a set of sense organs in the larva (see below).

An important piece of information about the function of the AS-C came from the molecular analysis of the complex, carried out in Modolell's laboratory (Campuzano et al. 1985). The complex spans 100 kb of DNA and comprises four independent transcription units that correspond to the genes described above. The transcribed regions are separated by large regions of non-transcribed DNA. This brings us to the core of the initial question: how is position encoded in the DNA? The *sc* mutations map outside the T4 transcribed region, along the 50 kb of DNA immediately downstream of the gene. Most of these mutations are rearrangements with breakpoints that physically separate the *sc* gene from part of its adjacent, nontranscribed region. All *sc* breakpoints follow two general rules: first, mutations that alter the same region of DNA remove the same set of bristles, and second, the closer the breakpoint to the gene, the stronger the phenotype. These observations led to the following explanation of the ability of the *sc* gene to promote the formation of sensory bristles at specific locations (Ruiz-Gómez and Modolell, 1987). This specificity results from the existence of control

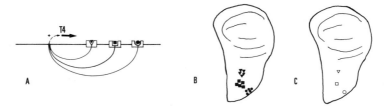

Fig. 1. Simplified view of the mechanisms that specify the determination of adult sensory organs at given positions. (a) Different regulatory sites in the AS-C DNA respond to positional cues and promote the expression of the *sc* gene in different regions of the epidermis. Positional cues may be the localized presence of the product of a regulatory gene, or of a combination of products of regulatory genes. Symbols in panels A and B may therefore represent either the distribution of a single "cueing" gene product, or overlap between the distribution of two or more "cueing" gene products, each of which may have a much wider distribution. (b) The *sc* gene is expressed in clusters of cells, each cluster probably depending on activation of *sc* gene by a specific regulatory site. (c) Only one cell within the cluster will be determined (SMC), as is reflected by individual cells expressing the *lac* gene in a transformant line.

sites in the nontranscribed DNA, each of which responds to positional cues and promotes the expression of the gene at given locations of the epidermis (Fig. 1A and B). Breakpoints disconnect a set of control sites from the transcription unit, resulting in the inactivity of the gene at the corresponding locations and therefore in the absence of a specific set of bristles. Mutations that affect the same control sites are expected to have similar phenotypes. As more control sites are disconnected by a breakpoint closer to the transcribed region, more bristles will be absent and the phenotype will be stronger.

The problem now is to imagine how a one-cell accuracy is achieved, that is, how to go from B to C in Figure 1. A crucial piece of information comes from the mosaic experiments of Stern (1954). In order to investigate if AS-C was involved in the establishment of a general positional system, Stern made mosaic flies in which part of the thorax was normal and part was mutant for one AS-C gene, *ac*. If *ac* had been involved in setting up a global system, for example a gradient that would specify a bristle at some point, then this system would be disturbed whenever part of the thorax is mutant, leading to disturbances in the pattern of *ac*-dependent bristles. What he found was that the presence or absence of a bristle in one region depends on the genotype of the cells in that region only, demonstrating that ac+ is required only at the position where *ac* bristles will form. There are interesting exceptions to this rule, however. When the normal site is within mutant territory, no bristle usually forms unless there is some wild type territory nearby: in some of those cases he found a bristle formed by wild type cells at a slightly displaced position. This result led Richelle and Ghysen (1979) to define a model which accounts for the generation of bristle patterns in normal flies, in mutants and in ac mosaics as shown by computer simulations. In this model the commitment of a precursor cell is a progressive process involving the initial expression of *ac* in extensive regions of epidermis, an averaging mechanism (diffusion or cellular interactions) that results in the determination of a cell in the middle of each region, and finally a process of lateral inhibition. This model makes several predictions about the distribution of sc transcripts: (1) we should find clusters of cells expressing the gene, and neither generalized expression nor single expressing cells, (2) the gene should be expressed early, before cells become determined, and (3) the gene should be expressed in regions where sensory structures will appear. The distribution of *sc* RNAs has very recently been described in the larval progenitor of the adult thorax (Romani et al., 1989). The result is that the *ac* and *sc* genes are expressed in clusters of cells. Moreover, the distribution of these clusters prefigures the distribution of adult sensory structures, supporting the idea that the local expression of AS-C is responsible for the decision to form a sense organ (Fig. 1). Thus it has been proposed to call the AS-C genes "proneural" as they define a state that occurs previous to and leads to the commitment of a cell to become a SMC.

In the formation of a sense organ, does cell type depend on lineage or on interactions?

There are two parts to this question: first, the specification of the type of SO (as a whole), second, the differentiation of its specialized cells. The SMC is already specified with respect to the type of SO it will form, including the morphology of the sensory structure (bristle, campaniform sensillum, chordotonal organ...), the number and modality of the neuron(s) (mechanosensory, chemosensory...), and the projection within the CNS. This early specification results at least in part from the particular combination of genes expressed in this cell. Since most of these genes seem to be transcriptional regulators, their different combinations may specifically activate or repress different programmes of differentiation.

The four different cells that derive from the SMC will each assume a unique fate (Blagburn and Bacon, 1990, this volume). This may depend strictly on the lineage, i.e., DNA replication or cell division may trigger changes in developmental programmes (Braisted and Raymond, 1990, this volume). The mechanism by which this result could be achieved is totally obscure. Alternatively, the fixed patterns of cell divisions may simply ensure the presence of the appropriate number of cells, while interactions between these cells are responsible for assigning the differentiation programmes. Cell interactions may specify the fates of the interacting cells in different ways. They may be instructive, specified cells telling naive surrounding cells what to do. An example is the development of the fly retina (Braisted and Raymond, 1990, this volume) and of the optic ganglion in *Daphnia*. Interactions may also be restrictive, limiting the number of cells that can adopt a preferred fate. An example are the "equivalence groups" demonstrated in the leech and in the nematode, and probably, the neurogenic genes of the fly (Jimenez and Campos-Ortega, 1990, this volume). In no case, however, do we know the molecular mechanisms in any detail. In the case of the fly sense organs, there is circumstantial or preliminary evidence in favor of both mechanisms (strictly lineage-dependent or interaction-dependent controls of cell fate). Thus the question remains completely open.

The Larval System

A complete analysis of the PNS of the *Drosophila* embryo, and a correlation of neurons with sense organs have been described (Bodmer and Jan, 1987; Dambly-Chaudière and Ghysen, 1986). The PNS of the larva includes different types of neurons innervating both external sense organs (es neurons) and internal sense organs, e.g., the chordotonal stretch receptors (ch neurons). All peripheral neurons are clearly identifiable and are arranged in very reproducible patterns which may differ from one segment to the next, for example, between the thoracic and the abdominal segments. Dambly-Chaudière and Ghysen (1987) assessed the role of the AS-C and of its different genes on the larval pattern. They found that embryos deficient for AS-C lack all es organs, much as do adults, confirming the essential function of AS-C. They also found that the *ac* and the *ase* genes affect two complementary subsets of sense organs (this is different from the adult, where the important genes are *ac* and *sc*). Looking carefully at the *ac* and *ase* subsets they were able to detect homologies between SO in the thoracic and abdominal segments, and concluded that different AS-C genes act repetitively in all segments to define an "archetype" of larval PNS, which later will be modified to generate the different segmental patterns. The existence of a common archetype in all segments was beautifully demonstrated by Ghysen and O'Kane (1989) making use of a transformant line of *Drosophila* that expresses the bacterial gene *lacZ* in the SMC (as well as in all their progeny). This permitted the study of the first steps in the generation of the PNS, and revealed that the SMCs appear very early during embryogenesis and are initially arranged in a similar pattern in all segments.

Another gene involved in PNS formation, *daughterless* (da), has been identified recently (Caudy et al.,1988). Whereas the maternal activity of the gene is required for proper sex determination in female embryos, its zygotic activity is essential both in male and in female embryos for the formation of the PNS, which is totally absent from embryos deficient for *da*. Using the *lac* transformant described above, it has been shown that no SMC ever develops in this mutant. The sequencing of the *da* gene has revealed that the *da* protein contains a conserved helix-loop-helix motif which was initially discovered in the four genes of the AS-C (Alonso and Cabrera, 1988), and which is also present in the oncogene *c-myc*, the gene *Myo-D*, and two human enhancer-binding proteins. This motif would play a role in DNA binding and dimerization. This strongly suggests that these products are regulatory transcription factors which can associate to form homo- or heterodimers. Thus it is likely that this motif defines a family of regulatory proteins which, by their ability to form heterodimers, can modulate each other's activity or specificity.

In this context there are two loci, *extramacrochaetae (emc)* and *hairy (h)*, that have been described as negative regulators of the *sc* and *ac* genes of the complex in the adult (Garcia Bellido, 1981). However, there are no differences in the amount or distribution of AS-C transcripts in *emc* or *h* mutants (Romani et al., 1989). Recently both genes have been cloned and sequenced, and it has been found that their products share the same helix-loop-helix motif found in the AS-C genes. This makes very attractive the idea of negative regulation by product interactions: the heterodimers *emc-sc* or *h-ac* could make *sc* and *ac* products less effective or otherwise modify their binding specificity.

Other known genes that affect the PNS are the "neurogenic" genes (Jimenez and Campos-Ortega, 1990, this volume). All neurogenic mutants are characterized by an hyperplasic PNS in late, fully differentiated embryos (Hartenstein and Campos-Ortega, 1986). However, the early pattern of SMC as seen with the *lac* transformant described above is completely normal in mutants of at least one of the neurogenic genes, *Notch* (N). The expression of *lac* soon extends to groups of cells instead of remaining restricted to one SMC, suggesting that the PNS hyperplasia results from a defect in the process of lateral inhibition .

In summary, there are two principles at work in the generation of a pattern of sense organs. First, accuracy is achieved stepwise, by first making a rough sketch that will later be sharpened (simplified in Fig. 2). Second, complexity is also achieved stepwise, by first building a basic pattern (archetype) and then introducing modifications to generate an array of derived patterns (segmental diversification). Both principles are probably very general in development and evolution. They both reflect the third and most general principle (of evolution and of everything), that apparently unmanageable complexity is most easily achieved as the cumulative result of a number of manageably complex steps.

Is there an analogy between genetic networks and neural networks?

The simple answer is yes, in the sense that both are decision-making devices in which the pattern of connections between elements plays a crucial role. This multiply connected structure is very different from the linearly organized systems we are familiar with, for example the sequence of genes responsible for a metabolic pathway, or the sequence of neurons responsible for a single reflex. Networks are obviously much more interesting since they underlie the ability of cells to choose between alternative states, an essential feature both in the development of the organism and in the functioning of the brain. Networks are also much more difficult to analyze than linear systems and their analysis is still in its infancy, both in developmental genetics and in neurobiology: we are dealing with complex systems with emerging systemic properties that depend on the structure of the system and cannot be derived from the analysis of the individual components.

Because our understanding of both genetic and neural networks is so limited it is difficult to say how far the analogy between the two can be pushed. I would suggest, however, that genetic networks may be both more complex and more flexible than neural networks. Complexity: neural networks generally comprise many more elements than genetic networks. Genetic networks, however, are active simultaneously in all cells: each cell of a developing organism is busily computing its developmental programme and exchanging information about it with the other cells, a striking case of parallel processing where intercellular communication ensures the coordination of the action of all the units. Flexibility: as described in the text, some genes can be involved in networks underlying very different choices, e.g., *da* in sex determination and PNS development, or *h* in segmentation and PNS development (see also chapter by Blagburn and Bacon). We do not know whether this duality reflects some meaningful feature of the system, or simply an opportunistic tendency of the organism to use again and again efficient genes or a set of genes. This brings us to a third and important difference between neural and gene networks, the time scale: neural networks respond in milliseconds and are adaptive at the level of ontogeny; gene networks respond in hours or days and are adaptive at the level of

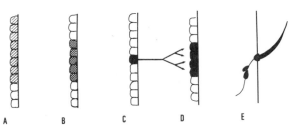

Fig. 2. Steps in the generation of sense organs. (a) Different regulatory genes are expressed in different positions of the body. (b) This promotes the activation of different combinations of proneural genes (*da*, AS-C genes, others?) in each region (= a cluster of proneural cells). (c) By a process of lateral inhibition mediated by genes involved in cell to cell communication, only one cell within the cluster will be singularized as a SMC. (d) The SMC by two differentiative mitoses will give rise to the four cells (e) that will differentiate the various components of the sense organ.

phylogeny. Whether these differences are essential or superficial is for future work to answer.

THE DIFFERENTIATION OF SENSORY ORGANS

Choice of Axonal Path from Neuron to CNS

Once a sensory neuron differentiates it must send its axon towards the CNS. In the case of the larval PNS two peripheral axonal pathways are established in each segment. The anterior pathway is pioneered partly by a central and partly by a peripheral axon. The two pioneers join and fasciculate about halfway. The growth of the axons is probably directed by dorsal-ventral cues, as there is no evidence of stepping stones in this pathway. The distance that the central and peripheral axons must travel before joining each other is so small (less than 100 μm) that the orientation need not be very precise. The same holds in the case of the posterior pathway, where the distances are even smaller, so it is reasonable to suggest that the establishment of the early pattern of peripheral nerves in the embryo is probably achieved by a simple mechanism. Later on condensation of CNS leads to a complication of this pattern, which becomes accentuated during larval growth and even more during metamorphosis. Thus, the complex pattern of peripheral adult nerves derives from a very simple pattern that is established early in the embryo.

In the adult, peripheral axons have to travel over large distances in order to reach the CNS. How is this achieved? At least two sources of guidance, which are thought to orient axonal growth in grasshoppers, are also used in *Drosophila*: the strong tendency of axons to join other neurons and to fasciculate with other axons, and the ability of axons to respond to directional cues. Based on these two mechanisms of axonal guidance, different strategies of pathway formation are used in different appendages, depending on the location and birthdate of pioneer neurons. Consider two examples: the leg and the wing, formed by undifferentiated larval precursors, the leg disc and the wing disc, respectively. The leg discs have a concentric organization, with the future tip of the leg situated in the center and more proximal segments in the more peripheral annuli. Early during metamorphosis, the leg disc unfolds to form the adult leg. Several larval neurons are present in the leg disc; their axons join a larval nerve that runs along the disc and connects it to the CNS. Most of these larval neurons have their cell bodies in the center of the disc and they are pulled out with the tip of the leg as the disc everts, so that their axons simply elongate and thereby form a guidance pathway that extends from the tip to the base of the leg and on to the CNS (Jan et al., 1985). Thus adult neurons do not have to navigate freely along the rapidly extending leg. Contrary to the leg disc, the wing disc contains no larval neurons. Very soon after the onset of metamorphosis, two pairs of neurons, one proximal and the other distal, differentiate in the middle region of the wing. During the next few hours the neurons send their axons proximally and shortly after, the axons from the distal pair of neurons reach the proximal pair,whose axons have by now reached the base of the wing. This establishes one of the major wing pathways. Experiments carried out in cultured wing disc fragments have shown that the distal pair of neurons continues growing proximally even in the absence of the proximal pair, leading to the proposition that axons follow proximo-distal positional cues in their travel along the wing surface (Blair et al.,1987). These positional cues could be provided by epidermal cells or by the basal lamina they produce.

The basic principle of contact guidance of axons by other axons originated with the classic experiments of Wigglesworth, who demonstrated that in another insect, *Rhodnius*, newly developing axons are guided towards the CNS along preexisting axon pathways. By analogy we assume that in the fly differentiating adult axons follow larval nerves. To test this idea Ghysen and Deak (1978) analyzed different experimental situations that induce morphological abnormalities in the larva (X-ray irradiation, surgical operations and homeotic mutations) to deprive the adult axons from their normal guide. The results indicate that when the larval nerve that the adults axons normally follow is absent or broken, the growing axons follow a different larval nerve, eventually entering the CNS at an inappropriate site. These results fully support the idea of contact guidance, but emphasize that it is a nonspecific guidance mechanism.

Here again the "stepwise" principle is at work. The tremendous complexity of the final pattern, in this case the adult peripheral nerve net, can be understood in terms of the cumulative effect of a number of elementary steps, each of which relies on simple mechanisms to transform a given landscape into a slightly more complex (heterogeneous) one.

Are the same operations involved in the development of the PNS and of the CNS?

Certainly the same genes are involved in the segregation of sensory mother cells (in the PNS) and of neuroblasts (in the CNS) from the ectoderm. This does not mean, however, that the same developmental operations are involved. A good example of this is provided by the case of h^+, which defines seven stripes early during embryogenesis, defines the number of bristles formed during metamorphosis, and specifies some central neurons. When expressed too early in a female, it alters the process of sex determination in her progeny. The common feature of these effects of h^+ is the molecular function of the gene product, which is probably a transcriptional regulator. The differences reflect the involvement of h^+ in different operations at different stages, or at different times. Likewise the molecular function of at least some of the neurogenic genes is probably related to cell communication; this tells us nothing of the operations where these genes will be involved, and indeed neurogenic mutants show defects not only in the segregation of SMC and of neuroblasts but also in the formation of wing veins, in non-neural eye cells, and possibly in the lineage of sense organs. Here again the gene provides a mechanism, or part of a mechanism, which may be used in different operations in different developing systems. What, then, is a developmental operation, and what are the relations between genes and operations? An operation could be defined, by analogy with the mathematical "operators", as a procedure which, when applied to a landscape, transforms it into a more complex (more defined, more structural) landscape. An excellent example is the process of segmentation of the fly embryo which implies several operations whereby the original graded landscape is consecutively transformed into three domains, then into seven stripes, then into fourteen segments. Interestingly, each operation depends on a particular set of genes, respectively the maternal A/P genes, the gap genes, the pair-rule genes and the segment-polarity genes. Also interestingly, the different genes of each set seem to form a highly connected network with only a minimal connection between the different networks.

To come back to the original question, it may be that some genes are involved in the same operations in the PNS and CNS; for example, the cell interactions mediated by the neurogenic genes may be involved in lateral inhibition in both cases. In the absence of solid evidence, however, and as long as we do not understand these processes completely, it is probably best not to rely on common genes to infer common operations.

Choice of Axonal Pathway within CNS

It is obvious that the function of the nervous system resides in the establishment of appropriate connections between nerve cells, but the problem is to know what are the mechanisms by which these connections are established, that is, the mechanisms by which neurites find their way to their synaptic targets. Sensory axons entering the CNS as a bundle make different projections within the CNS, according to which sensory neurons they come from. What has to be explained is how this is achieved. To answer these questions Ghysen (1978) carried out a series of experiments in which he forced adult sensory axons to enter the CNS at inappropriate places. The result was that even if the axons enter the CNS at a wrong place as a consequence of genetic (homeotic mutation) or experimental manipulation, they are able to establish the appropriate projection. In some cases axons had to follow the pathway in a direction opposite to the normal one. The interpretation was that there are specific pathways within the CNS that are recognized and followed by growing axons regardless of where the first contact is made. Furthermore these pathways have to be differentially labelled, since different sensory axons can specifically recognize and follow different CNS pathways. The existence of these marked pathways would ensure that growing axons will be led to the proximity of their specific target. The existence of marked pathways was also postulated by Goodman (1982) on the basis of an analysis of the behavior of growth cones in the grasshopper CNS. Later work in the fly has led to the identification of several molecules, the fasciclins, which may be involved in pathway labeling (Bastiani, et al., 1987). The choice of which labeled pathway a given sensory axon will recognize is correlated with the type and developmental origin of the sensory structure; the same is probably true for central neurons (see the chapter by Blagburn & Bacon, this volume). In particular the segmental origin of neurons influences their projections (Ghysen et al., 1983, Teugels and Ghysen, 1985). The position and time of birth of the neuron may also play a role in the decision (Ghysen, 1980, Murphey, et al., 1983, Palka, et al., 1986). After the axon has been guided towards the vicinity of its target a different mechanism must allow it to recognize the target and make specific synapses. Virtually nothing is known of this last step, which remains a major challenge in our understanding of how connectivity develops in the fly and how it is coded for by the genome.

What is the role of the target in defining the axonal pathway?

There is no evidence in the fly (and little evidence in any other organism) that the target acts at a distance to orient the growth of the axon. On the contrary, the discovery that fly sensory axons are able to recognize and follow specific pathways in the CNS, and the subsequent demonstration that a scaffold of labeled pathways is erected early during the development of the CNS, leave little doubt that in insects it is the pathway that guides the axon to the target, and not the target which defines the pathway of the axon. Whether a similar scaffold is erected early in vertebrate neurogenesis, and is used to set up the basic connectivity of the CNS is still an open question (see, however, the chapters by Metcalfe and Westerfield and by Ross and Easter).

Short distance effects of the target on the axonal projection are widespread both in vertebrates and in invertebrates. Most of those proximity effects are mediated by physical contact; however, short range diffusion of trophic or growth factors might also be involved. Whatever the case, this influence of the target is important in defining the final shape of the axon terminals. Depending on the extent of the projection, the role of the target may appear minimal (for axons that cover long distances) or essential (for axons that project locally). Furthermore, in cases where synaptic contact with the target is required to stabilize a particular branch, competition effects (long assumed to be unimportant in insects) may profoundly affect axonal morphology. To this extent the target may in some cases play a role in defining the final projection even though it had no role in defining the pathway initially followed by the axon.

How is it that an axon will unfailingly select the pathway that brings it close to its target, if the target itself has no role in this choice? This question must be seen in the light of evolution. The recognition properties of the growing axon depend on the development of particular membrane molecules which depend on the presence of particular regulatory molecules which depend on the location and history of the sensory mother cell. It is also to be presumed that a recognition programme that would lead an axon along a totally "useless" pathway (ie., one that does not bring the axon close to a decent target) has not been of particular value for the animal, and therefore that programme changes. Mechanisms that allow the recognition of a pathway that turns out to be "useful" have long been favored by selection.

ACKNOWLEDGEMENTS

I am most grateful to A. Ghysen and C. Dambly-Chaudière for critical reading of the manuscript. I also thank L. Leyns for assistance on the preparation of the manuscript. I am the recipient of a postdoctoral fellowship from Ministerio de Educación y Ciencia and Consejo Superior de Investigaciones Científicas.

REFERENCES

Alonso, M. C., and Cabrera, C. V., 1988, The *achaete-scute* gene complex of *Drosophila melanogaster* comprises four homologous genes, *EMBO J.*, 7:2589.

Bastiani, M. J., Harrelson, A. L., Snow, P. M.,and Goodman, C. S., 1987, Expression of *fasciclin* I and II glycoproteins on subsets of axon pathways during neuronal development in the grasshopper, *Cell*, 48:745.

Blair, S. S., Murray, S. A., and Palka, J.,1987, The guidance of axons from transplanted neurons through aneural *Drosophila* wings, *J. Neurosci.*, 7:4165.

Bodmer, R., and Jan, Y. N., 1987, Morphological differentiation of the embryonic peripheral neurons in *Drosophila* , *Wilhelm Roux's Arch. Dev. Biol.*, 196:69.

Campuzano, S., Carramolino, L., Cabrera, C. V., Ruiz-Gómez, M., Villares, R., Boronat, A., and Modolell, J., 1985, Molecular genetics of the *achaete-scute* gene complex of *D. melanogaster*, *Cell*, 40:327.

Caudy, M., Grell, E., Dambly-Chaudière, C., Ghysen, A., Jan, L. Y., and Jan, Y.N., 1988, The maternal sex-determination gene *daughterless* has zygotic activity necessary for the formation of peripheral neurons in *Drosophila*, *Genes Dev.*, 2:843.

Dambly-Chaudière, C., and Ghysen, A., 1986, The sense organs in the *Drosophila* larva and its relation to the embryonic pattern of sensory neurons, *Wilhelm Roux's Arch. Dev. Biol.*, 195:222.

Dambly-Chaudière, C., and Ghysen, A., 1987, Independent subpatterns of sense organs require independent genes of the *achaete-scute* complex in *Drosophila* larvae, *Genes Dev.*, 1:297.

García-Bellido, A., 1981, From the gene to the pattern: chaetae differentiation, in: "Cellular Controls in Differentiation", C. W. Lloyd and D. A. Rees, eds., Academic Press, New York.

Ghysen, A., 1978, Sensory axons recognize defined pathways in *Drosophila* central nervous system, *Nature*, 274:869.

Ghysen, A., 1980, The projection of sensory neurons in the central nervous system of *Drosophila* : choice of the appropriate pathway, *Dev. Biol.*, 78:521.

Ghysen, A., and Deak, I., 1978, Experimental analysis of sensory nerve pathways in *Drosophila*, *Wilhelm Roux's Arch. Dev. Biol.*, 184:273.

Ghysen, A., Janson, R.,and Santamaria, P., 1983, Segmental determination of sensory neurons in *Drosophila*, *Devel.Biol.*, 99:7.

Ghysen, A., and O'Kane, C., 1989, Detection of neural enhancer-like elements in the genome of *Drosophila* , *Development*, 105:35.

Goodman, C. S., Raper, J. A., Ho, R. K., and Chang, S., 1982, Pathfinding by neural growth cones during grasshoppers embryogenesis, *Symp. Soc. Dev. Biol.*, 40:275.

Hartenstein, V., and Campos-Ortega, J., A., 1986, The peripheral nervous system of mutants of early neurogenesis in *Drosophila melanogaster*, *Wilhelm Roux's Arch Dev. Biol.*, 195:210.

Jan, Y., N., Ghysen, A., Christoph, I., Barbel, S., and Jan, L., Y., 1985, Formation of neuronal pathways in the imaginal discs of *Drosophila*, *J. Neurosci.*, 5:2453.

Murphey, R., K., Johnson, S., E., and Sakaguchi, D., S., 1983, Anatomy and physiology of supernumerary cercal afferents in crickets: implications for pattern formation, *J. Neurosci.*, 3:312.

Palka, J., Malone, M. A., Ellison, R. L., and Wigston, D. G., 1986, Central projection of identified *Drosophila* sensory neurons relative to their time of development, *J. Neurosci.*, 6:1822.

Richelle, J., and Ghysen, A., 1979, Bristle determination and pattern formation in *Drosophila* . I. A model, *Dev. Biol.*, 70:418

Romani, S., Campuzano, S., Macagno, E., and Modolell, J., 1989, *Genes Dev.*, (in press).

Ruiz-Gómez, M., and Modolell, J., 1987, Deletion analysis of the *achaete-scute* locus of *Drosophila melanogaster*, *Genes Dev.*, 1:1238.

Stern, C., 1954, Two or three bristles, *Amer. Sci.*, 42:213.

Teugels, E., and Ghysen, A., 1985, Domains of action of *bithorax* genes in *Drosophila* central nervous system, *Nature,* 314:558.

Wigglesworth, V. B., 1940, Local and general factors in the development of pattern in *Rhodnius prolixus*, *J. Exp. Biol.*, 17:180.

GENETIC AND CELLULAR INTERACTIONS IN NEUROGENESIS OF *DROSOPHILA MELANOGASTER* [*]

Fernando Jiménez (scribe)

Centro de Biologia, CSIC
Universidad Autonoma
Facultad de Ciencias, Canto Blanco
Madrid, SPAIN

José A. Campos-Ortega (lecturer)

Institut für Entwicklungsphysiologie
Universität zu Köln
 Köln, FRG

INTRODUCTION

One of the main problems of developmental biology is the origin of cell diversity: how are different cell types of a multicellular organism generated from initially equivalent progenitor cells? Early neurogenesis of insects is a convenient model to study the origin of cell diversity. In insects, neurogenesis is initiated by the separation of individual neural progenitor cells, or neuroblasts (NBs), from a sheet of epidermal progenitor cells, or epidermoblasts (EBs; Poulson, 1950; Hartenstein and Campos-Ortega, 1984). In *Drosophila melanogaster*, NBs and EBs develop from the neurogenic region (NR), where these cells are intermingled before the separation of lineages takes place (Hartenstein and Campos-Ortega, 1984; Technau and Campos-Ortega, 1985). Work on grasshoppers has shown that cell interactions are involved in generating different classes of NBs (Taghert et al., 1984; Doe and Goodman, 1985). Below, various results will be discussed which suggest that, in *Drosophila*, the separation of NBs from EBs also depends on cellular interactions. The simplest hypothesis to account for the current experimental data states that communication between the cells of the NR is necessary to assume and to maintain a specific fate.

The NR of the *Drosophila* embryo contains approximately 2000 cells, of which 500 develop as NBs, whereas the remaining 1500 cells develop as EBs (Hartenstein and Campos-Ortega, 1985; Technau and Campos-Ortega, 1985). NBs segregate from the EBs in three pulses, which distinguish three subpopulations of NBs that are arranged according to a characteristic pattern (Hartenstein and Campos-Ortega, 1984; Hartenstein et al., 1987). Experimental evidence shows that although the final pattern is fairly constant and reproducible from animal to animal, the selection of specific fates by individual cells is not determined *a priori* (Technau and Campos-Ortega, 1986). When a single cell of the NR of one embryo (donor) is homotopically transplanted into the NR of another (host) embryo, the transplanted cell may develop either as a NB or as an EB. In some cases, the transplanted cell may undergo mitosis before the separation of lineages occurs, and daughter cells of both histotypes are found among its progeny.

---

[*]This chapter to be cited as: Jiménez, F., and Campos-Ortega, J. A., 1990, Genetic and cellular interactions in neurogenesis of *Drosophila Melanogaster*, in: "Systems Approaches to Developmental Neurobiology," P. A. Raymond, S. S. Easter, Jr., and G. M. Innocenti, eds., Plenum Press, New York.

REGULATORY SIGNALS IN THE NEUROGENIC REGION

The transplantation of ectodermal cells from the dorsal ectoderm of the donor into the dorsal ectoderm of the host never yields neural progenies. However, following heterotopic transplantation into the NR, dorsal cells may occasionally adopt a neural fate (Technau and Campos-Ortega, 1986). This result may be interpreted to mean that the surrounding neuroectodermal cells impose upon the transplanted dorsal cell the capacity to produce neural progeny. Intercellular influences which might actively prevent neurogenesis in the dorsal region during development cannot be demonstrated, since ventral cells transplanted dorsally sometimes adopt a neural fate in such heterotopic locations. Hence, these results suggest that a signal with neuralizing character passes from cell to cell within the neuroectoderm.

The existence of epidermalizing signals in the NR has been established by two different lines of evidence. Transplanting NBs back into the NR of younger embryos in some cases results in development of these cells as EBs (Technau and Campos-Ortega, 1987; Technau et al., 1988), suggesting that the NBs are responsive to epidermalizing influences from their neighboring cells. The other line of evidence derives from the analysis of mutants (see below).

Is there any evidence for mesodermal induction of neural fate in ectodermal cells during gastrulation in Drosophila?

No. In fact, there is suggestive evidence to the contrary. There are mutants that do not produce mesoderm and yet they develop CNS. I want to emphasize an important point: neurogenesis in insects is very different from the process in vertebrates. There is induction in insects but the difference is that the inductive process is not a function of mesodermal cells but of ectodermal cells which, by means of interactions mediated by the neurogenic genes, induce the fate of their neighbors. Perhaps similar genes exist in vertebrates.

What do you think is the primary event that signals a particular cell to initiate the neural fate?

Thanks to the work of Ch. Nüsslein-Volhard and K. Anderson we know that in *Drosophila* there is a gene system which regulates pattern formation along the dorso-ventral axis of the embryo. Genes of this system which are maternally expressed are responsible for the distribution of positional values along this axis. This includes the regionalization of the ectoderm in the dorsal epidermal anlage and the ventral neurogenic region. We are presently testing whether the function of this gene system confers to the neuroectodermal cells a primary neurogenic fate.

Is it necessary to assume a neuralizing signal? Could all ectodermal cells be predisposed to make NBs, and when cells are transplanted from the dorsal to the ventral ectodermal region, they are released from some inhibitory interaction present dorsally and are free to develop as NBs?

One argument against this possibility is that if you transplant ventral cells dorsally, they will in some cases develop neural progeny, indicating that there is nothing dorsally that actively inhibits neuralization.

BLAST CELLS ARE NOT FIRMLY COMMITTED TO THEIR FATES

At the time of transplantation, 10 to 12 minutes after the onset of gastrulation, the ectodermal cells in the experiments described above were not irreversibly committed to their fates. In order to test whether irreversible commitment occurs at a later age, heterochronic transplantations were carried out using increasingly older NBs and EBs removed from donors up to 170 min after gastrulation and individually transplanted into the NR of younger embryos (Technau et al., 1988). Surprisingly, the transplanted cells frequently switched their fate, e.g., from EBs to NBs, or *vice versa*, irrespective of their age, even though the oldest transplanted cells had already divided several times in the donor embryos and produced several epidermal or neural progenies, respectively, prior to transplantation. These results suggest that irreversible commitment to either of the two fates does not occur as long as the cells are capable of dividing and, moreover, the cells are able to react to the putative regulatory signals for a long time.

THE PRODUCTS OF THE NEUROGENIC GENES MAY PROVIDE AN EPIDERMALIZING SIGNAL

The analysis of a group of genes called the neurogenic genes strongly supports the existence of epidermalizing signals. Complete lack of function of any one of these genes causes all cells of the NR to adopt the neural fate; hence, no EBs develop from the NR and the mutants die as embryos with a highly hyperplasic CNS and a very defective, strongly reduced epidermal sheath (Poulson, 1937; Lehmann et al., 1983). All the neurogenic genes are likely to be involved in the same function, since the loss of any one of them always yields equivalent phenotypic defects. Indeed, the results of genetic experiments show that six of the neurogenic genes are arranged in an epistatic series, whereas the seventh gene *big brain* (*bib*), although participating in the same function, acts independently from others. Accordingly, six of the neurogenic genes form a sort of functional chain or network, the last link of which is the *Enhancer of split* [*E(spl)*] locus (de la Concha et al., 1988). All these results support the hypothesis that the products of the neurogenic genes mediate production of a signal that leads to epidermal development of the receiving cell.

Genetic mosaics indicate that the products of the neurogenic genes, perhaps with the exception of *bib*, are not able to diffuse over long distances (Dietrich and Campos-Ortega, 1984; Hoppe and Greenspan, 1986). However, if single cells from the NR of mutants lacking the genes *almondex* (*amx*), *Notch* (*N*), *bib*, *master mind* (*mam*), *neuralised* (*neu*) or *Delta* (*Dl*) , are transplanted into the NR of wildtype hosts, the mutant cells behave in the same manner as cells with a wildtype genotype (Technau and Campos-Ortega, 1987), and give rise to progeny of either epidermal, neural or mixed histotypes, irrespective of their genotype. Hence, the expression of mutations in any of these six neurogenic genes is not cell autonomous. In contrast, cells that lack *E(spl)*⁻ give rise to neural progenies only; in other words *E(spl)* expresses its phenotype in a cell autonomous manner.

One possible interpretation of these results is that cells lacking the *E(spl)* locus cannot react to the regulatory signals and, consequently, cannot take on the epidermal fate. Since the genes are functionally related, this result suggests that *E(spl)*⁻ cells have defective receptor mechanisms, whereas cells lacking any of the other six genes have normal receptive capabilities, but a defective signal source (Technau and Campos-Ortega, 1987).

GENES NECESSARY FOR NEURAL DEVELOPMENT

Another group of genes, including the genes of the *achaete-scute* complex (AS-C), *ventral nervous system condensation defective* (*vnd*), *embryonic lethal, abnormal visual system* (*elav*), located in the subdivision 1B of the X-chromosome, and *daughterless* (*da*), in the second chromosome, are known to be required for neural development (Jiménez and Campos-Ortega, 1979, 1987; White, 1980; Campos et al., 1985; Caudy et al., 1988a). Loss of function of these genes results in conspicuous hypoplasic defects in both the central and peripheral nervous systems. This phenotype is opposite to those of the neurogenic mutations discussed above. The current phenotypic analysis of the subdivision 1B mutants (Jimenez and Campos-Ortega, 1987) indicates that CNS defects can be attributed to [the deletion of lethal of scute *l'sc*, and *vnd*].

The origin of the phenotype of this group of mutants has not yet been firmly established. However, two different processes are certainly involved. First, the complement of NBs is defective in mutants of the subdivision 1B (F. Jiménez and J.A. Campos-Ortega, unpublished observations) and in *da* mutants (M. Brand and J.A.Campos-Ortega, unpublished observations). Neurogenesis is initiated in these animals by fewer NBs than in the wild-type. Second, there is increased cell death in the primordia of both CNS and PNS (Jiménez and Campos-Ortega, 1979). These results suggest that the function of these genes under discussion is required for NB development.

How do you interpret cell death in AS-C and da mutants?

There are many possible interpretations. One is that cell death is a consequence of regulation of epidermal size. Cells which normally would have developed as neural progenitors would now, in the absence of those genes, become EBs. However, since the epidermis of the embryo has a limited spatial capacity, the extra cells cannot be incorporated into the epidermal sheath and they die. Alternatively, the imposition of a new fate may lead to death of the mutant cells because of incompatiblity with other physiological functions.

THE GENES OF THE AS-C AND *da* INTERACT WITH THE NEUROGENIC GENES

The abnormal phenotype of homozygous neurogenic mutants can be considerably reduced if a homo- or hemizygotic mutation of the AS-C or of *da* is present in the same genome. This reduction in phenotypic severity of the double mutant strongly suggests functional interrelationships between the gene groups (Brand and Campos-Ortega, 1988). At least some of the interactions between neurogenic and AS-C genes are likely to involve modifications in the pattern of transcription of these genes. Changes in the pattern of transcription of the genes *T3* and *T5* (*l'sc* and *ac*; refer to Romani et al., 1987; Cabrera et al., 1987) have been observed in embryos carrying any of several neurogenic mutations (Brand and Campos-Ortega, 1988). In these mutant embryos, more cells express T3 and T5 than in wild-type embryos. However, the early pattern of expression of *T3* and *T5* in NG mutants is indistinguishable from the wildtype, and these transcriptional interactions seem not to operate, or at least do not become evident, until the time when segregation of lineages is taking place. These results suggest that cellular interactions mediated by the neurogenic genes are responsible for the refinement of the territories of *T3-T5* expression in the wildtype, and that the neurogenic genes exert this function by suppressing the transcription of *T3* and *T5* in some of the neuroectodermal cells.

The expansion of the territories of transcription of the AS-C genes that is observed in NG mutants raises the question of whether this phenomenon is causally related to the misrouting of all neuroectodermal cells into the neurogenic pathways. If in the wildtype a combination of the products of AS-C, and other similar genes, were necessary for a neuroectodermal cell to take on the fate of a NB, one could imagine that an increase in the number of cells transcribing AS-C genes may be responsible for the appearance of additional NBs.

MOLECULAR ANALYSIS OF THE NEUROGENIC GENES

The molecular analysis of the neurogenic genes confirms and extends the conclusion that these genes participate in a cell-cell communication (Artavanis-Tsakonas et al., 1983; Kidd et al., 1983; Wharton et al., 1985; Kidd et al., 1986; Vässin et al., 1987; Knust et al., 1987). The *N* locus (Artavanis-Tsakonas et al., 1983; Kidd et al., 1983) is expressed in all cells of the embryo during the critical developmental stages (Hartley et al., 1987); thus, its function is likely to be required in other processes in addition to neurogenesis. The complete sequence of the *N* transcript has been determined, and the conceptual translation indicates a transmembrane protein, the extracellular domain of which consists mainly of 36 tandem repeats with homology to various proteins, among them the epidermal growth factor (EGF) (Wharton et al., 1985; Kidd et al., 1986). This proposed structure, along with all other data from embryology and genetics, immediately suggests a role in cell communication processes.

The *Dl* locus exhibits a complex regulation, producing several overlapping RNAs (Vässin et al., 1987; Kopczynski et al., 1988). *In situ* hybridization shows that the distribution of *Dl* transcripts conforms with the expectation for a neurogenic gene. In contrast to *N*, which is ubiquitously expressed, *Dl* is selectively expressed in territories with neurogenic capacities, like the NR or the anlagen of sensory organs. After an initial phase during which the gene is transcribed in all cells in these territories, transcription becomes restricted to the cells that adopt the neural fate, e.g., the NBs. The sequence of the largest <u>Dl</u> transcript has been established and the encoded protein possesses some similarity to the *N* protein (Vässin et al., 1987; Kopczynski et al., 1988), including a transmembrane region with a putative extracellular domain containing 9 EGF-like repeats.

Data from both transmission and molecular genetics indicate that *E(spl)* is actually not a single gene, but rather a complex of several related genes clustered in neighborhood (Knust et al., 1987; Ziemer et al., 1988; Klämbt et al., 1989). Several transcription units have been found to be affected in *E(spl)* mutants (Knust et al., 1987; Preiss et al., 1988, Klämbt et al., 1989). They encode at least eleven major RNAs (*m1* to *m11*), four of which (*m4, m5, m7* and *m8*) are particularly interesting, for they exhibit similar spatial patterns of expression that conform to the assumed epidermalizing function of *E(spl)*. There is direct evidence that *m8* encodes *E(spl)* functions: wild-type flies transformed with the *m8* transcription unit from the dominant mutant allele $E(spl)^D$, which encodes a modified protein, express the adult phenotype characteristic of the mutant (Klämbt et al., 1989). The sequences of the proteins encoded by the *m5, m7* and *m8* transcripts are very similar to each other, which suggests some functional redundancy (Klämbt et al., 1989). In addition, these proteins contain a region similar to one in the *T3, T4, T5* and *T8* proteins of the AS-C gene complex (Villares and Cabrera, 1987; Alonso and Cabrera, 1988) and of the gene *da* (Caudy et al., 1988b). This homologous part of the sequence of *Drosophila* genes is also similar to a region in the nuclear oncogene *myc*, suggesting that the corresponding proteins may exert regulatory functions in the cell nucleus. Hartley et al (1988) have determined the sequence of the protein encoded by the transcription unit *m9-m10* and found that it has homologies with the ß-subunit of transducin, a G-protein. This observation suggests that the protein encoded by *m9-m10* might participate in membrane-related communication processes.

How can you directly address the question of the molecular mechanisms by which the neurogenic genes operate in neurogenesis?

What we have up to now is circumstantial and indirect evidence. What we are trying to do next is to develop a heterologous transformation system. We are looking for cells which normally do not express those genes, with the aim of transforming them with the genes, to see whether phenotypic changes occur. This experiment would allow us to test the various hypotheses about the mechanism of action.

CONCLUSIONS

The evidence that the products of the neurogenic genes form a functional network that mediates postulated cell interactions during development is rather indirect. Yet, this hypothesis best explains all the available data, at least with respect to a cell's decision to follow the neural or the epidermal pathways. We would like to propose that within the neuroectodermal cells the *N* protein, the *Dl* protein and protein(s) encoded by the *E(spl)* gene complex interact with each other. Sequencing data suggest that the latter proteins may be responsible for transducing and/or relaying the signal into the genome of the receiving cell.

It is not known whether a neuralizing signal is operative during normal development, for its existence is supported only by the results of heterotopic transplantations. Several pieces of evidence derived, for example, from laser ablations (Taghert et al., 1984; Doe and Goodman, 1985), from normal embryology (Hartenstein and Campos-Ortega, 1984) and cell transplantations (Technau and Campos-Ortega, 1986), and from the phenotype of neurogenic mutants (Lehmann et al., 1983), point to a primary neural fate for all the neuroectodermal cells. It is possible, however, that a neuralizing signal is required to reinforce the primary neural fate in those cells that definitively adopt the neural fate.

In any case, the functions of the genes of the AS-C and neighboring loci (Garcia-Bellido, 1979; Jimenez and Campos-Ortega, 1979; 1987; Carramolino et al., 1982) and the *da* locus (Caudy et al., 1988a; 1988b), are likely to be responsible for the neural pathway of development. Two main arguments support this contention: the phenotype of loss-of-function mutations, that are in part caused by NB defects, and the distribution of some of the AS-C transcripts that are clearly correlated with NB segregation (Romani et al., 1987; Cabrera et al., 1987). Interactions among the neurogenic genes indicate that the genes of the subdivision 1B and *da* may be functionally related as intermediate links between the products of the neurogenic genes and the genome of the presumptive NBs.

ACKNOWLEDGEMENTS

Most of the results reported here have been obtained in collaboration with our colleagues of the Institut für Entwicklungsphysiologie. We thank the Deutsche Forschung Gemeinschaft (SFB 74) for financial support.

REFERENCES

Alonso, M.C., and Cabrera, C.V., 1988,. The achaete-scute gene complex of *Drosophila melanogaster* comprises four homologous genes, *EMBO J.* , 7:2585.

Artavanis-Tsakonas, S., Muskavitch, M.A.T., and Yedvobnick, B., 1983, Molecular cloning of *Notch* , a locus affecting neurogenesis in *Drosophila melanogaster*, *Proc. Natl. Acad. Sci. USA*, 80:1977.

Brand, M., and Campos-Ortega, J.A., 1988, Two groups of interrelated genes regulate early neurogenesis in *Drosophila melanogaster*, *Wilhelm Roux`s Arch. Dev. Biol.*, 197:457.

Cabrera, C.V., Martinez-Arias, A., and Bate, M., 1987, The expression of three members of the *achaete-scute* gene complex correlates with neuroblast segregation in *Drosophila*, *Cell*, 50:425.

Campos, A.R., Grossman D., and White K., 1985, Mutant alleles at the locus *elav* in *Drosophila melanogaster* lead to nervous system defects. A developmental-genetic analysis, *J. Neurogenet.*, 2:197.

Carramolino, L., Ruiz-Gomez, M., Guerrero, M.C., Campuzano, S., and Modolell, J., 1982, DNA map of mutations at the *scute* locus of *Drosophila melanogaster*, *EMBO J.*, 1:1185.

Caudy, M., Grell, E.H., Dambly-Chaudière, C., Ghysen, A., Jan, L.Y., Jan, Y.N., 1988a, The maternal sex determination gene daughterless has zygotic activity necessary for the formation of peripheral neurons in *Drosophila*, *Genes Dev.*, 2:843.

Caudy, M., Vässin, H., Brand, M., Tuma, R., Jan, L.Y., Jan, Y.N., 1988b, *daughterless,* a gene essential for both neurogenesis and sex determination in *Drosophila*, has sequence similarities to *myc* and the *achaete-scute* complex, *Cell*, 55:1061.

de la Concha, A., Dietrich, U., Weigel, D., and Campos-Ortega, J.A., 1988, Functional interactions of neurogenic genes of *Drosophila melanogaster*, *Genetics*, 118:499.

Dietrich , U., and Campos-Ortega, J.A., 1984, The expression of neurogenic loci in imaginal epidermal cells of *Drosophila melanogaster*, *J. Neurogenet.*, 1:315.

Doe, C.Q. and Goodman, C.S., 1985, Early events in insect neurogenesis. II. The role of cell interactions and cell lineages in the determination of neuronal precursor cells, *Dev. Biol.*, 111:206.

Garcia-Bellido, A., 1979, Genetic analysis of the *achaete-scute* system of *Drosophila melanogaster*, *Genetics*, 91:491.

Hartenstein, V., and Campos-Ortega, J.A., 1984, Early neurogenesis in wildtype *Drosophila melanogaster*, *Wilhelm Roux`s Arch. Dev. Biol.*, 193:308.

Hartenstein, V. ,and Campos-Ortega, J.A., 1985, Fate mapping in wildtype *Drosophila melanogaster*. I. The pattern of embryonic cell divisions, *Wilhelm Roux`s Arch. Dev. Biol.*, 194:181.

Hartenstein, V., Rudloff, E., and Campos-Ortega, J.A., 1987, The pattern of proliferation of the neuroblasts in the wildtype embryo of *Drosophila melanogaster*, *Wilhelm Roux`s Arch. Dev. Biol.*, 196:473.

Hartley, D.A., Xu, T., and Artavanis-Tsakonas, S., 1987, The embryonic expression of the *Notch* locus of *Drosophila melanogaster* and the implications of point mutations in the extracellular EGF-like domain of the predicted protein, *EMBO J.*, 6:3407.

Hartley, D.A., Preiss, A., and Artavanis-Tsakonas, S., 1988, A deduced gene product from the *Drosophila* neurogenic locus *Enhancer of split* shows homology to mammalian G-protein ß subunit, *Cell,* 55:785.

Hoppe, P.E., and Greenspan, R.J., 1986, Local function of the *Notch* gene for embryonic ectodermal choice in *Drosophila, Cell,* 46:773.

Jiménez, F., and Campos-Ortega, J.A., 1979, A region of the *Drosophila* genome necessary for CNS development, *Nature,* 282:310.

Jiménez, F., and Campos-Ortega, J.A., 1987, Genes in subdivision 1B of the *Drosophila melanogaster* X-chromosome and their influence on neural development, *J. Neurogenet.,* 4:179.

Kidd, S., Lockett, T.J., and Young, M.W.,1983, The *Notch* locus of *Drosophila melanogaster, Cell,* 34:421.

Kidd, S., Kelley, M.R., and Young, M.W., 1986, Sequence of the *Notch* locus of *Drosophila melanogaster:*Relationship of the encoded protein to mammalian clotting and growth factors, *Mol. Cell Biol.,* 6:3094.

Klämbt, C., Knust, E., Tietze, K., and Campos-Ortega, J.A., 1989, Closely related transcripts encoded by the neurogenic gene complex *Enhancer of split* of *Drosophila melanogaster, EMBO J.,* (in press).

Knust, E., Tietze, K., and Campos-Ortega, J.A., 1987, Molecular analysis of the neurogenic locus *Enhancer of split* of *Drosophila melanogaster, EMBO J.,* 6:4113.

Kopczynski, C.C., Alton, A.K., Fetchel, K., Kooh, P.J., and Muskavitch, A.T., 1988, *Delta,* a *Drosophila* neurogenic gene, is transcriptionally complex and encodes a protein related to blood coagulation factors and epidermal growth factor of vertebrates, *Genes Dev.,* 2:1723.

Lehmann, R., Jiménez, F., Dietrich, U, and Campos-Ortega, J. A., 1983, On the phenotype and development of mutants of early neurogenesis in *Drosophila melanogaster, Wilhelm Roux's Arch. Dev. Biol.,* 192:62.

Poulson, D.F., 1937, Chromosomal deficiencies and embryonic development of *Drosophila melanogaster, Proc. Natl. Acad. Sci. USA .,* 23:133.

Poulson, D.F., 1950, Histogenesis, organogenesis and differentiation in the embryo of *Drosophila melanogaster,* in:"Biology of *Drosophila,"* M. Demerec, ed., Hafner, New York, p. 268.

Preiss, A., Hartley, D.A., and Artavanis-Tsakonas, S., 1988, The molecular genetics of *Enhancer of split,* a gene required for embryonic neural development in *Drosophila, EMBO J.,* 7:3917.

Romani, S., Campuzano, S., and Modolell, J., 1987, The *achaete-scute* complex is expressed in neurogenic regions of *Drosophila* embryos, *EMBO J.,* 6:2085.

Taghert, P.H., Doe, C.Q., and Goodman, C.S., 1984, Cell determination and regulation during development of neuroblasts and neurones in grasshopper embryos, *Nature,* 307:163.

Technau, G.M., Becker, T., and Campos-Ortega, J.A., 1988, Reversible commitment of neural and epidermal progenitor cells during embryogenesis of *Drosophila melanogaster, Wilhelm Roux's Arch. Dev. Biol.,* 197:413.

Technau, G.M., and Campos-Ortega, J.A., 1985, Fate mapping in wildtype *Drosophila melanogaster.* II. Injections of horseradish peroxidase in cells of the early gastrula stage, *Wilhelm Roux's Arch. Dev. Biol.,* 194:196.

Technau, G.M., and Campos-Ortega, J.A., 1986, Lineage analysis of transplanted individual cells in embryos of *Drosophila melanogaster.* II. Commitment and proliferative capabilities of neural and epidermal cell progenitors, *Wilhelm Roux's Arch. Dev. Biol.,* 195:445.

Technau, G.M., and Campos-Ortega, J.A., 1987, Cell autonomy of expression of neurogenic genes of *Drosophila melanogaster, Proc. Natl. Acad. Sci. USA.,* 84:4500 .

Vässin, H., Bremer, K. A., Knust, E., and Campos-Ortega, J.A.,1987, The neurogenic locus *Delta* of *Drosophila melanogaster* is expressed in neurogenic territories and encodes a putative transmembrane protein with EGF-like repeats, *EMBO J.,* 6:3431.

Villares, R., and Cabrera, C.V., 1987, The *achaete-scute* gene complex of *Drosophila melanogaster:* conserved domains in a subset of genes required for neurogenesis and their homology to *myc, Cell,* 50:415.

Wharton, K.A., Johansen, K.M., Xu, T., and Artavanis-Tsakonas, S., 1985, Nucleotide sequence from the neurogenic locus *Notch* implies a gene product that shares homology with proteins containing EGF-like repeats, *Cell,* 43:567.

White, K., 1980, Defective neural development in *Drosophila melanogaster* embryos deficient for the tip of the X-chromosome, *Dev. Biol.,* 80:322.

Ziemer, A., Tietze, K., Knust, E., and Campos-Ortega, J.A., 1988, Genetic analysis of *Enhancer of split,* a locus involved in neurogenesis in *Drosophila melanogaster, Genetics,* 119:63.

LINEAGE VERSUS ENVIRONMENT AS A DETERMINANT OF NEURONAL PHENOTYPE [*]

Janet E. Braisted (scribe), Pamela A. Raymond (lecturer)

Department of Anatomy and Cell Biology
University of Michigan Medical School
Ann Arbor, Michigan, USA

INTRODUCTION

How do neurons and glial cells acquire their distinct identities? What determines cell fate during neural development? What constraints are placed on the developing nervous system by genetic and environmental factors, and how do these two influences interact? The answers to these questions are essential to understanding how the highly ordered nervous system, characterized by extreme cellular diversity, develops from a seemingly homogeneous population of neuroectodermal cells.

The control of cell determination is a problem of general importance in developmental biology, not just the nervous system. But because of the enormous diversity of neuronal cell types, and the importance of the highly specific morphological and physiological properties of individual cells on which the very function of the nervous system depends, the processes that determine cell identity are especially critical. For purposes of argument, it is useful to set up a dichotomy between lineage-dependent programming and lineage-independent mechanisms, two hypotheses that have been proposed to underlie cell determination. Lineage-dependent programming predicts that the differentiated fate of a cell depends on predetermined or intrinsic instructions passed from progenitor cells to their progeny, carried out, for example, by asymmetric partitioning of cellular determinants. We could paraphrase this hypothesis as: "You are who you are because of ancestry". Lineage-independent mechanisms imply that cells are intrinsically equipotent (i.e., can potentially select a number of different developmental pathways), and cell fate is determined by environmental or positional factors such as position-dependent cell interactions: or "Who you are depends on who your neighbors are". Any particular developing system is likely to involve a combination of these two extreme alternative mechanisms, but with a variable contribution from each.

Our challenge is to learn which factors are important at each stage in development of the nervous system and how they might interact. Two model systems will be discussed which hold the promise of providing useful clues to understanding the relative roles of lineage and environment in the determination of neuronal phenotype. The first model is the compound eye of *Drosophila*, and the second is the vertebrate retina. Although the insect compound eye and the vertebrate eye evolved independently, both have a highly ordered structure and a limited number of discrete cell types, properties which are favorable for an analysis of cell determination. The *Drosophila* eye has the additional important advantage of being amenable to genetic analysis.

---

[*] This chapter to be cited as: Braisted, J. E., and Raymond, P. A., 1990, Lineage versus environment as a determinant of neuronal phenotype, in: "Systems Approaches to Developmental Neurobiology," P. A. Raymond, S. S. Easter, Jr., and G. M. Innocenti, eds., Plenum Press, New York.

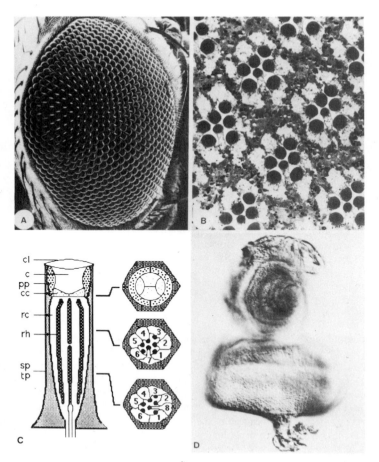

Fig. 1. (A) A smooth array of 700-800 ommatidia forms a *Drosophila* compound eye. Anterior is to the right. Small mechanosensory bristles project between ommatidia. (B) A tangential section of the eye; anterior is to the right. In any cross section, ommatidia present an asymmetric, trapezoidal pattern of seven rhabdomeres. (C) A schematic ommatidium; anterior is to the right. Below the corneal lens (**cl**) is a second lens element, the pseudocone (**c**), which is a refractile extracellular secretion of the four underlying cone cells (**cc**). The accessory cone cells meet in the center occluding the principal cone cells from contact. The cone cells are collared by the two primary pigment cells (**pp**). Photoreceptors, or retinula cells (**rc**), are elongated sensory neurons that carry rhabdomeres (**rh**), dense stacks of rhodopsin-loaded microvilli. Rhabdomeres of photoreceptors **R1-R6** extend the depth of the ommatidium. The rhabdomere of **R7** lies above that of **R8** on the central axis. A sheath of secondary and tertiary pigment cells (**sp, tp**) optically insulates each ommatidium. (D) A late third instar eye-antennal disc; anterior is to the top. The upper portion is the antennal disc which is folded into a series of concentric rings, and below it is the broad, slightly cupped eye disc. The morphogenetic furrow runs dorsoventrally across the eye disc. Ommatidial patterning occurs posterior to the furrow. At the posterior of the eye disc is the optic stalk which carries axons to the brain (not shown). (Reprinted with permission from Tomlinson and Ready, 1987b.)

EVIDENCE FOR POSITIONAL CUES AS REGULATORS OF CELL DETERMINATION IN *DROSOPHILA* RETINA

The compound eye of *Drosophila* consists of 700-800 repeating units or facets called ommatidia (Fig. 1A). Each ommatidium contains 8 individual photoreceptor cells, R1 to R8, arranged in a stereotyped array (Fig. 1B). Overlying each cluster of photoreceptors are four cone cells which secrete a lens that acts as a tiny focusing apparatus for each ommatidium (Fig. 1C).

The developing retinal epithelium, or eye disc, begins as an undifferentiated neuroepithelium (Ready, 1989). Ommatidial development starts at the posterior pole of the eye disc and progresses anteriorly. The transition between undifferentiated cells anteriorly and differentiating retina posteriorly is marked by a groove in the neuroepithelium called the morphogenetic furrow, and the various cells of the ommatidia differentiate behind it (Fig. 1D). This highly regular and stereotyped spatiotemporal pattern of development allows one to visualize the entire range of ommatidial cell differentiation in a single developing eye disc.

Mosaic Analysis

In 1976, Ready and colleagues (Ready et al., 1976) asked the question, are *Drosophila* photoreceptor cells related by lineage? In order to answer this, they created mosaics of wild type and a recessive, pigment-deleting mutant, white. This is done by x-ray irradiation of embryonic flies heterozygous for white; this manipulation causes chromosomal breaks and reunions in mitotic cells, and in some cases daughter cells homozygous for white are generated. The clonal progeny of the white daughter cells populate a patch of the growing eyes and along the border of white and wild type regions are mosaic ommatidia. A careful analysis of phenotypes in mixed populations of wild type and mutant cells comprising single ommatidia revealed that there were no consistent lineage relationships among photoreceptor cells in each ommatidium. This result suggested that cell identity was determined instead by cell position in the ommatidium. The isolation and characterization in Seymour Benzer's laboratory of a mutant, *sevenless* (Harris et al., 1976), which lacks the UV sensitive R7 photoreceptor cells, allowed this hypothesis to be tested directly.

The *Sevenless* Mutation

During ommatidial development in wild type flies, neuroepithelial cells rise to the apical surface, then sink back down as they differentiate into photoreceptors (Fig. 2, top panel). In the *sevenless* mutant, the putative R7 photoreceptor cell rises to the apical surface of the neuroepithelium, but it never sinks back down to the basal surface (Fig. 2, bottom panel). Instead, the putative R7 cell remains at the apical surface and differentiates into a cone cell (Tomlinson and Ready, 1986). Although the putative R7 becomes a cone, only four cone cells are found in each ommatidium, as in the wild type, and it is not known what happens to the cell that would normally have become the fourth cone cell.

In order to test whether the mutant R7 cell is unable to respond to environmental cues which would instruct or allow it to become a photoreceptor, mosaics of wild type and *sevenless* were analyzed (Harris et al., 1976; Tomlinson and Ready, 1987a). Both groups found that cells with wild type genotype in the R7 position of an ommatidium otherwise composed of cells with *sevenless* genotype differentiated as R7, but never was an R7 cell with *sevenless* genotype found. The conclusions are that the *sevenless* mutation is cell-autonomous, and the mutant R7 cell lacks some factor which allows it to "read" its environment.

The *sevenless* gene has recently been isolated and cloned (Hafen et al., 1978). It codes for a putative transmembrane protein with a large extracellular domain and a tyrosine kinase domain, features common to both the EGF receptor and certain viral oncogenes. These observations are consistent with the suggestion that the *sevenless* gene product codes for a receptor which allows the R7 cell to read positional information which directs it to select the R7 developmental pathway. Other cells besides R7, both inside and outside the eye, express the *sevenless* gene product (Tomlinson et al., 1987; Bowtell et al., 1988), but the role of *sevenless* in these cells, if any, is presently not known.

LACK OF EVIDENCE FOR LINEAGE-DEPENDENT MECHANISMS IN VERTEBRATE RETINA

The vertebrate retina has a number of advantages for the analysis of cell determination in the CNS. It is a highly ordered, laminated structure with a limited number of cell types, arranged in a

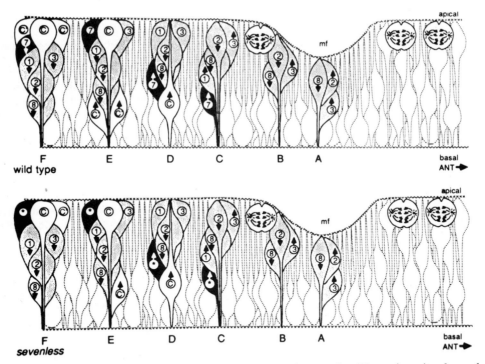

Fig. 2. Schematic longitudinal view of ommatidial assembly as it occurs in wild type (upper) and *sevenless* (lower) third instar eye discs. Many of the cells (including **R1** and **R6**, **R2** and **R5**, **R3** and **R4**, anterior and posterior cone cells) behave as pairs and only a single member of these pairs is shown. Ommatidial assembly begins in the morphogenetic furrow (**mf**) where the nuclei of all cells are compacted into the basal regions. (A,B) Five nuclei, those of photoreceptors **R2, R3, R4, R5,** and **R8,** begin to rise into the apical regions as all other cells undergo division. Cells are progressively added to this five-cell unit, and as a cell becomes incorporated into the cluster its nucleus rises into the apical regions. To accommodate the newly rising nuclei, those already in the apical regions begin to move basally. Arrows indicate nuclear movement at each stage, those shown for A and B are inferred and are not known precisely. (C) The first cells to become added to the five are the remaining photoreceptors **R1, R6,** and **R7, R7** being delayed somewhat compared to the other two. (D) By the symmetrical cluster stage, the nucleus of **R7** is still comparatively basal. (E) As the nucleus of **R7** completes its apical migration the nuclei of the anterior and posterior cone cells (**c**) also rise. (F) The nucleus of **R7** now falls; the nuclei of the equatorial and polar cone cells (**c'**) rise (F). In *sevenless* the process occurs identically (A-E), but the nucleus of the cell in the **R7** position (asterisk) does not withdraw basally but remains in the apical regions as the equatorial cone cell. (Reprinted with permission from Tomlinson and Ready, 1987a.)

repeating pattern that is conserved throughout vertebrate evolution. Development takes place in an orderly spatiotemporal progression that begins in the posterior eye cup and sweeps anteriorly. Distinct cell types can be identified not only by their morphology and laminar position but also by the use of cell-specific antibodies (Barnstable, 1980). In addition, numerous specific RNA/DNA probes are available for certain retinal cell types, especially photoreceptors (Lerea et al., 1986; Nathans et al., 1986).

32

Retinal Development

The structure and morphological development of the vertebrate eye is well known. The retina is an outgrowth of the brain, and consists of an outer layer, the retinal pigmented epithelium or **RPE**, and an inner layer, the neural retina. Between these two layers there is a presumptive space, filled with cell processes, called the subretinal space; this is actually the remnant of the optic ventricle, a cavity originally continuous with the ventricular spaces in the brain, which collapsed during development. The **RPE** consists of a single layer of cuboidal cells filled with melanin granules that function to absorb scattered light entering the eye. The neural retina consists of 3 nuclear layers, the outer nuclear layer (**ONL**), the inner nuclear layer (**INL**), and the ganglion cell layer (**GCL**). The **ONL** consists of the nuclei of the photoreceptor cells, the rods and cones, whereas the **INL** contains the nuclei of various interneurons.

A simplified scheme of retinal development is shown in Fig. 3. The developing vertebrate retina is a simple pseudostratified epithelium of dividing neuroepithelial cells (Fig. 3A). The dividing neuroepithelial cells, like neuroepithelial cells elsewhere in the developing central nervous system, undergo a process known as interkinetic nuclear migration (Barnstable, 1987; Stone, 1988). The first evidence of differentiation occurs when a neuroepithelial cell stops dividing, loses contact with the apical surface, then migrates to the basal surface and begins to differentiate (Fig. 3B). The first cells in the neural retina to differentiate are the ganglion cells, and (in mammals and fish) the photoreceptor cells of the **ONL** are among the last to differentiate (Raymond and Rivlin, 1987; Stone, 1988)

Retinal Cell Lineage

Many investigators have asked whether specific lineage relationships exist among the various retinal cells. Recent work includes two elegant studies in the amphibian retina (Holt et al., 1988; Wetts and Fraser, 1988). Holt and Harris injected HRP into individual neuroepithelial cells of embryonic *Xenopus* at the optic vesicle stage. The HRP was passed from mother to daughter cells, and the clone of labeled cells was later visualized histochemically in the adult retina. Wetts and Fraser performed similar experiments, but instead injected fluorescently-labeled dextran into individual neuroepithelial cells. Both groups found radially elongated clones composed of many combinations of neurons and sometimes Müller glial cells. Therefore, single neuroepithelial cells have the capacity to produce multiple types of retinal cells. This observation suggests that lineage-dependent mechanisms may not be very important in the determination of cell phenotype in the amphibian retina.

A different technique for clonal analysis was pioneered by Cepko and colleagues in the rat retina (Price et al., 1987; Turner and Cepko, 1987). This technique uses retroviral vector-mediated gene transfer. The vector, which contains a reporter gene, the bacterial enzyme B-galactosidase, is injected into the early postnatal rat retina. Only those host cells that are undergoing mitosis stably incorporate the introduced genes into their genome, and pass them on to their progeny. If an appropriately low concentration of the vector is injected, isolated clusters (presumed clones) of cells can be detected using a histochemical stain to demonstrate B-galactosidase activity. Results in the rat were similar to those in frogs, in that clones were radially distributed, with little lateral dispersion of labeled cells, and most clones consisted of multiple cell types, somtimes including Müller glial cells along with neurons. This again suggests that retinal precursor cells are not committed to predetermined pathways, and that lineage relationships are not important for determining cell type in the vertebrate retina.

If lineage is not related to the determination of neuronal phenotype in the vertebrate retina, then perhaps positional cues are important, as in the *Drosophila* retina.

THE SEARCH FOR POSITIONAL CUES INVOLVED IN CELL DETERMINATION IN VERTEBRATE RETINA

The teleost fish retina possesses a number of unique features that make it especially useful for investigating the role of cell interactions in determining cell fate in the vertebrate retina. Most important is the fact that the retina in fish continues to grow even in the adult by the proliferation of precursor cells (Raymond, 1985). Some precursor cells are found in an undifferentiated germinal zone at the circumferential margin of the retina. Complete rings of new retina are added throughout

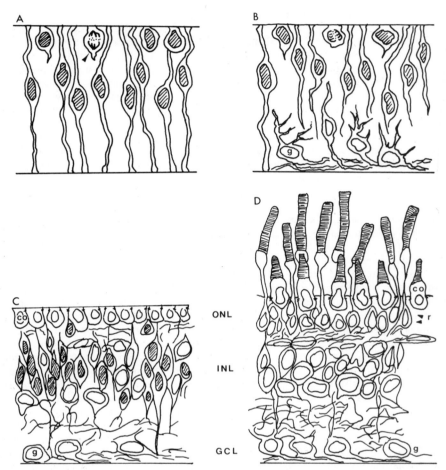

Fig. 3. Retinal histogenesis. (A) The primitive retinal epithelium is a homogeneous sheet of dividing neuroepithelial cells. These are spindle-shaped cells which typically span the width of the epithelium. During mitosis the basal process is withdrawn, the nucleus moves to the apical surface and the cell rounds up to divide (arrowhead). (B) Cells with hatched nuclei are immature neuroepithelial cells still actively proliferating. Open nuclei are post-mitotic differentiating neurons or glia. The first neurons to differentiate are ganglion cells (g). As a young neuron leaves the mitotic cycle it detaches from the apical surface and the nucleus moves down the basal process until it reaches the appropriate level, which for the ganglion cells is next to the inner (basal) surface. While the nucleus is still migrating an axon begins to grow out, as can be seen in the post-mitotic cell directly beneath the mitotic figure. (C) With further development the cells of the neuroepithelium are partitioned into the three definitive strata of the differentiated retina, the ganglion cell layer (**GCL**), the inner nuclear layer (**INL**), and the outer nuclear layer (**ONL**). In teleost fish and also in primates, rods are at first under-represented in the layer of photoreceptor nuclei (the outer nuclear layer). At this early stage, the outer nuclear layer consists of a single layer of immature cone nuclei. This drawing equally well depicts the immature mammalian retina, or the larval teleost retina. (D) In the mature teleost retina there is a single layer of cone nuclei (**co**) and multiple layers of rod nuclei (**r**) in the outer nuclear layer. A similar organization is found in most mammalian retinas. (Modified from Raymond, 1985.)

adult life, like the rings in a growing tree trunk. In addition, specialized neuronal precursors are scattered within differentiated regions of retina, and these play a special role in retinal neurogenesis, as described below.

Development of Photoreceptors in the Fish Retina

In teleost fish, there is a temporal segregation of rod and cone birthdates in the developing retina. Raymond showed that in larval goldfish, during the early stages of retinal differentiation, the ONL consists of a single row of postmitotic cells, all of which subsequently differentiate into cones (Johns, 1982; Raymond, 1985). Rods are added at a later stage. A similar sequence occurs in other teleosts, including zebrafish (Branchek and BreMiller, 1984). At the time of hatching, photoreceptor cells are immature, and in particular they lack outer segments (elongated processes that extend apically into the subretinal space and that contain the visual pigments). Maturation of photoreceptors proceeds quickly, so that within a couple of days after hatching, a monolayer of young cones with well developed outer segments is present apically in the ONL. Rod nuclei are inserted into the ONL basal to the cone nuclei after a slight temporal delay, and rod, but not cone nuclei accummulate in the central retina over a very prolonged period, as the eye continues to enlarge throughout the animal's lifetime.

What are the visual consequences of this temporal segregation of cone and rod differentiation? Why do early larval fish have a cone-dominated retina?

Blaxter and Staines (1970) described a similar sequence of photoreceptor development in a number of marine teleost fish. Some of these fish have a very slow rate of development; for example, in herring and sole the larval stage can last for several months. During the larval period these fish possess an "all-cone" retina. Rods are not added until metamorphosis. A rationale for this curious developmental sequence is that the larval fish are visual predators and hunt moving prey near the surface of the water column where the light intensity is high. Since cones are specialized for photopic vision, an "all-cone" retina is suitable during this stage in the animal's life. At metamorphosis the fish move into deeper water where less light penetrates, and therefore they benefit from the increased visual sensitivity imparted by rods.

In the early 1980's it was discovered that specialized rod precursor cells located within differentiated regions of retina produce new rods that are inserted into the fixed mosaic of cones (Sandy and Blaxter, 1980; Johns and Fernald, 1981). Studies with tritiated thymidine autoradiography to label mitotic cells and their progeny demonstrated that mitotically-active rod precursor cells are initially located in the INL in larval goldfish (Johns, 1982). These precursor cells migrate to the ONL as the retina differentiates; there they persist and continue to divide producing new rods even in adult fish (Fig. 4; Johns, 1982). With serial EM autoradiography, Raymond and Rivlin (1987) demonstrated that clusters of undifferentiated precursor cells are associated with radial fibers of Müller glial cells, and they argued that the precursor cells use the glial fibers as guides to assist in their migration from the INL to the ONL. The lineage relationship between the undifferentiated precursors and the Müller glia is not certain, but the clonal experiments in amphibian and rat retina suggest the possibility that Müller glia and the associated clusters of undifferentiated cells destined to become rod precursors in the ONL might be clonally related.

The question of most importance to the present discussion is whether rod precursor cells are committed to the rod pathway. Recent work by Raymond and colleagues suggests that this may not be the case. If neurons in adult goldfish are killed either with ouabain, a neurotoxin which inhibits Na/K ATPase, or by ischemia, the neural retina subsequently regenerates (Raymond et al., 1988; Raymond, unpublished observations). With tritiated thymidine autoradiography, local foci of dividing cells associated with the apical surface were shown to give rise to regenerated retina. Since the only cells consistently surviving after either of these treatments were glial cells, dividing cells (both rod precursors and neuroepithelial cells in the marginal germinal zone) and vascular cells, including microglia, one of these cell types is likely to be the source of cells for the new retina. The weight of evidence suggests that it is the mitotically-active rod precursors in the ONL that produce the new retina (Raymond et al., 1988). If, as the data suggest, the rod precursors are the source of cells for the regenerate, then the developmental potential of the rod precursors is intrinsically greater than the developmental fate that they normally express. This conclusion is again consistent with the idea that retinal cell fate is independent of lineage.

Could electrical activity play a role in retinal cell differentiation?

Branchek (1984) showed in the zebrafish retina that electrical activity is correlated with the first appearance of photoreceptor outer segments and ribbon synapses in photoreceptor cells, on the third day post-fertilization. At about the same time, retinal ganglion cell axons reach the optic tectum (Stuermer, 1988). These initial electrical responses (ERGs) are small in amplitude and require a high intensity stimulus. On the eighth day rod nuclei are present, and not until day twelve are rod outer segments seen with light microscopy, long after electrical activity is detected in the retina. It is therefore possible that early electrical activity could influence the differentiation of rods.

Possible Positional Cues

In order to examine position-dependent cell interactions that might be involved in regulating cell determination in the vertebrate retina, we must first describe the anatomical relationships among cells at various stages of development. Based on a number of earlier studies of retinal histogenesis (Stone, 1988), several different developmental pathways that give rise to the various retinal cell types can be recognized. Three of these are shown in Figure 4; the cone, the rod, and the ganglion cell pathways. All three pathways start with undifferentiated neuroepithelial cells. At the apical surface, the cells are connected to one another by junctional complexes. Those cells that are destined to become cones (left panel) retract their basal process and round up at the apical surface. At the basal end of the cell synaptic vesicles accumulate and a short axon sprouts, and on the apical side an elongated ciliated appendage penetrates the subretinal space and matures into an inner and outer segment.

The rod pathway is quite different (Fig. 4, center panel). After the ONL becomes distinguishable as a single row of post-mitotic cones, some neuroepithelial cells whose nuclei are located in the INL lose their attachments at both apical and basal surfaces, and partially withdraw their processes. In the developing fish retina, clusters of these spindle-shaped cells in the INL migrate into the ONL in association with radial Müller fibers. In the ONL they generate a layer of rod nuclei basal to the layer of preexisting cone nuclei, as described above. Differentiation of the newly-forming rods is similar to cones in that they extend axons toward the basal surface and apical processes into the subretinal space beyond the layer of cone outer segments.

Cells differentiating as ganglion cells detach from the apical surface after the last round of cell division, then migrate basally as they differentiate (Fig. 4, right panel). Their axons turn and grow along the basal surface, and subsequently exit the eye in the developing optic nerve.

With these descriptive observations as a base, we can now begin to formulate hypotheses about what environmental cues might possibly influence the choice of developmental pathway that a given neuroepithelial cell makes. For example, differentiating cells in the cone pathway do not lose contact with the apical surface nor do they lose junctional contacts with their neighbors. These positional relationships might be important in triggering cone cell differentiation. In contrast, differentiating rods detach from both the apical and basal surfaces, are in intimate contact with Müller cells, and are surrounded by a variety of other differentiating cell types. While in the INL, rod precursors continue to divide and migrate; when they reach the ONL, they may divide and some begin to differentiate. Which, if any, of these associations are important in determining the rod developmental pathway is not yet clear. There is some evidence that when dissociated cells from neonatal rat retina are placed in culture, photoreceptors differentiate, as evidenced by the formation of outer segments and the expression of specific gene products, but only when specific junctions are formed with Müller glial cells (Barnstable, 1987). This observation tends to support the proposal that cell-cell interactions are important in photoreceptor determination. Finally, environmental cues important for ganglion cell

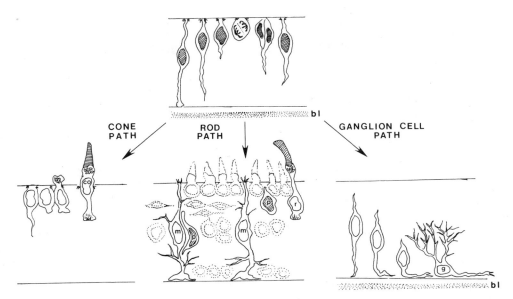

Fig. 4. Schematic view of three developmental pathways that give rise to differentiated neurons in the vertebrate retina. The upper panel illustrates the undifferentiated state common to all three developmental pathways. The lower panels illustrate the three different developmental pathways that give rise to cones (left), rods (middle), and ganglion cells (right). In each panel, apical is above, and basal is below. For details, see text. (**bl**=basal lamina, **m**=Müller glial cell, **p**=rod precursor, **r**=rod; all other abbreviations as in Fig. 3.)

differentiation might be related to their early detachment from the apical surface (perhaps the cells get "pushed" out?), or their close contact with the basal lamina.

It is interesting to ask whether known differences in the molecular environment of the apical and basal surfaces might be involved in determining cell fate in the retina. The composition of the extracellular matrix has been shown to influence neural development in other systems, most notably neural crest migration and formation of neuromuscular junctions (Sanes, 1989). A thick basement membrane, called Bruch's membrane, lies adjacent to the retinal pigmented epithelium (RPE), on the side distant from the neural retina. On the basal surface of the neural retina lies another basement membrane, the inner limiting membrane or ILM. Reh and colleagues (Reh et al., 1987) looked at the composition of extracellular matrix molecules in these two membranes in the amphibian eye and determined that Bruch's membrane has a substantially lower laminin content than the ILM. Laminin is known to be a good substrate for axonal outgrowth, and in the layer of cells immediately adjacent to the ILM there are retinal ganglion cells, the only retinal neurons with long projecting axons. It is tempting to speculate that contact with the ECM components of the ILM, such as laminin, might be causally related to determination of the ganglion cell phenotype. Suggestive evidence in support of this notion comes from recent *in vitro* studies again by Reh and colleagues (Reh et al., 1987). When RPE cells were cultured on a laminin-poor substrate, they retained their differentiated phenotype. However, when the RPE cells were instead placed on a substrate with a high concentration of laminin, they divided, lost their pigment and began to express neuronal cell markers. Reh had earlier demonstrated that in the regenerating amphibian retina, RPE cells lose contact with Bruch's membrane and participate in phagocytosis of the degenerating retina. As the retinal debris is removed, the RPE cells come to lie adjacent to the ILM, at which point they appear to transdifferentiate into neuroepithelial-like cells, which subsequently produce new neural retina (Reh and Nagy, 1987). Thus it appears that the composition of Bruch's membrane and the ILM may regulate or stabilize the commitment to neuronal versus epithelial phenotype in this system.

By analogy, we might consider ECM components in searching for molecular clues involved in the choice of the photoreceptor developmental pathways in developing retinae. For example, there is a specialized extracellular matrix sheath found around cone outer segments in the differentiated retina (Johnson et al., 1986). This cone sheath can be selectively stained with the lectin, peanut agglutinin (Johnson et al., 1986), but the composition of the cone sheath and its possible role in the determination of cell fate are not presently known. Recently, however, it was shown that the cone sheath is present very early in development, even before the cone outer segments appear (Anderson et al., 1989), and it is therefore ideally suited to be an environmental cue perhaps signalling cells to differentiate as cones.

A working hypothesis that evolves out of these considerations is that the apical surface of the neural retina is special, and contact with it is important in directing or allowing cells to choose the photoreceptor pathway of differentiation. If a neuroepithelial cell finds itself in this location at a particular stage in development, it becomes a photoreceptor. But what regulates the choice to become a rod or a cone? The cone pathway seems to be the preferred choice, since a complete layer of cones lines the apical surface before any rods are added. The rod pathway seems to be chosen secondarily, and the cellular environment and positional relationships of neuroepithelial cells that chose this pathway must be altogether different from those that might regulate cone differentiation.

SUMMARY

The conclusion seems inescapable that positional cues are important for cell determination in the vertebrate retina. There is good evidence that lineage-dependent mechanisms are not involved, so positional factors are strongly implicated. So far there is no hard evidence for positional factors but there are a lot of interesting possibilities that await to be tested. In the insect compound eye there is strong evidence against lineage and strong evidence in support of extrinsic, position-dependent cell interactions as the determinate of photoreceptor cell identities. Only with further research will we learn whether vertebrate eyes and insect eyes obey similar rules for determination of cell fate.

REFERENCES

Anderson, K., Hageman, G. S., Blanks, J. C., and Spee, C., 1989, Developmental expression of human cone matrix sheath-specific molecules, *Invest. Ophthalmol. Vis. Sci. Suppl.*, 30:490.

Barnstable, C. J., 1980, Monoclonal antibodies which recognize different cell types in the rat retina, *Nature*, 286:231.

Barnstable, C. J., 1987, A molecular view of vertebrate retinal development, *Mol. Neurobiol.*, 1:9.

Blaxter, J. H. S., and Staines, M., 1970, Pure cone retinae and retinomotor responses in larval teleosts, *J. Mar.Biol. Assoc. UK*, 50:449.

Bowtell, D. D. L., Simon, M. A., and Rubin, G. M., 1988, Nucleotide sequence and structure of the *sevenless* gene of *Drosophila melanogaster*, *Genes Dev.*, 2:620.

Branchek, T., 1984, The development of the photoreceptors in the zebrafish, *Brachydanio rerio*. II. Function, *J.Comp. Neurol.*, 224:116.

Branchek, T., and BreMiller, R., 1984, The development of the photoreceptors in the zebrafish, *Brachydanio rerio*. I. Structure, *J. Comp. Neurol.*, 224:107.

Hafen, E., Basler, K., Edstroem, J. E., and Rubin, G. M., 1978, *Sevenless*, a cell-specific homeotic gene of *Drosophila*, encodes a putative transmembrane receptor with a tyrosine kinase domain, *Science*, 236:55.

Harris, W. A., Stark, W. S., and Walker, J. A., 1976, Genetic dissection of the photoreceptor system in the compound eye of *Drosophila melanogaster*, *J. Physiol.(London)*, 256:415.

Holt, C. E., Bertsch, T. W., Ellis, H. M., and Harris, W. A., 1988, Cellular determination in the *Xenopus* retina is independent of lineage and birth date, *Neuron*, 1:15.

Johns (Raymond), P., 1982, The formation of photoreceptors in the growing retinas of larval and adult goldfish, *J.Neurosci.*, 2:178-198.

Johns (Raymond), P., and Fernald, R. D., 1981, Genesis of rods in teleost fish retina, *Nature*, 293:141.

Johnson, L. V., Hageman, G. S., and Blanks, J. C., 1986, Interphotoreceptor matrix domains ensheath vertebrate cone photoreceptor cells, *Invest. Ophthalmol. Vis. Sci.*, 27:129.

Lerea, C. L., Somers, D. E., Hurley, J. B., Klock, I. B., and Bunt-Milam, A. H., 1986, Identification of specific transducin a subunits in retinal rod and cone photoreceptors, *Science*, 234:77.

Nathans, J., Thomas, D., and Hogness, D. S., 1986, Molecular genetics of human color vision: the genes encoding blue, green, and red pigments, *Science*, 232:193.

Price, J., Turner, D., and Cepko, C., 1987, Lineage analysis in the vertebrate nervous system by retrovirus-mediated gene transfer, *Proc. Natl. Acad. Sci. USA*, 8:156.

Raymond, P. A., 1985, Cytodifferentiation of photoreceptors in larval goldfish: delayed maturation of rods, *J.Comp. Neurol.*, 236:90.

Raymond, P. A., Reifler, M. J., and Rivlin, P. K., 1988, Regeneration of goldfish retina: rod precursors are a likely source of regenerated cells, *J. Neurobiol.*, 19:431.

Raymond, P. A., and Rivlin, P. K., 1987, Germinal cells in the goldfish retina that produce rod photoreceptors, *Dev. Biol.*, 122:120.

Ready, D. F., 1989, A multifaceted approach to neural development, *Trends Neurosci.*, 12:102-110.

Ready, D. F., Hanson, T. E., and Benzer, S., 1976, Development of the *Drosophila* retina, a neurocrystalline lattice, *Dev. Biol.*, 53:217.

Reh, T. A., and Nagy, T., 1987, A possible role for the vascular membrane in retinal regeneration in *Rana catesbienna* tadpoles, *Dev. Biol.*, 122;471.

Reh, T. A., Nagy, T., and Gretton, H., 1987, Laminin promotes transdifferentiation of retinal pigment epithelial cells to neurons, *Nature*, 330:68.

Sandy, J. M., and Blaxter, J. H. S., 1980, A study of retinal development in larval herring and sole, *J. Mar. Biol. Assoc. UK*, 60:59.

Sanes, J. R., 1989, Extracellular matrix molecules that influence neural development, *Annu. Rev. Neurosci.*, 12:491.

Stone, J., 1988, The origins of the cells of vertebrate retina, *Prog. Retinal Res.*, 7:1.

Stuermer, C. A. O., 1988, Retinotopic organization of the developing retinotectal projection in the zebrafish embryo, *J. Neurosci.* 8:4513.

Tomlinson, A., Bowtell, D. D. L., Hafen, E., and Rubin G. M., 1987, Localization of the *sevenless* protein, a putative receptor for positional information, in the eye imaginal disc of *Drosophila*, *Cell*, 51:143.

Tomlinson, A., and Ready, D. F., 1986, *Sevenless*: a cell-specific homeotic mutation of the *Drosophila* eye, *Science*, 231:400.

Tomlinson, A., and Ready, D. F., 1987a, Cell fate in *Drosophila* ommatidium, *Dev. Biol.*, 123:264.

Tomlinson, A., and Ready, D. F., 1987b, Neuronal differentiation in the *Drosophila* ommatidium, *Dev. Biol.*, 120:336.

Turner, D. L., and Cepko, C. L., 1987, A common progenitor for neurons and glia persists in rat retina late in development, *Nature*, 328:131.

Wetts, R., and Fraser, S. E., 1988, Multipotent precursors can give rise to all major cell types of the frog retina, *Science*, 239:1142.

PRIMARY MOTONEURONS OF THE ZEBRAFISH [*]

Walter K. Metcalfe (scribe), Monte Westerfield (lecturer)

Institute of Neuroscience
University of Oregon
Eugene, Oregon, USA

INTRODUCTION

We are interested in understanding how cell fate is determined in the nervous system. That is, we want to learn how neurons acquire their particular size, shape, and pattern of connections. This lecture reviews our current state of understanding of rules that govern the embryonic development of a specific set of neurons, the primary motoneurons of the spinal cord in zebrafish (*Brachydanio rerio*). Primary motoneurons are a subset of a larger class of early-developing neurons called primary neurons (Coghill, 1913; Kimmel and Westerfield, 1989).

PRIMARY NEURONS

What is a Primary Neuron?

Primary neurons include a specific subset of neurons from all three functional classes: (1) sensory neurons, such as the tactile-sensitive trigeminal and Rohon-Beard cells, and the vibration-sensitive lateral line (Metcalfe et al., 1985) and auditory neurons, (2) interneurons, including the reticulospinal neurons (Kimmel et al., 1982; Metcalfe et al., 1986) and spinal interneurons (Kuwada, 1986; Roberts and Clarke, 1982). At least some of these reticulospinal neurons (i.e. the Mauthner cell) receive inputs directly from primary sensory neurons, and finally (3) motoneurons, such as the primary motoneurons of the spinal cord (Myers, 1985; Westerfield et al., 1986), which receive input from the reticulospinal neurons and project axons directly to the axial muscle of the fish.

Primary neurons arise early in development (Mendelson, 1986b). They have birthdays (exit the mitotic cycle) near the end of gastrulation, during a short period of time that is distinct from the birthdays of the later-developing secondary neurons. The primary neurons are also the first neurons in the embryo to grow axons; primary neurons are defined as those neurons that grow axons during the first day after fertilization (Kimmel and Westerfield, 1989). Primary neuronal somata are large, and these cells have long axons that interconnect to form a functional circuit that mediates the embryonic behavior of the animal. This circuit of primary neurons may also mediate the adult escape response (Kimmel et al., 1974).

---

[*] This chapter is to be cited as: Metcalfe, W. M., and Westerfield, M., 1990, Primary motoneurons of the zebrafish, in: "Systems Approaches to Developmental Neurobiology," P. A. Raymond, S. S. Easter, Jr., and G. M. Innocenti, eds., Plenum Press, New York.

Primary Neurons are Segmentally Arranged

In the spinal cord and hindbrain, there is a segmentally arranged pattern of organization of the primary neurons. For example, the primary reticulospinal neurons of the hindbrain (Metcalfe et al., 1986) and primary motoneurons of the spinal cord (Eisen et al., 1986) are arranged at similar segmental intervals, suggesting that the spinal cord and hindbrain may be patterned by a common mechanism in the early embryo (Metcalfe et al., 1986; Hanneman et al., 1988).

Genetic Analysis of Development

Zebrafish development is amenable to genetic mutational analysis. George Streisinger pioneered methods of screening directly for recessive mutations in the progeny of fish that had been exposed to gamma rays (Streisinger et al., 1981; Walker and Streisinger, 1983; Chakrabarti et al., 1983). Such screens are performed directly on haploid or diploid offspring. Haploid offspring are derived from eggs that are activated by sperm that carry no genetic information. Such sperm result from ultraviolet irradiation, which destroys the DNA. Homozygous diploid offspring are created from eggs that are activated as above, and in which the first mitotic division is suppressed by hydrostatic pressure. Interesting mutations that affect primary neurons, or the muscle targets of primary motoneurons, are recognized by a lack of function, such as changes in motility in the early embryos, when behavior is dominated by primary neurons. Such mutations, most of which are lethal in homozygous form, are maintained in heterozygous form by crossing the parent lines with wild-type stock. In one such mutation, called *Ned-1*, the primary neurons are specifically spared, while all other (secondary) neurons undergo early cell death (Grunwald et al., 1988). The presence of this mutation suggests that primary neurons are a genetically distinct population of neurons; they may require a different set of genes for their development or maintenance than the later-developing secondary neurons.

Development of Identified Primary Neurons

This simple system of primary neurons provides an unusual opportunity to study details of the life history of identified neurons in a vertebrate. Identified primary neurons are present in reproducible positions, and because of the optical clarity of the embryo, these neurons can be observed directly as they develop in the live embryo. In addition, fluorescent lineage tracer dyes have been used to label blastomere precursors of identified neurons (Kimmel and Law, 1985; Eisen et al., 1986). The dye is distributed to the descendants of the injected cell, resulting in labeled neurons. This technique appears to be nondestructive, since the labeled neurons sprout axons and appear to grow normally. In this way, continuous or repeated observations can be made of the same neuron in intact embryos during their development.

Observations of labeled neurons have enabled a detailed examination of the time course of development and pathway selection by primary motoneurons of the spinal cord (Eisen et al., 1986; Myers et al., 1986). There are three identified primary motoneurons on each side of each spinal segment, and each grows in a stereotyped manner (Westerfield et al, 1986). The caudal motoneuron (CaP) is the first to sprout an axon. The axon grows to the horizontal myoseptum (a special region that separates the dorsal and ventral muscles in each segment), pauses, and then grows to the ventral muscle of its own segment. Similarly, the rostral (RoP) and middle (MiP) primary motoneurons sprout axons in turn, and each follows the common pathway to the horizontal myoseptum, then makes cell-specific divergent pathway choices to innervate spatially separate regions of the muscle in their own segment. Thus, unique, individual neurons have unique developmental programs that include time of origin, time of axonal outgrowth, and axonal pathway.

The resulting circuits of primary neurons form the neural basis for the behavior of the embryo, and remain functional in the adult (Liu and Westerfield, 1988). The primary neurons may also have a special function as pioneers in the embryo, establishing the initial axonal pathways that are subsequently followed by the later-developing secondary neurons (Kuwada, 1986).

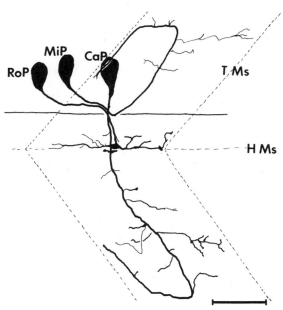

Fig. 1. Lateral view of the three individually identifiable primary motoneurons that innervate each myotome. These motoneurons innervate non-overlapping regions of the myotome. **RoP** (for Rostral Primary) innervates the intermediate muscles in the region of the horizontal myoseptum (dashed line labeled **H Ms** that separates the dorsal and ventral muscles of a segment), **MiP** (Middle Primary) innervates the dorsal muscles, and **CaP** (Caudal Primary) innervates the ventral muscles. The peripheral fields of these primary motoneurons do not cross myotomal boundaries, which are delineated by the transverse myosepta (T Ms). This pattern of motoneurons is repeated in each spinal segment. Scale bar = 25 μm. (Redrawn from Myers et al., 1986.)

HOW IS CELL IDENTITY DETERMINED?

How do the primary motoneurons (CaP, MiP, and RoP) become different from one another, and make divergent cell-type specific pathway choices? There are several potential mechanisms of cell specification including lineage, birth date, time of axonal outgrowth, and cell body position.

Cell Lineage

In many organisms, especially invertebrates, cell fate is determined primarily by cell lineage. In vertebrates, however, the role of cell lineage is not well understood. The blastomere labeling methods described above have allowed us to examine directly the patterns of cell lineages that give rise to the primary motoneurons in zebrafish. If cell lineage plays an important role in specifying cell fate, then perhaps we should expect a specific pattern of cell divisions for each cell type. However, the division patterns giving rise to primary motoneurons are variable (Kimmel and Warga, 1987).

Time of Origin

Is cell fate determined by the time that a cell becomes postmitotic? One possibility would be that the first neuron to become postmitotic in a spinal segment is assigned the fate of CaP, the next MiP, and so on. However, Paul Myers determined the birthdays of primary motoneurons and found variable patterns; CAP may or may not be the first postmitotic neuron in a segment, although it is always the first motoneuron to grow an axon (Myers et al., 1986).

Time of Axonal Outgrowth

Does the temporal sequence of axonal outgrowth specify cell fate? Perhaps the first motoneuron to grow an axon, which is always the CaP motoneuron, will grow to the ventral musculature and acquire the CaP fate. This idea was tested by laser ablation of individual CaP motoneurons before they grew axons. This hypothesis predicts that another primary motoneuron will acquire the CaP cell fate, since it will then become the first to grow an axon out of the cord. However, labeling the remaining primary motoneurons (MiP and RoP) with lucifer yellow showed that they developed normally, i.e., as MiP and RoP, and that they never projected axons into the CaP target region (Eisen et al., 1989; Pike and Eisen, 1990).

Cell Body Position

Each of the primary motoneurons occupies a cell-specific position in the spinal cord. Perhaps this position determines cell fate and specifies the path that the axon will take. To test this, Judith Eisen has begun to transplant identified primary motoneurons to new locations in the spinal cord (Eisen, 1989). She has observed that when CaP is moved to the MiP position before it has begun to grow an axon, it acquires the MiP fate. Thus, the fate of primary motoneurons may be determined at least in part by a position-dependent mechanism.

THE PERIPHERAL PATHWAY

Having considered factors that may determine which motoneuron will project its axon along a particular peripheral pathway, the peripheral pathway itself is now examined. What forms the pathway?

Acetylcholine Receptors

Growing motor axons appear to interact functionally with their muscle target cells as they grow. Eric Hanneman showed that muscle fibers in individual segments twitch at the time that growth cones grow out from the corresponding spinal segment (Hanneman and Westerfield, 1989). Intracellular electrical recordings from the muscle cells revealed spontaneous and evoked potentials that could be blocked by curare (Grunwald et al., 1988). Thus, it appears that acetylcholine (ACh) is released by the growth cones as they navigate in the periphery, and that the muscle cells respond to this released transmitter.

In a study using labeled alpha-bungarotoxin, Dennis Liu found that ACh receptor clusters appear on the surface of muscle cells within minutes of the time of arrival of the CaP axon (Liu and Westerfield, 1989). This raised the possibility that receptor clusters could precede the growth cones and direct the peripheral growth of the axon. In agreement with this idea, zebrafish muscle cells *in vitro* , like other vertebrate muscle cells, will form clusters of ACh receptors independently of innervation. To test this idea experimentally, the distribution of ACh receptors was studied in embryos in which the CaP neuron had been ablated. If the receptor clusters precede the axons, we would expect them to be distributed normally. Instead, it was found that the receptor clusters were missing. Thus, the CaP axon does not simply follow a trail of receptor clusters that labels its pathway.

Does a lack of ACh receptors influence the axonal path? To answer this, a mutant that lacks functional ACh receptors was examined (Liu and Westerfield, 1989). The mutant was identified by its lack of movement in a standard mutant screen as described earlier (Westerfield et al., 1987). Intracellular records showed no spontaneous or evoked activity in the mutant muscle cells nor any response to exogenously applied neurotransmitter. However, the muscle could contract with direct electrical stimulation, and electron microscopy revealed apparently normal synapses between the nerve and mutant muscle cells. However, studies with labeled alpha-bungarotoxin showed that clustered ACh receptors are missing in the mutant, and monoclonal antibodies directed against ACh receptor subunits showed clustered receptors only in wild-type embryos, not in the mutant. Thus, while the mutant muscle cells appear normal in many respects, they fail to make ACh receptor clusters. Since the primary motoneuronal axons make normal pathway choices in these mutants, neither receptor clusters nor functional communication are necessary to specify the peripheral pathway.

The Extracellular Matrix

As the axons of the primary motoneurons grow in the periphery, they are restricted to their own segment. They initially grow along the middle region of their myotome, and later extend in the region of the segment boundary. Deanna Frost examined the temporal and spatial distribution of the extracellular matrix components laminin and fibronectin in the zebrafish embryo and found that their presence is correlated with the path of the primary motoneuronal axons (Frost and Westerfield, 1986; Westerfield, 1987). When the axons initially begin to grow, laminin is present on the surface of cells throughout the myotome. Later, the intensity of laminin staining increases, particularly in the region of the segment cell boundary, when the axons are growing there. On the other hand, fibronectin is located in the region of the segment boundaries early, when axons avoid this area. Later, as the axons grow into this region, fibronectin is no longer evident.

These results suggest a model in which laminin may be a permissive substrate for axons to grow on, while fibronectin may inhibit axonal growth. Frost tested this model by growing cells on different substrates *in vitro*. As predicted, quantitative analysis of outgrowth showed good axonal outgrowth on a laminin substrate, and inhibition on a fibronectin substrate. To demonstrate that these *in vitro* results may apply to normal development, Bettina Debu injected laminin into embryos and found no effect on axonal outgrowth, while injection of fibronectin resulted in abnormal axonal outgrowth (Debu, et al., 1989). These observations do not explain the cell specific choices taken by individual axons, but suggest that laminin and fibronectin distributions may be important for the segmental restriction of axonal pathways in the periphery.

Primary Muscle Fibers

As mentioned earlier, all three primary motoneurons of each segment follow a common path to the region of the horizontal myoseptum before they make cell specific divergent pathway choices. What is special about this region? It has been noted previously that the earliest muscle cells differentiate in this location (Myers et al., 1986, Hanneman and Westerfield, 1989). These three to four muscle fibers in each segment form a special class of fibers; they are the first to twitch, the first to express ACh receptor clusters and a cell surface antigen recognized by the zn-5 monoclonal antibody, and their nuclei specifically become immunolabeled with an antibody directed against the *engrailed* gene product (Debu et al., 1989). The presence of such special muscle fibers in the region where all of the primary axons grow suggested the possibility that they may play a role in the establishment of the normal peripheral axonal pathways.

A mutation in zebrafish provides support for the idea that these early muscle fibers may play a role in axonal pathfinding. In this mutant, called *spadetail* (Kimmel et al., 1989), the early muscle fibers fail to differentiate in most trunk segments (as revealed by the absence of *engrailed* antibody labelling). The axonal paths of primary motoneurons are severely disturbed in segments lacking the early muscle fibers, but the axons grow quite normally in segments with the early muscle fibers (Debu et al, 1989). However, since the mutation could have affected the axons directly, a laser was used to ablate the early muscle fibers in normal embryos. Under those conditions, the axons grew in a disturbed manner. Thus, it appears that these special muscle cells are important, and may be required for normal axonal pathfinding in the periphery.

SUMMARY AND CONCLUSIONS

The work described here has focused on the CaP motoneuron. CaP is an identified primary neuron that is present in each of the spinal segments of the zebrafish embryo. It develops early and its axon grows to the ventral muscle cells within its segment. Experimental studies have suggested that the CaP cell fate may be determined by its position in the spinal cord, but that cell lineage, time of origin, and time of axonal outgrowth are not directly involved in the specification of its fate.

Examination of the peripheral axonal pathway has led to the suggestion that a small and special subset of the peripheral muscle cells is required for normal pathfinding, and that the distribution of laminin and fibronectin may also play important roles. On the other hand, neither activity nor the pattern of acetylcholine receptor clusters appears to direct axonal outgrowth.

It is not known how general these principles are. Specifically, does cell position determine cell fate for other primary neurons? Are axonal pathways generally determined by the distribution of extracellular matrix molecules and special cells in their pathway? Do these principles apply to other later-developing neurons? It is possible that these principles are very general. However, primary neurons could play a special role in development. Perhaps they form a framework for the nervous system, laying down the initial pathways that later developing neurons follow. Finally, it remains for the future to determine whether there is a similar system of primary neurons in other vertebrates.

ACKNOWLEDGEMENTS

The work described in this lecture includes contributions from B. Debu, J. Eisen, D. Frost, E. Hanneman, C. Kimmel, D. Liu, B. Mendelson, W. Metcalfe, P. Myers, S. Pike, and B. Trevarrow, all of whom have studied zebrafish development at the University of Oregon.

REFERENCES

Chakrabarti, S., Streisinger, G., Singer, F., and Walker, C., 1983, Frequency of gamma-ray induced specific locus and recessive lethal mutations in mature germ cells of the zebrafish, *Brachydanio rerio, Genetics*, 103:109.

Coghill, G. E., 1913, The primary ventral roots and somatic motor column of *Amblystoma*, *J. Comp. Neurol.*, 23:121.

Debu, B., Frost, D. M., Westerfield, M., and Eisen, J. S., 1990, Exogenous fibronectin interferes with pathway navigation by primary motoneurons in zebrafish embryos, (in preparation).

Debu, B., Pike, S. H., Bremiller, R., Kimmel, C. B., and Eisen, J. S., 1989, A small subpopulation of myocytes may be required for proper morphogenesis of identified motoneurons in embryonic zebrafish, *Soc. Neurosci. Abs.*, 15:877.

Eisen, J. S., 1989, Soma position determines identity of primary motoneurons in developing zebrafish embryos, *Soc. Neurosci. Abs.*,15:1262.

Eisen, J. S., Pike, S. H., and Debu, B., 1989, The growth cones of identified motoneurons in embryonic zebrafish select appropriate pathways in the absence of specific cellular interactions, *Neuron*, 2:1097.

Eisen, J. S., Myers, P. Z., and Westerfield, M., 1986, Pathway selection by growth cones of identified motoneurons in live zebrafish embryos, *Nature*, 320:269.

Frost, D., and Westerfield, M., 1986, Axon outgrowth of embryonic zebrafish neurons is promoted by laminin and inhibited by fibronectin, *Soc. Neurosci. Abs.*, 12:1114.

Grunwald, D. J., Kimmel, C. B., Westerfield, M., Walker, C., and Streisinger, G., 1988, A neural degeneration mutation that spares primary neurons in the zebrafish, *Dev. Biol.*, 126:115.

Hanneman, E., Trevarrow, B., Metcalfe, W. K., Kimmel, C. B., and Westerfield, M., 1988, Segmental pattern of development of the hindbrain and spinal cord of the zebrafish embryo, *Development*, 103:49.

Hanneman, E., and Westerfield, M., 1989, Early expression of acetylcholinesterase activity in functionally distinct neurons of the zebrafish, *J. Comp. Neurol.*, (in press).

Kimmel, C. B., Kane, D. A., Walker, C., Warga, R. M., and Rothman, M. B., A mutation that changes cell movement and cell fate in the zebrafish embryo, *Nature*, 337:358.

Kimmel, C. B., and Law, R. D., 1985, Cell lineage of zebrafish blastomeres: III. Clonal analysis of the blastula and gastrula stages, *Dev. Biol.*, 108:94.

Kimmel, C. B., Patterson, J., and Kimmel, R. O., 1974, The development and behavioral characteristics of the startle response in the zebrafish, *Dev. Psychobiol.*, 7:47.

Kimmel, C. B., Powell, S. L., and Metcalfe, W. K., 1982, Brain neurons which project to the spinal cord of young larvae of the zebrafish, *J. Comp. Neurol.*, 205:112.

Kimmel, C. B., and Warga, R. M., 1987, Indeterminate cell lineage of the zebrafish embryo, *Dev. Biol.*, 124:269.

Kimmel, C. B., and Westerfield, M., 1989, Primary neurons of the zebrafish, in: "Signals and Sense," Edelman, G. M., and Cowan, M. W., eds., Wiley Interscience, New York.

Kuwada, J. Y., 1986, Cell recognition by neuronal growth cones in a simple vertebrate embryo, *Science*, 233:740.

Liu, D. W., and Westerfield, M., 1988, Function of identified motoneurons and coordination of primary and secondary motor systems during zebrafish swimming, *J. Physiol.* (Lond), 403:73.

Liu, D. W., and Westerfield, M., 1989, Primary motoneurons instruct muscle acetylcholine receptor placement, but receptors don't instruct motoneuronal synapse placement, in live zebrafish, *Soc. Neurosci. Abs.*, 15:1262.

Mendelson, B., 1986a, Soma position is correlated with time of development in three types of identified reticulospinal neurons, *Dev. Biol.*, 112:489.

Mendelson, B., 1986b, Development of reticulospinal neurons of zebrafish. II. Early axonal outgrowth and cell body position, *J. Comp. Neurol.*, 251:172.

Metcalfe, W. K., 1985, Sensory neuron growth cones comigrate with posterior lateral line primordial cells in zebrafish, *J. Comp. Neurol.*, 238:218.

Metcalfe, W. K., Kimmel, C. B., and Schabtach, E., 1985, Anatomy of the posterior lateral line system in young larvae of the zebrafish, *J. Comp. Neurol.*, 233:377.

Metcalfe, W. K., Mendelson, B., and Kimmel, C. B., 1986, Segmental homologies among reticulospinal neurons in the hindbrain of the zebrafish larva, *J. Comp. Neurol.*, 251:147.

Myers, P. Z., 1985, Spinal motoneurons of the larval zebrafish, *J. Comp. Neurol.*, 236:555.

Myers, P. Z., Eisen, J. S., and Westerfield, M., 1986, Development and axonal outgrowth of identified motoneurons in the zebrafish, *J. Neurosci.*, 6:2278.

Pike, S. H., and Eisen, J. S., 1990, Identified primary motoneurons in embryonic zebrafish select appropriate pathways in the absence of other primary motoneurons, *J. Neurosci.*, (in press).

Roberts, A., and Clarke, J. D. W., 1982, The neuroanatomy of an amphibian embryo spinal cord, *Phil. Trans. R. Soc. Lond. B.*, 296:195.

Streisinger, G., Walker, C., Dower N., Knauber, D., and Singer, F., 1981, Production of clones of homozygous diploid zebra fish *(Brachydanio rerio)*, *Nature*, 291:293.

Walker, C., and Streisinger, G., 1983, Induction of mutations by gamma-rays in pregonial cells of zebrafish embryos, *Genetics*, 103:125.

Westerfield, M., 1987, Substrate interactions affecting motor growth cone guidance during development and regeneration, *J. Exp. Biol.*, 132:161.

Westerfield, M., Kimmel, C. B., and Walker, C., 1987, Normal pathfinding by pioneer motor growth cones in mutant zebrafish lacking functional acetylcholine receptors, *Soc. Neurosci. Abs.*, 13:5.

Westerfield, M., and Eisen, J. S., 1988a, Neuromuscular specificity: Pathfinding by identified growth cones in a vertebrate embryo, *Trends Neurosci.*, 11:18.

Westerfield, M., and Eisen, J. S., 1988b, Common mechanisms of growth cone guidance during axonal pathfinding, in: "From Message to Mind: Directions in Developmental Neurobiology", Easter, S. S., Barald, K., and Carlson, B. M., eds., Sinaur Assoc., New York.

Westerfield, M., McMurray, J. V., and Eisen, J. S., 1986, Identified motoneurons and their innervation of axial muscles in the zebrafish, *J. Neurosci.*, 6:2267.

EARLY EVENTS IN THE FORMATION OF THE VERTEBRATE BRAIN [*]

Linda S. Ross (scribe), Stephen S. Easter , Jr. (lecturer)

Department of Biology
University of Michigan
Ann Arbor, Michigan, USA

INTRODUCTION

For many years Dr. Easter's research has focused on the development of the retinotectal pathway in fish and amphibians. Because these animals grow throughout life and continue to add new cells to the retina, they are more accessible and easier to examine than embryos. Dr. Easter's previous investigations have suggested that retinal axons added late in life probably use the optic fibers that preceded them as guides to the optic tectum. In an attempt to understand the origin of the first axons, Dr. Easter and his colleagues have examined embryonic neural development, and that work is described here. This chapter first covers work done in collaboration with Dr. Jeremy Taylor in the laboratory of Dr. Michael Gaze on the early development of the optic pathway and its microenvironment in *Xenopus laevis* (Easter and Taylor, 1989). Second, the early neuronal scaffolding in the zebrafish brain, work done in collaboration with Drs. Stephen Wilson and Linda Ross and Mr. Timothy Parrett (Wilson et al., 1990), is described.

In the past, examinations of ordered projections such as the retinotectal pathway have relied almost exclusively on electrophysiological mapping. More recently, Gaze's group has popularized anatomical approaches, first using cobalt (Steedman et al., 1979), then HRP (Gaze and Fawcett, 1983), to visualize the optic axons. These two tracing techniques work very well on whole-mounted brains, as the labeled fibers appear in high contrast on a featureless background, in three dimensions without serial reconstruction. The limitation of the whole-mount preparation is the fact that it reveals nothing of the labeled axons' microenvironment.

Harris and his colleagues have exploited the whole-mount technique in a series of provocative papers on the development of the retinotectal pathway (Harris, 1986, 1989; Harris et al., 1987). Before their work, one had to infer the details of axonal growth from axons stained after they had reached their target. Harris has combined the whole-mount technique with experimental manipulations to visualize axons as they are growing rather than after they have reached their target.

In one study, Harris used *Xenopus* embryos of early stages, prior to axon outgrowth, and transplanted the eye vesicle to an ectopic location (Harris, 1986). The optic axons were then labeled with HRP before their arrival on the tectum; most tended to grow toward the tectum. From these data, Harris formulated two possible explanations; ectopic axons are capable of navigating on the basis of either local cues or long range target attraction cues. However, like most experimental embryology, Harris' study produced variable results. In particular, when eyes were transplanted to caudal locations, some axons grew caudally, away from the tectum and toward the spinal cord, confirming

---

[*] This chapter to be cited as: Ross, L. S., and Easter, S. S., 1990, Early events in the formation of the vertebrate brain, in: "Systems Approaches to Developmental Neurobiology," P. A. Raymond, S. S. Easter, Jr., and G. M. Innocenti, eds., Plenum Press, New York.

the observations of Constantine-Paton and Capranica (1976) and Katz and Lasek (1978; 1979). The two mechanisms of axonal navigation that Harris proposed do not explain these data. Easter introduced the idea that much of what Harris saw might not be due to axons navigating "across country", but rather may be due to new axons encountering and joining pre-existing axonal pathways.

A search of the neuroembryological literature provided some support for that interpretation. Herrick (1938) described the tracts and commissures in the embryonic brain of the urodele amphibian, *Ambystoma tigrinum*. Among the first to develop was the postoptic commissure, a ventral commissure just caudal to the optic stalk. Herrick (1938) claimed that the optic chiasm and tract developed later, in close association with it. Very little of this kind of work has been done on embryonic vertebrate brains since then. This is surprising, in view of the advent of very powerful axon-tracing methods over the past few years. Most recent studies of very early development have been restricted to invertebrates, particularly insects (Bastiani et al., 1985; Harrelson and Goodman, 1988).

XENOPUS RETINOFUGAL PROJECTION

The need for a more contemporary analysis lead Easter and Taylor (1989) to study the early development of the retinofugal pathway to address such questions as: What is the state of the *Xenopus* brain at the time of optic axon outgrowth? What sort of microenvironment do the optic axons encounter on their way to the optic tectum? A combination of techniques was used: whole-mounts of various stages of normal brains with HRP labeled optic axons, serially sectioned brains, three-dimensional computer reconstructions of the brain, and electron microscopy.

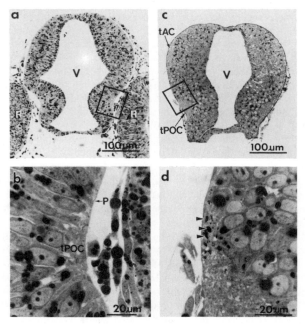

Fig. 1. Sections from brains of *Xenopus* embryos. (a) Horizontal semithin section of the brain of a Stage 32 embryo at low magnification. Rostral is up. (b) More highly magnified view of the nucleus-free region indicated by the box in a. (c) Horizontal semithin section of the brain of a Stage 35 embryo at low magnification. The tract of the postoptic commissure is evident. (d) More highly magnified view of the region indicated by the box in d, showing labeled optic fibers (arrowheads) cut transversely. Abbreviations: P, presumptive pia; R, retina; tAC, tract of the anterior commissure; tPOC, tract of the postoptic commissure; V, ventricle. (From Easter and Taylor, 1989.)

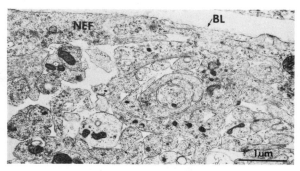

Fig. 2. Electron micrograph of the tract of the postoptic commissure of a Stage 32 embryo. The basal lamina surrounding the brain is underlain by neuroepithelial cell processes. Nuclei are excluded. Many processes are cut transversely and are probably axons. Abbreviations: BL, basal lamina; NEF, neuroepithelial endfoot. (From Easter and Taylor, 1989.)

At embryonic Stage 32, prior to optic axon outgrowth, the brain of *Xenopus* is filled with a uniform population of neuroepithelial cells (Fig. 1a). The nuclei of the cells are closely packed together, but there are a few nucleus-free zones directly next to the pia (Fig. 1b). The texture of the nucleus-free zones is granular, resembling a transversely cut tract or neuropil at the light microscopic level. Electron microscopy confirmed this interpretation (Fig. 2). The basal lamina in the nucleus-free zones is separated from the nuclei by neuroepithelial endfeet, and the nucleus-free zones are filled with round and elliptical membrane-bound processes containing microtubules and other elements characteristic of axons. An exhaustive search through the presumptive fore- and midbrain revealed that all the axons were in this superficial location.

In three-dimensional reconstructions of the Stage 32 brain, nucleus-free zones line up on the surface of the brain as a vertical strip, that extends across the ventral surface of the brain, suggesting that it forms a commissure across the ventral midline (Fig. 3a). Its location corresponds to the postoptic commissure (Herrick, 1938). Easter's terminology differed slightly from that of Herrick, who referred to the entire stirrup-shaped structure as a "commissure". Easter reserves that term for the portion of the axonal bundle that crosses the midline, and calls the segment of the structure that extends away from the midline the "tract of the commissure".

By Stage 35 the brain is more complex in various ways. In particular, the tract of the postoptic commissure is larger. At this stage the first optic axons have exited the eye and are enroute to the optic tectum. HRP-labeled optic axons join the postoptic commissure (Figs. 1c,d; 3b) or at least run very closely alongside it. They occupy a position at the anterior edge of the tract of the postoptic commissure, in a superficial position between the pia and the cell bodies which lie deeper.

At the electron microscopic level, the tract of the postoptic commissure does not differ greatly from that of Stage 32. More axons are present, but they remain located either immediately adjacent to the pia or adjacent to other axons in the same tract. Other commissures, such as the anterior, the posterior and perhaps the habenular, have appeared in the brain, but all axons are still located superficially in nucleus-free zones. The anterior and postoptic commissures are the only substantial ventral commissures with dorsoventral tracts in the fore- and midbrain.

At Stage 39 there are still only two ventral commissures, and both have increased in size (not illustrated). More optic axons are present, and they continue to join the tract of the postoptic commissure superficially in an anterior position, closely apposed to other processes (Fig. 4). By this stage some optic axons have reached the tectum, extended over its surface, and arborized.

The neuropil regions at Stage 39 continue to enlarge, with the bulk of the new axons adding to the pre-existing tracts. All existing tracts are still superficial, so that the brain takes the form of a fibrous exterior and a nuclear core, with no axons in deep locations.

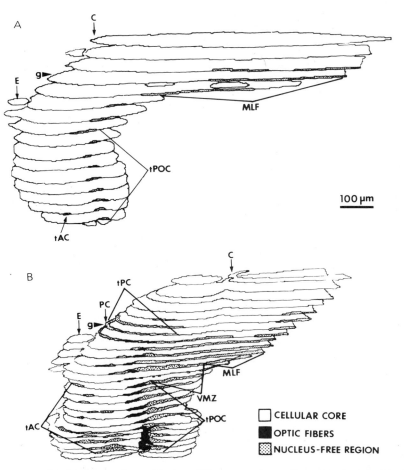

Fig. 3. Computer assisted reconstructions of brains of *Xenopus* embryos. Rostral to the left, dorsal up. (a) Stage 32 embryo. The outer boundary of the brain and the nucleus-free regions are shown. The latter line up to form the tract of the postoptic commissure. A longitudinal nucleus-free region, more caudally, is presumed to be the forerunner of the medial longitudinal fasciculus. (b) Stage 35 embryo. The regions occupied by labeled optic fibers is also shown. Abbreviations: C, cerebellum; E, epiphysis; MLF, medial longitudinal fasciculus; PC, posterior commissure; tAC, tract of the anterior commissure; tPC, tract of the posterior commissure; tPOC, tract of the postoptic commissure; VMZ, ventral marginal zone. (From Easter and Taylor, 1989.)

With one exception, the same trends are apparent in the Stage 46 brain (not illustrated). The tracts of the anterior and postoptic commissures are still the major dorsoventral tracts in the fore- and midbrain. The optic axons remain in the anterior portion of the postoptic commissure, and the nucleus- free zones increase in size. At Stage 39 the posterior commissure occupies a superficial position on the dorsal surface of the midbrain. By stage 46, it has been enveloped by cell nuclei; it is the first deep tract to be seen.

This study of the formation of the optic pathway in the early brain of *Xenopus* has led to two empirical generalizations regarding the origin of axonal tracts. First, all tracts are initially superficial, between the nuclear core and the presumptive pia. Deep tracts present at later stages of development may result as the superficial tracts are secondarily enveloped by nuclei migrating outward from the periventricular zone. Second, the most common behavior of early axons is to join a pre-existing tract. The number of these primary tracts is quite small.

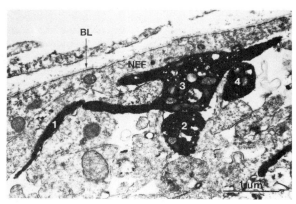

Fig. 4. Electron micrograph of HRP labeled axons and growth cones of a Stage 39 *Xenopus* embryo. Four elements are labeled. Presumably established optic axons (numbers 2 and 4) are present. A presumed growth cone (number 3) with three lamellopodia is making intimate contact with a neuroepithelial endfoot and other unidentified processes. Number 1 is an isolated filopodium or lamellipodium, possibly attached to 3. Abbreviations: BL, basal lamina; NEF, neuroepithelial endfoot. (From Easter and Taylor, 1989.)

With regard to the optic pathway, this study has suggested that the optic fibers are not pioneers; instead they join a pre-existing tract, that of the postoptic commissure. Furthermore, when they join this pathway, the optic fibers do not mix freely with the other fibers but stay tightly bundled superficially in the anterior portion of the tract. It is impossible to say whether or not the first optic axons are following cues in the neuroepithelium (and just happened to be adjacent to the postoptic commissure) or whether they are following cues on the axons in this early tract. The fact that an initial axonal scaffolding is present in the embryonic brain, coupled with the fact that optic axons readily join a pre-existing pathway, suggests an alternative explanation for the variable results of the experiments of Harris. Those axons of ectopic eyes that reach the tectum could be using one of the early tracts, most probably, the tract of the postoptic commissure, to reach the vicinity of the tectum. Likewise, those axons of caudally placed eyes may be misdirected down the spinal cord by joining a different component, one of the pre-existing longitudinal tracts.

If this interpretation is correct, then it suggests that the nature of the axons may be less important than just the fact that they are axons. This idea that axons provide a good substrate for other axons' growth is an old one. Paul Weiss (1941) showed that when ganglia were placed in tissue culture, axons grew out in all directions. If a target tissue was co-cultured with the ganglia, some of the randomly growing axons reached the target tissue and others did not. Those fibers that found the target were subsequently reinforced by the addition of other fibers, producing a fasciculated pathway. This "selective fasciculation" by new fibers on some, but not all, of their predecessors suggested that the early axons that found the target were thereby changed to be more hospitable to later outgrowing axons.

What is the difference between these generalizations and the blueprint hypothesis?

They are quite different, but not necessarily incompatible. The blueprint hypothesis was formulated to explain the guidance of the longitudinal axonal tracts in the hindbrain and spinal cord (Nordlander, 1984; Nordlander and Singer, 1982a;b; Singer et al., 1979). The essential feature of the blueprint hypothesis was that there were extracellular spaces along the pathway that preceded the axons. It is not known whether spaces precede the formation of the initial axonal scaffolding in the brain. In the earliest stage examined, Stage 32, even though there was slightly more space in the nucleus- free zones, axons were already present in the space. Although one might suspect that some mechanical feature like a fold might define the site of the first tract, nothing like that is obvious; the boundary of the brain seems to be smooth with no signs of a fissure. Others who have labeled antibodies to general substrate adhesion molecules such as N-CAM (Silver and Rutishauser, 1984) have never seen specific pathways traced out. So the cue - be it mechanical or something else - that causes the early axons to grow in this particular region of the neural tube is unknown.

Evidence for the preferential growth of axons on other axons also comes from data of regeneration experiments. If the optic nerve of goldfish is crushed, the fibers will regenerate and innvervate the tectum. An electron microscopic examination of the nerve revealed that near the front of the regenerating axons there are very few solitary axons; most are in clusters. Within the cluster,axonal growth cones are in immediate and extensive contact with other axons, not with glia or degenerating axons, suggesting that axons are the preferred substrate (Easter, 1987). Regenerating optic axons will also join other axonal tracts to reach their target. Normally, goldfish retinal axons take the standard route to the contralateral optic tectal lobe. However, if one tectal lobe is ablated, and those optic axons that innervated it are thereby severed, the regenerating axons cross the midline to innervate the remaining tectal lobe. To reach it, they join other commissural pathways that are already present in the brain but that would normally contain no optic fibers (Easter et al., 1978). The regenerates do not grow through uncharted territory, but along a relatively few selected paths.

These examples provide support for the idea that much of the so-called pathfinding in the developing brain may be the result of following pre-existing pathways. If this does prove to be true, then interpretations of axonal pathfinding require caution, as supposed examples of pioneering may actually prove to be merely axons following other axons.

In insects, the whole idea of pioneer axons has changed over the years because as people have ablated pioneer neurons in more systems, they found that the "followers" could pioneer the pathway perfectly well. Is it the same in *Xenopus*?

The term "pioneer" is a loaded one. Originally, it was used to describe the first axon to grow along a particular route. Later, the pioneer was alleged to have properties that the later, follower axons did not have; that is, the pioneer was supposed to be able to navigate in ways that the followers could not. Ablation of the pioneers left the followers to navigate on their own, and it turned out that they could, so the special skills of the pioneer were not so special after all, but were also properties of the later axons. More recently, some "pioneers" have in fact been shown to be essential for tract formation (Bastiani et al., 1985; Harrelson and Goodman, 1988; Kuwada, 1986). The question in the context of *Xenopus* development is really two questions, in experimental terms. One is: What would happen if we could wipe out the axons in the tract of the postoptic commissure? Would the optic axons still be able to find their way? The second question is: If you put the eye in a different location, with no axons around, would they still find their way? We don't have answers to either question. The main reason for setting this particular problem in that context was to make a larger point. So many experimental undertakings are misleading when there is no description of the normal development of the system with which to interpret one's results. In order to differentiate between true cases of pioneering and cases of axons following other axons it is necessary to know what pathways are present at early stages of development. This is a plea for not leaping into experimental manipulations necessarily until you have an idea of what the normal case is. It is a plea for renewed respectability for so-called descriptive studies.

The work on *Xenopus* was followed up with a related study on the embryonic fore- and mid-brains of the zebrafish, *Brachydanio rerio* (Wilson et al., 1990). This descriptive study has used a variety of contemporary techniques. Regions of neuronal differentiation have been demonstrated using acetylcholinesterase histochemistry as a marker for differentiated cells. Immunocytochemistry with antibodies to HNK-1 (supplied by Dr. C. Stern) and acetylated alpha-tubulin (supplied by Dr. G. Piperno) have both been used to stain early axons in whole-mount preparations, providing an outline of the early axonal scaffolding. The HNK-1 antibody is directed against a molecule involved in cell adhesion and stains axons as early as 20 hours of development. By 48 hours the staining for HNK-1 in whole-mounts is reduced, so an antibody to acetylated alpha-tubulin, a cytoskeletal component, has been used for the analysis of the brain at 48 hours. Applications of HRP to the brain have been used to assess connectivity and morphology within the axonal scaffolding, and many of the observations have been checked electron microscopically.

Recently, staining for acetylcholinesterase (AChE) has been used as a marker for differentiated cells in the brain (Layer, 1983; Layer et al., 1988; Moody and Stein, 1988). Additional evidence in *Drosophila* indicates that it does play a role in neuronal development (Wolfgang and Forte, 1989). In *Drosophila* there is a single gene for AChE, and when this gene is deleted, neuronal development is abnormal. Staining for AChE in the zebrafish brain was used to examine correlations between the location of differentiated cells and the location of axonal tracts.

At 24 hours, positive staining for AChE is restricted to well defined regions of the brain corresponding to regions where the early tracts arise (described below). In the forebrain the rostral telencephalon and postoptic region of the ventral diencephalon stain darkly. Cells within the anlagen of the pituitary and epiphysis are labeled, and in the midbrain cells along the rostral margin of the tectum and in the ventral portion of the midbrain are labeled. All of these regions that stain for AChE are also labeled by the antibody to HNK-1 at 24 hours, as described below.

At 24 hours, the labeling with antibodies defines a limited number of axonal tracts and commissures (Fig. 5a,b). All are superficial, and they correspond to the ones described in *Ambystoma* by Herrick (1938) and in *Xenopus* above. The three commissures are the anterior, postoptic, and posterior. As in *Xenopus* and *Ambystoma*, the anterior and postoptic commissures are the only two ventral commissures present in the early brain. The posterior commissure is a dorsal commissure that arises from a cluster of cells at the rostral margin of the presumptive tectum that project both dorsally across the midline, and ventrally, through the tract of the posterior commissure to join the tract of the postoptic commissure. Four dorsoventral tracts are present: the tracts of three commissures, and the dorsoventral diencephalic tract, made up of axons from cells near or within the anlage of the epiphysis. Two longitudinal tracts are present: the supraoptic (linking the tracts of the anterior and postoptic commissures) and the caudal part of the tract of the postoptic commissure which merges with a complex of midbrain tracts that continue through the hindbrain to the spinal cord.

One gets the impression that the early tracts are generally organized as mostly dorsoventral or anteroposterior pathways. Do you think this is accomplished with simple dorsoventral and anteroposterior cues, or is that too simple-minded?

Although it is tempting to describe this network as an orthogonal arrangement of dorsoventral and anteroposterior tracts, one must be cautious, as the direction of the neuraxis in the fore- and mid-brains is not clear. A particularly ambiguous tract is that of the postoptic commissure which starts off dorsoventrally and then curves over to merge with a tract that is anteroposterior.

Labeling with the HNK-1 antibody identifies a second dorsal commissure at 36 hours, the habenular commissure. The tract of the habenular commissure projects ventrally from the dorsal midline to the telencephalon and ventral diencephalon. The labeling by the acetylated tubulin antibody

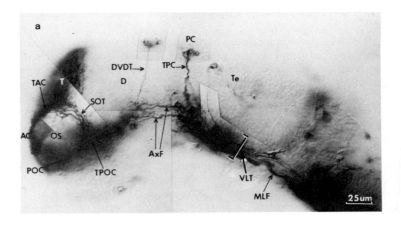

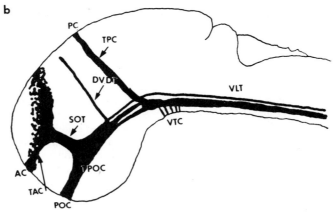

Fig. 5. Axon tracts in the 24 hour zebrafish brain. (a) HNK-l labeling of the brain. (b) Schematic summary
diagram of HNK-l labeled tracts. Abbreviations: AC, anterior commissure; AxF, axon fascicles; D,
diencephalon; DVDT, dorsoventral diencephalic tract; MLF, medial longitudinal fasciculus; OS, optic
stalk; PC, posterior commissure; POC, postoptic commissure; SOT, supraoptic tract; T,
telencephalon; TAC, tract of the anterior commissure; Te, tectum; TPC, tract of the posterior
commissure; TPOC, tract of the postoptic commissure; VLT, ventral longitudinal tract; VTC, ventral
tegmental commissure. (From Wilson et al., 1990.)

antibodies and one other, the olfactory nerve, the projection between the olfactory placode and the
telencephalon (the olfactory placode is normally dissected away in immunolabeled whole-mounts, and
therefore was not seen with the immunocytochemical probes). With HRP injections it was possible to
identify the projection between the olfactory placode and the telencephalon. The olfactory nerve
projects from the olfactory placode to the mid to dorsal rostral telencephalon where it forms
glomerulus-like terminations. The olfactory nerve projection is present at 24 hours. The retinotectal
projection develops later, at about 36 hours of development, confirming Stuermer (1988). The optic
axons in the zebrafish also join the postoptic commissure in the same anterior position as seen in
Xenopus embryos.

One general observation was made from the HRP material. In all cases, the axons contributing to
a tract are located right next to it, and therefore the segments of axons outside a tract are quite short
(less than a few cell diameters). At 24 hours, most axons are quite short, with one notable exception.
HRP applied to the tract of the postoptic commissure labeled a cell in the hindbrain at about the level
of the otocyst. This cell's axon was traced in isolation, all the way to the commissure, so there is no
question that it was a real projection. It was the only axonal link between hindbrain and forebrain.

Do you see any signs of growth cone selectivity along these tracts such as changes in growth cone morphology or pausing at choice points?

We could see no pauses, as we never followed the axons in real time. We have labeled growth cones, but we have not studied their morphologies systematically. The HRP-labeled axons clearly made choices at the intersection of one tract with another. For example, there is a great wash of fibers emerging from the telencephalon, and they must choose whether to enter the tract of the anterior commissure or the supraoptic or both. Labeled axons from the dorsal telencephalon enter both the tract of the anterior commissure and the supraoptic tract, but it is impossible to tell whether a single axon is branched or individual axons took different routes. There is another choice point at the intersection between the dorsoventral diencephalic tract and the tract of the postoptic commissure, where axons must choose whether to run rostrally or caudally. Invariably the axons turn rostrally towards the postoptic commissure. As the axons in the dorsoventral diencephalic tract leave the midline they are very tightly fasciculated, but when they reach the tract of the postoptic commissure, they disperse and run separately from one another. These two examples demonstrate axonal selection, and we hope to investigate this further.

This study has shown that the early system of tracts of the zebrafish brain is rather simple at 24 hours. Most of the axons added over the next 24 hours join them rather than form new ones. Now that the initial framework has been defined, it will be possible to examine earlier stages to determine the pioneer neurons that produce this scaffolding. Additionally, this description of early axonal tracts will also provide the background to aid interpretation of manipulative experiments.

ACKNOWLEDGEMENTS

This research was supported by a research grant from NIH to S.S.E. (EY-00168), and by fellowships to S.S.E. (from the Royal Society), and to L.R. (from NIH: HD-07274).

REFERENCES

Bastiani, M.J., du Lac, S., and Goodman, C.S., 1985, The first neuronal growth cones in insect embryos. Model system for studying he development of neuronal specificity, in "Model Neural Networks and Behavior", A.I. Selverston, ed., Plenum Press, New York, p. 149.

Constantine-Paton, M. and Capranica, R.R., 1976, Axonal guidance of transplanted eye primordia. *J. Comp. Neurol.*, 170:17.

Easter, S.S., 1987, Retinal axons and the basal lamina, in: "Mesenchymal-Epithelial Interactions in Neural Development," J.R. Wolff, J. Sievers, and M. Berry, eds., Springer-Verlag, Berlin , p. 385.

Easter, S.S. and Taylor, J.S.H., 1989, The development of the *Xenopus* retinofugal pathway: optic fibers join a pre-existing tract, *Development* (in press).

Easter, S.S., Schmidt, J.T., and Leber, S.M., 1978, The paths and destinations of the induced ipsilateral retinal projection in goldfish, *J. Embryol. Exp. Morph.*, 45:145.

Gaze, R.M. and Fawcett, J.W., 1983, Pathways of *Xenopus* optic fibres regenerating from normal and compound eyes under various conditions, *J. Embryol. Exp. Morph.*, 73:17.

Harrelson, A.L. and Goodman, C.S., 1988, Growth cone guidance in insects: Fasciclin II is a member of the immunoglobulin superfamily, *Science*, 242:700.

Harris, W.A., 1986, Homing behavior of axons in the embryonic vertebrate brain, *Nature,* 320:266.

Harris, W.A., 1989, Local positional cues in the neuroepithelium guide retinal axons in embryonic *Xenopus* brain, *Nature,* 339:218.

Harris, W.A., Holt, C.E., and Bonhoeffer, F., 1987, Retinal axons with *Xenopus* embryos: a time-lapse video study of single fibre *in vivo, Development,* 101:123.

Herrick, C.J., 1938, Development of the cerebrum of *Amblystoma* during the early swimming stages, *J. Comp. Neurol.*, 68:203.

Katz, M.J. and Lasek, R.J., 1978, Eyes transplanted to tadpole tails send axons rostrally in two spinal cord tracts, *Science*, 109:202.

Katz, M.J. and Lasek, R.J., 1979, Substrate pathways which guide growing axons in *Xenopus* embryos, *J. Comp. Neurol.*, 183:817.

Kuwada, J., 1986, Cell recognition by neuronal growth cones in a simple vertebrate embryo, *Science*, 233:740.

Layer, P.G., 1983, Comparative localization of acetylcholinesterase and pseudocholinesterase during morphogenesis of the chicken brain, *Proc. Natl. Acad. Sci. USA*, 80:6413.

Layer, P.G., Rommel, S., Bulthoff, H., and Hengstenberg, R., 1988, Independent spatial waves of biochemical differentiation along the surface of chicken brain as revealed by the sequential expression of acetylcholinesterase, *Cell Tissue Res.*, 251:587.

Moody, S.A. and Stein, D.B., 1988, The development of acetylcholinesterase activity in the embryonic nervous system of the frog, *Xenopus laevis*, *Dev. Brain Res.*, 39:225.

Nordlander, R.N., 1984, Developing descending neurons of the early *Xenopus* tail spinal cord in the caudal spinal cord of early *Xenopus*, *J. Comp. Neurol.*, 228:117.

Nordlander, R.H., and Singer, M., 1982a, Spaces precede axons in the embryonic spinal cord, *Exp. Neurol.*, 75:221.

Nordlander, R.H. and Singer, M., 1982b, Morphology and position of growth cones in the developing *Xenopus* spinal cord, *Dev. Brain Res.*, 4:181.

Silver, J., and Rutishauser, U., 1984, Guidance of optic axons by a preformed adhesive pathway on neuroepithelial endfeet, *Dev. Biol.*, 106:485.

Singer, M., Nordlander, R.H., and Egar, M., 1979, Axonal guidance during embryogenesis and regeneration in the spinal cord of the newt: the blueprint hypothesis of neuronal pathway patterning, *J. Comp. Neurol.*, 188:1.

Steedman, J.G., Stirling, R.V., and Gaze, R.M., 1979, The central pathways of optic fibres in *Xenopus* tadpoles, *J. Embryol. Exp. Morph.*, 50:199.

Stuermer, C.A.O., 1988, Retinotopic organization of the developing retinotectal projection in the zebrafish embryo, *J. Neurosci.*, 8:4513.

Weiss, P., 1941, Nerve patterns: mechanics of growth, *Growth*, 5:163.

Wilson, S.W., Ross, L.S., Parrett, T., and Easter, S.S.,Jr., 1990, The development of a simple scaffold of axon tracts in the brain of the embryonic zebrafish, *Brachydanio rerio*, *Development* (in press).

Wolfgang, W.J., and Forte, M.A., 1989, Expression of acetylcholinesterase during visual system development in *Drosophila*, *Dev. Biol.*, 131:321.

IN VIVO AND *IN VITRO* GUIDANCE OF AXONS [*]

Timothy Allsopp (scribe), Friedrich Bonhoeffer (lecturer)

Max Planck Institut fur Entwicklungsbiologie
Abteilung Physikaliche Biologie
Tüebingen, FRG

INTRODUCTION

The brain of a vertebrate contains in one cubic millimeter about 10^5 neurones, 10^9 times more than this in the number of synapses, and about a kilometre in the length of axons and dendrites. The neurones, axons, dendrites and synapses are arranged and connected in a highly specific and ordered manner, though relatively little is known about how this complicated system develops. Developing connections between neurones are established via the neuronal growth cone, which has to navigate through an environment crowded with cellular and extra-cellular signals. The growth cone is a structure exquisitely designed for motility and this environmental exploration; it possesses a dynamic cytoskeleton and surface molecules essential for its recognition of, and recognition by, target cells.

The visual system of the chick embryo is a favoured model system for studying events underlying the specificty of neuronal connections. It is a classical example of a long distance topographic projection of neurones from one part of the brain to another. This lecture first summarises the developmental anatomy, then reviews theoretical considerations and experimental results of assays designed to elucidate cellular mechanisms of growth cone guidance in this system.

ANATOMY AND DEVELOPMENT OF THE CHICK RETINOTECTAL SYSTEM

In the chick embryo the first retinal ganglion cells become post-mitotic at embryonic day (E) 2, and their axons leave the retina at E3. Eight classes of ganglion cell have been morphologically characterised, though the time sequence of their development is unknown. They have been classified according to their soma size, and the extent and type of dendritic arborisation. Soma sizes vary from 60 to 277 μm^2, while dendritic extent from 5 to 77 μm^2. The inner plexiform layer branching patterns of these cells varies also in their level of stratification. The displaced ganglion cell has the largest soma, positioned in the inner nuclear layer, and the largest dendritic tree which extends deep into the inner plexiform layer (J. Vanselow, unpublished observations).

The retina develops in a centrifugal manner, ganglion cells from all the four quadrants of the retina contributing the first axons to the optic nerve. The mature retinotectal connection is entirely crossed, but at E4, when the growing axons are traversing the optic chiasm, about 15% of these early

---

[*] This chapter to be cited as: Allsopp, T., and Bonhoeffer, F., 1990, *In vivo* and *in vitro* guidance of axons, in: "Systems Approaches to Developmental Neurobiology," P. A. Raymond, S. S. Easter, Jr., and G. M. Innocenti, eds., Plenum Press, New York.

central axons grow ipsilaterally. The ipsilaterally growing axons arrive at the ventro-anterior tectum one day later (at E7) than their contralateral counterparts. This transient ipsilateral projection reaches its maximum in numbers of axons at E9, though the projection never consists of more than 1% of the total number of axons at this time. The ipsilateral projection is organised retinotopically along the dorsoventral axis and consists of axons from all four retinal quadrants. Dye-labelling shows them not to be collaterals from the contralateral projection. By E15, no axons ipsilateral in origin can be detected on the tectum.

Retinal axons invade the developing tectum at its anterior margin and advance over the surface as the stratum opticum (SO), covering the whole tectal surface by E13. The SO increases in thickness by the addition of newly arriving axons from more peripherally placed retinal areas. These later arriving axons grow on top of the axons from the central retinal areas. Approximately 3 days after invading the tectum, the first axons can be seen to leave the SO and invade the *stratum griseum et fibrosum superficiale* (SGFS), in whose layers they branch and arborise to form their specific connections with tectal cells. This sequence of events first occurs in the area centralis of the tectum, situated in the anterio-dorsal tectal quadrant about 1mm away from the anterior tectal margin. Between E13 and E16 the extension of terminal arbors increases in both the anterior-posterior and dorsal-ventral dimensions by a factor of about 1.5, while the number of branch points per axonal tree increases by a factor of 3.5 between E13 and E18. The mature retinotectal connection is topographically organised, with the retinal dorso-ventral axis being inverted on the tectum, nasal half-retina projecting to posterior (caudal) tectum, and temporal half-retina to anterior (rostral) tectum.

Retinal axons within the contralateral optic tract have collaterals which are directed towards the underlying retino-receptive pretectal nuclei. These collaterals leave the SO perpendicular to axon fascicles, and give rise to dense retinal projections to the nucleus ecto- mammillaris, the nucleus externus and the tectal grey, which are situated at the anterior margin of the tectum. In addition to the pretectal nuclei, there is a transient projection from the contralateral retina to the mesencephalic isthmo-optic nucleus (ION). This prominent nucleus gives rise to centrifugal fibres which develop subsequent to this transient retino-ION projection, and which innervate the amacrine and displaced ganglion cells of the contralateral retina in a topographic manner. The ION also provides a transient projection to the ipsilateral tectum with collaterals projecting to the contralateral retina (Fig 1. A.Wizenmann unpublished observations). In addition, dye-labelling has revealed stellate-like arrangements of cells which appear transiently in the developing tectum at a time when invading retinal axons can be observed to undergo course corrections. The pattern produced by these corrections often reiterates this stellate arrangement.

What are the phylogenetic implications of the projections in the developing chicken visual system, and what function might the transient connections serve?

There is a sharp line of division between nasal and temporal half-retina and a transient ipsilateral projection to the tectum. One cannot exclude the possibility that this might indicate that birds once had a functional bilateral projection, which they have now effectively lost. The other transient projections may also have their origins in the fact that they were once functional permanent projections. One could speculate that transient projections serve to guide permanent projections. For example, during development axons project to their target organ and may not be correctly guided. But if the target area were to send out axons which contain a positional marker, then this might help the later arriving axons to find the correct spot. The projection from the ION to the retina could be guided in this way; the axons from the ION could be sorted to project in a topographic manner to the amacrine cells based on the order of the retinal axons. Additionally, the connection from the ION to the ipsilateral tectum may serve to guide the developing connection from the tectum to the ION.

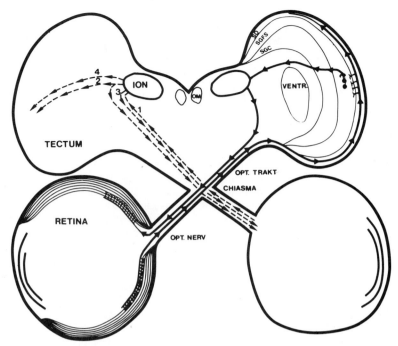

Fig. 1. The developing visual system has transient axonal projections. Drawing showing the permanent projections (continuous lines) from the bird's right retina to the contralateral tectum, from the tectum to the ipsilateral **ION** and from the **ION** to the contralateral retina. Transient projections (dashed lines) are numbered **1** to **4** and are for the bird's left retina to the contralateral **ION** and tectum. Arrowheads represent anterograde direction. (**ventr**; ventricle, **SGC**; stratum griseum centrale, **OM**; nucleus oculomotoreus, other abbreviations as in text).

DIRECTIONAL CUES FOR RETINAL AXONS IN THE TARGET ORGAN

The topographic representation of the avian retina onto the tectum is one which reflects a spatial order of axonal origin in the order of axonal terminals. Physiologically, this preserves spatial relationships within the visual field. The simplest way of achieving topographic representations would be an interaction between spatial markers carried by axons -- ones that specify a position of origin -- and spatial complementary markers in the tectum. This derives from a model proposed by Sperry (1963). One version of this model proposes that each axon arising in a given area of retina carries some specific molecule on its surface which is complementary to position-specific substances in the target. Alternatively, only a few substances would suffice if these could be distributed in a graded manner in the target organ. This graded distribution, in combination with an axonal position-dependent marker which helps the growing axon interpret the gradient, could give directional cues. However, many additional or alternative factors may be involved, such as the timing of neuronal birth and axonal outgrowth (Rager, 1980), a pre-ordering of axons in the nerve, or direct and indirect axon-axon interactions in the target organ (Willshaw and von der Malsburg, 1979).

Experimental Evidence for Directional Cues

1) In goldfish, rotation of the tectum led to a rotation of the projection (Yoon 1973), suggesting that axons are guided by spatial markers on the tectum, at least in part. This rotation of the projection has also been seen in *Xenopus*, following a rostral-caudal rotation of the embryonic dorsal midbrain precursor (Taylor and Stirling, 1989).

2) Misrouting of regenerating axons in the newt, did not prevent axons relocating their correct tectal target area (Fujisawa et al., 1982). In many cases they seemed to do this through a progressive branching and selective stabilisation of branches until the correct site was reached. It appeared that position-dependent properties on the retinal and tectal cells determined the selective loss or stabilisation.

3) Transplantation of embryonic chick retinal pieces to the virgin tectum in anopthalmic embryos (Thanos and Duetting, 1987), showed that both nasal and temporal axons recognise their position along the anterior-posterior axis, as they corrected the direction of their outgrowth towards their appropriate projection area.

4) Misrouting axons in their trajectory to the tectum, and on the tectal surface, via N-CAM mediated defasciculation at the optic fissure (Thanos et al., 1984) showed that ectopically growing axons fasciculated with other axons in the normal anterior-posterior axis, but then were able to turn at right angles to reach their target area. Mechanical disruption of the normal anterior-posterior growth across the tectum, showed that axons correct their trajectories with smooth curving tracts to their target, as if sensing directional cues in both axes on the tectum (Thanos and Bonhoeffer, 1986). These corrections in trajectory were always most pronounced for the earliest axons growing in close contact to the tectal surface; later arriving ectopic axons followed the route of the initial axons.

Theoretical Considerations for Gradients and Retinotopography

The experiments suggest that in part the projecting axons are guided by spatial cues on the tectum, and as they are able to approach their targets over considerable distances and via non-random routes, that these markers are graded and not highly localised. Many factors most likely play a part in the mechanism of guidance, but the evidence implies that graded distributions of directional cues in the target are prominent in establishing the primary projection.

Guidance of growth cones by gradients has been the subject of intense mathematical analysis (Gierer, 1981;1987). Gradient guidance suggests that the growth cone is able to detect a spatial distribution of a cue in its environment, and responds by growing in the direction of the maximum slope of this distribution. However, a single gradient on the tectum would therefore guide all axons to one tectal margin, instead of generating a topographic projection. Guidance to a defined tectal area could occur if this area was a maximum or minimum resulting from the combined effect of two antagonistic gradients, or if it were the resultant of two antagonistic effects of the same gradient- one attracting and one repelling effect. A characteristic of a topographic projection is the dependence of the target position on the position of axonal origin. Thus the axonal components involved must be graded with respect to their position of origin in the retina, and these axonal components affect the influence of the target-derived antagonistic gradients on the final choice of target area. Models incorporating these ideas allow for the correction of misrouted axons where the target position can be approached from any point at which the search is initiated, either at the margin of the target tissue or at a position within the region where a searching axon departs from a fasciculated bundle. The results of experiments in amphibians (Fujisawa et al.,1982) and goldfish (Stuermer, 1986) appear to fit these predictions extremely well, where the observed axonal trajectories are ones of directed growth from ectopic positions. In the region of the growth cone the axonal components translate the graded distribution of target components. This leads to directed growth by an amplified change in the concentration gradient of intra-growth cone components.

Actual Gradients in the Retina and on the Tectum

Gradients have been detected in both the retina and the tectum in chicken. There exists a dorsal-ventral gradient of adhesion within the retina (Gottlieb and Glaser, 1976), with highest cell soma affinities exhibited between cells derived from extremes of the gradient. These experiments with dissociated retinal cells do not distinguish ganglion cells from the many other types, nor are they a direct measure of a ganglion cell's axonal affinity for a tectal target. Trisler and colleagues have identified gradients of an antigen called TOP in the developing retina and tectum. In the dorsal retina there appears to be an approximately 30-fold higher amount of the membrane-associated antigen than there is in the ventral retina, with a smooth and continuous transition in between. In the tectum the TOP gradient is inverted, with highest amounts being detectable in ventral regions up to a developmental time when retinal axons are invading (Trisler and Collins, 1987). The significance of the TOP retinotectal gradients for the formation of a topographic projection are not clear. Though gradients of molecules have been difficult to show for the developing projection, distinct 'step-like' transitions seem more common. Along the nasal-temporal axis of the retina there is a stepwise change of axonal adhesiveness; nasal axons allow a strong adhesion of tectal membranes, while temporal axons appear less adhesive (Halfter et al., 1981). Dräger and colleagues (Rabacchi et al., 1988) have identified a 'dorsal eye antigen' which appears to be closely related to a high-affinity laminin receptor, and antibodies to this molecule label the dorsal retina in several species including chicken. Though the antigen is not restricted to retinal neurones, it appears transiently in high levels on axons from the dorsal retina.

IN VITRO ASSAYS FOR RETINAL GANGLION AXON GUIDANCE

Manipulations of the developing projection *in vivo* are useful for providing descriptive information, particularly of the time sequence of development for the projection, however many different effects may complicate interpretation of the results, and the system is not amenable to an ultimate analysis of the process at a cellular or molecular level. Alternatively, to reduce the system to a series of logistically simpler encounters of developing retina and tectum *in vitro* involves problems associated with a dependable reproduction of the events. For example, the markers necessary for specifying a projection may not be stable or fully expressed in an *in vitro* assay.

However, evidence for the existence of one gradient in the tectum that could be directly related to the axon preference for the tectal target area has been found through a co-explantation experiment involving embryonic retinal and tectal tissue. When growing axons *in vitro* are presented with a choice of two cell monolayers (each monolayer derived from either the anterior or posterior tectum and the cells arranged as opposable surfaces between which the axons grow) temporal axons prefer to grow on the anterior tectal cells, which is in accordance with their natural target. By subdividing tectal cells, or their membranes, the relatively more anterior substratum is always preferred to the relatively more posterior one. This would tend to suggest that the tectal guidance cue for temporal axons is graded in its distribution, and exists independently of tectal innervation. This type of *in vitro* assay did not show a preference of nasal axons for posterior tectum, nor did it reveal any positional cues along the dorsal- ventral axis.

The opposable monolayer assay, though conceptually very simple, was extremely tedious to perform with biochemical investigations. An easier and more amenable assay was developed, one that could be associated with biochemical tests concerning the graded component. Axons in this type of assay are given the choice to grow on tectal membrane components which are presented to them in a 2-dimensional, rather than 3-dimensional, array. Dye-labelled axons grow on the alternating stripes of anterior and posterior tectal membranes which are supported on a Nucleopore filter. The membrane-containing filters (carpets) are prepared by first filtering one set of membrane particles onto the filter by suction through a series of narrow (about 90 µm) parallel channels, and then the remaining lanes on the filter are plugged through suction onto the carpet of a different set of membrane particles.

The first findings from the use of such carpets were that the temporal axons indeed preferred to grow on anterior tectal membranes when given the choice of anterior and posterior membranes (Fig. 2a), but when given a carpet of only one type of membrane then both nasal and temporal axons grow at about the same rate (Walter et al., 1987a). Thus nasal and temporal axons do not differ in their general ability to grow on either anterior or posterior membranes. The preference of temporal axons to grow on anterior membranes seems not to be graded across the retina; the nasal-temporal transition occurs within a zone 200 µm in width with the orientation of the fissure. As in previous assays, no preference of nasal axons for posterior membranes, dorsal axons for lateral tectum nor ventral axons for medial tectum was found. The choice of temporal axons seems restricted to the period when the retinotectal projection is developing.

The results suggest that the posterior membranes contain a repulsing cue, not that the anterior membranes contain an attractive cue, and this is emphasised by the results of experiments which alter the protein constituents of the posterior membranes. Heat treatment of posterior membranes (63°C for 8 mins.) renders them incapable of initiating a temporal axon choice, and in fact heat treatment of anterior or posterior membranes slightly improves their overall ability to be chosen as a growth substratum (when presented simultaneously with untreated membranes) by nasal or temporal axons (Fig. 2b and Walter *et al.*,1987b). Exposure of posterior membranes to the phosphatidyl-inositol specific form of phospholipase C (PI-PLC) has a similar effect in that the decision made by axons is also lost (Fig. 2c and Walter *et al.*, 1989). One outcome of these results is that temporal axons can be observed to behave like nasal axons, that is, they do not respect the borders. A polyclonal antiserum, raised against embryonic tectal tissue, is also able to disrupt the decision in a manner which is qualitatively similar to that seen for PI-PLC treatment of the tectal membranes (Fig. 2d).

Given that there are morphologically many types of ganglion cells in the developing chick retina, does one know whether the pathways and choices made by the retinal axons *in vivo* and *in vitro* are represented by all these types, or is it one particular class or subclass that is being analysed, perhaps ones that are the first to develop?.

All the different types of ganglion cells that exist send out axons, and in *in vitro* experiments a lot of these axons are regenerating, while others are growing de novo. Axons growing from explant strips *in vitro* are representative of all the ganglion cell types, as has been shown by retrograde labelling. At the moment there is no indication that there is a particular cell type which behaves differently from the others in, for example, its ability to choose between anterior and posterior material. But the ratio of the different cell types and their distribution across the nasal and temporal halves of the retina are not known.

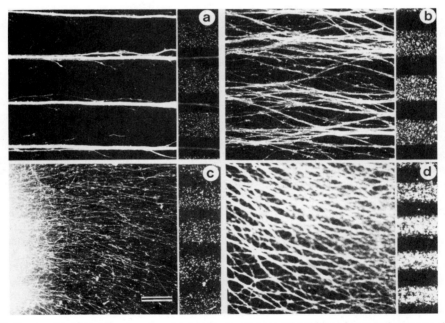

Fig. 2. Temporal axons prefer to grow on anterior membranes. The ability of temporal axons to choose growth on anterior instead of posterior membranes (a), is impaired if the posterior membranes are previously heat treated (b), PI-PLC treated (c) or antiserum treated (d). Axons are labelled with rhodamine; posterior membranes with fluorescein labelled microsphres (lanes of posterior membranes are shown to the right of each figure section). Bar is 30 μm in (c) and 20 μm in (a,b,d).

Additionally, these results are intriguing as they reveal a subtle difference between general growth and decision characteristics made by the growth cones. A good example of this discriminating process is revealed when individual encounters between temporal growth cones and the anterior-posterior border are analysed with high resolution fluorescence microscopy, using short exposure times of light illumination with time-lapse cinematography. In general, the population response of the growth cones seems to be a deflection away from the border, with no decrease in the growth rate of the growth cone for the period in which it is 'experiencing' the posterior material. (Fig. 3). It is not really known what growth cone structures are required for sensing the repulsing influence, nor how the growth cone is made to turn. It is possible that transient generation of a second messenger like calcium is involved, which directly or indirectly alters the dynamic cytoskeleton of the growth cone to initiate the turn.

The original observation of a choice made for anterior membranes by temporal axons would therefore seem to involve a repulsion of these axons by the posterior material. The interpretation is that the originally observed gradient consists of a repulsing cue.

How in molecular terms could the tectal gradients be established, and would there be enough information contained in gradients to explain the specificity and precision of growth cone guidance in the formation of the retinotectal map?

The active posterior material is a membrane-associated protein and is unlikely to constitute a diffusable gradient. It is more likely that tectal cells have been instructed to produce various amounts of this material on their membranes, and thus the posterior material could be graded across the tectum. This instruction might be a response to other events that have specified their position in the tectum, such as cell lineage or birth date. The gradient is probably not steep as dilution of posterior material with anterior by a factor of only five is enough to prevent the choice made by temporal axons. A weak gradient could be sufficient to signal information if amplification can occur in the growth cone. Slime moulds, for example, can detect very small concentrations of materials across the extent of the cell. This degree of sensitivity has not been seen for growth cones, but might be observed with an analysis of a growth cone response to a gradient of posterior material.

What is known about the cellular source of the posterior repulsive material, and what experiments can be designed to test the relationship of the *in vitro* observations to the *in vivo* situation?

Tectal glial cells may be the source of the posterior material. The ingrowing axons see the radial glial cells, and when the axons leave the SO to invade the SFGS they turn in a direction which is parallel to the glial processes. One could test the hypothesis that the glia express the necessary components by studying isolated radial glia. An antibody which disrupts the formation of the map *in vivo* by neutralising the activity of the posterior material, might be seen to bind to radial glia. One could slice the tectum into layers and establish which layer expresses the antigen. However, it is possible that all tectal cells have guidance components related to their position. For example, Trisler's marker is expressed on all tectal cells.

Inhibiting Growth Cones

The phenomenon of avoidance by a growth cone could be of general significance to mechanisms of growth cone guidance during development. There are many examples known where axons will fasciculate with homotypic axons, but fail to grow along the axons of another type. For example temporal axons will select other temporal axons to grow on rather than axons from the nasal half of

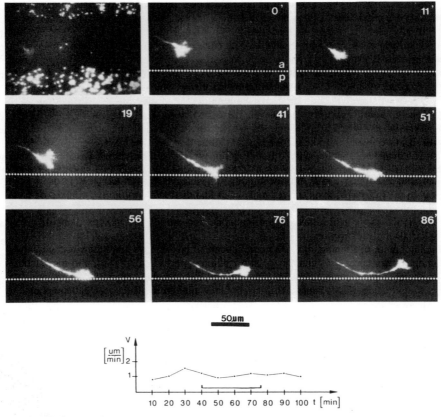

Fig. 3. Growth cones are repulsed by posterior membranes. Successive video frames depicting a border
   encounter of a labelled growth cone. The first frame shows the anterior to posterior (labelled)
   membrane margin. There is no obvious change in the morphology or the growth rate (see lower
   portion of figure) for the time period that the growth cone is growing along the border. Numbers
   represent time sequence in minutes.

the retina (Bonhoeffer and Huff, 1985). Axons from the PNS and CNS fail to mix when together in
the same culture dish; the axons establish territories as a result of many avoidance reactions that their
growth cones display when encountering heterotypic neurites. The growth cones of one tissue
encounter the neurites of the other tissue and hesitate, then collapse and retract. Subsequent
rechallenging by the growth cone is only associated with a successful crossing after a considerable
delay.

   From observations of the altered behavior of growth cones when avoiding an unfriendly contact
the phrase "growth cone collapse" has been coined, and it applies to the condensation of
lamellopodia, cessation in motility and resorbtion of the growth cone which accompanies such an
event. Several workers have now described systems in which they observe growth cone collapse in
response to membrane-associated components. Collapse has been seen for PNS growth cones which
encounter mature oligodendrocytes (Bandtlow et al. 1989; Fawcett et al., 1989). Raper and
Kapfhammer (1989) observe growth cone collapse when membrane particles of embryonic chick
CNS are sprinkled onto dorsal root ganglion neurons, and Cox et al. (1989) have observed growth
cone collapse for temporal axons when they are challenged with membrane particles isolated from
posterior tectum. The relevance of this temporal ganglion cell growth cone collapse to that of the
growth cone avoidance reaction on membrane carpets, and more importantly to that of the formation

of the retinotopic projection, are not fully understood. However, the growth cone collapsing activity can be found in the correct part of the tectum at the relevant developmental age.

In conclusion, *in vitro* assays show that the growth cones of ganglion cells from temporal retina can be guided by a repulsing membrane-associated component of posterior tectum. Several questions concerning the nature of this substance, how its graded distribution could be established and how it acts to guide growth cones will remain unanswered until its molecular investigation is complete.

Guidance By Diffusible Molecules; Diffusible Gradients in the Chick Tectum

The posterior tectal component would seem to fit into the category of a cell-surface guidance cue. However, there is evidence that the growth cones of some peripheral neurones respond to gradients of chemoattractant molecules emanating from their peripheral targets (Lumsden and Davies, 1983), and there is some evidence that chemotropism may operate to guide CNS axons in the absence of any preformed cellular, or extracellular pathway. A recent example of this is provided by evidence that commissural axon outgrowth in the developing spinal cord can be influenced *in vitro* by a factor secreted by the floor plate cells (Tessier-Lavigne et al., 1989). This factor appears to affect only commissural axons within the spinal cord, and it can orient their outgrowth. There is a possibility that the local guidance of retinal growth cones to their final tectal area could involve target cell-derived diffusible components like neurotransmitters or growth factors, which could be graded in their distribution.

REFERENCES

Bandtlow, C., Zachleder, T., and Schwab, M.E. 1989, Rapid and permanent inhibition of growth cone motility by oligodendrocytes, *Neuron*, (submitted).

Bonhoeffer, F., and Huff, J., 1985, Position-dependant properties of retinal axons and their growth cones, *Nature*, 315:409.

Cox, T., Mueller, B., Bonhoeffer, F., 1989, Axonal guidance in the chick visual system: Posterior tectal membranes induce collapse of growth cones from the temporal lobe, (submitted).

Fawcett, J. W., Rokos, J., and Bakst, I., 1989, Oligodendrocytes repel axons and cause axonal growth cone collapse, *J. Cell Sci.*, 92:93.

Fujisawa, H., Tani, N., Watanabe, K., and Ibata, Y., 1982, Branching of regenerating retinal axons and preferential selection of appropriate branches for specific neuronal connection in the newt, *Dev. Biol.*, 90:43.

Gieter, A., 1981, Developing projections between areas of the nervous system, *Biol. Cybern..*, 42:69.

Gierer, A. 1987, Directional cues for growing axons forming the retinotectal projection, *Development.*, 101:479.

Gottlieb, D.I., Rock, K. and Glaser, L., 1976, A gradient of adhesive specificity in the developing avian retina, *Proc. Natl. Acad. Sci. USA*, 73:410.

Halfter, W., Claviez, M., and Schwarz, V., 1981, Preferential adhesion of tectal membranes to anterior embryonic chick retina neurites, *Nature*, 202:67.

Lumsden, A.G.S., and Davies, A.M., 1983, Earliest sensory nerve fibres are guided to peripheral targets by attractants other than nerve growth factor, *Nature*, 306:786.

Rabacchi, S. A., Nere, R. L., and Dräger, U. C., 1988, Molecular cloning of the "dorsal eye antigen": Homology to the high affinity laminin receptor, *Soc. Neurosci. Abst.*, 14:769.

Rager, G.H., 1980, Development of the retinotectal projection in the chicken, in: "Advances in Anatomy, Embryology and Cell Biology", vol. 63, Brodal, A., van Luisbough, J., Ortmann, R. and Tondury, G., eds., Springer-Verlag, Berlin, p.1.

Raper, J.A., and Kapfhammer, J.P., 1989, The enrichment of a neuronal growth cone collapsing activity from embryonic brain. Submitted.

Sperry, R.W., 1963, Chemoaffinity in the orderly growth of nerve fiber patterns and connections, *Proc. Natl. Acad. Sci. USA*, 50:703.

Stuermer, C.A.O., 1986, Pathways of regenerated retinotectal axons in goldfish, *J. Embryol. Exp. Morph..*, 93:1.

Tessier-Lavigne, M., Placzek, M., Lumsden, A.G.S., Dodd, J., and Jessell, T.M., 1989, Chemotropic guidance of developing axons in the mammalian central nervous system, *Nature*, 336:775.

Thanos, S., and Deutting, D., 1987, Outgrowth and directional specificity of fibres from embryonic retinal transplants in the chick optic tectum, *Dev. Brain Res.*, 32:161.

Thanos, S., Bonhoeffer, F., and Rutishauser, U., 1984, Fibre-fibre interaction and tectal cues influence the development of the chicken retinotectal projection, *Proc. Natl. Acad. Sci. USA*, 81:1906.

Thanos, S. and Bonhoeffer, F., 1986, Course corrections of deflected retinal axons on the tectum of the chick embryo, *Neurosci. Lett.*, 72:31.

Trisler, D., and Collins, F., 1987, Corresponding spatial gradients of TOP molecules in the developing retina and optic tectum, *Science*, 237:1208.

Walter, J., Kern-Veits, B., Huf, J., Stolze, B., and Bonhoeffer, F., 1987a, Recognition of position-specific properties of tectal cell membranes by retinal axons in vitro, *Development*, 101:685

Walter, J., Henke-Fahle, S., and Bonhoeffer, F., 1987b, Avoidance of posterior tectal membranes by temporal retinal axons, *Development,* 101:909.

Walter, J., Mueller, B., and Bonhoeffer, F., 1989, Axonal guidance by an avoidance mechanism, *J. Physiol. (Paris),* in press.

Willshaw, D. J., and von der Malsburg, D., 1979, *Philos. Trans. R. Soc. Lond. [Biol.]*, 287:203.

Yoon, M. G., 1973, Retention of the original topographic polarity by the 180 degree rotated tectal reimplant in young adult goldfish. *J. Physiol. (Lond)*, 233:575.

THE CONSTRUCTION OF A VISUAL SYSTEM [*]

J. S. H. Taylor (scribe)

Dept. Human Anatomy
University of Oxford
Oxford, UK

R. M. Gaze (lecturer)

MRC Neural Development
and Regeneration Group
University of Edinburgh
Edinburgh, UK

INTRODUCTION

The work presented in this chapter concerns the development of the frog visual system, concentrating upon the specific connections which are formed between the retina and the primary visual center, the optic tectum. Topographic inter-connections between arrays of neurons, are commonly found in the vertebrate CNS and studies of their formation are thought to be central to our understanding of neural connectivity. The frog retinotectal projection, as an example of a topographically organized system, has been extensively used in such investigations. This system offers great advantages for developmental studies, since it continues to grow for many months, and throughout its development all parts of the system can be examined using a variety of methods of analysis. It is also possible to perform operations which perturb the system in a controlled fashion, either in the embryo, or at later stages when the regeneration of the retinal axons can be exploited. A further advantage, which arises naturally as a consequence of the extended period of growth of the system, is the continual and orderly alteration of the connections necessary for maintained function of the system during development.

THE FROG RETINOTECTAL PROJECTION

The connections between the ganglion cells of the retina and their target cells in the tectum are highly organized; neighboring cells in the retina connect with neighboring cells in the tectum, forming a topographic projection (Fig.1). The nature of this projection can be shown by recording electrophysiologically the responses in the tectum elicited by stimulation in the visual field or by using tracers such as HRP to selectively stain populations of retinal ganglion cells, their axons and their terminal arbors.

THE DEVELOPMENT OF THE PROJECTION

The retina starts to differentiate after about two days of embryonic life, and subsequently grows from a germinal epithelium lying around its periphery (Straznicky and Gaze, 1971). The growth of

---

[*] This chapter to be cited as: Taylor, J. S. H., and Gaze, R. M., 1990, The construction of a visual system, in: "Systems Approaches to Developmental Neurobiology," P. A. Raymond, S. S. Easter, Jr., and G. M. Innocenti, eds., Plenum Press, New York.

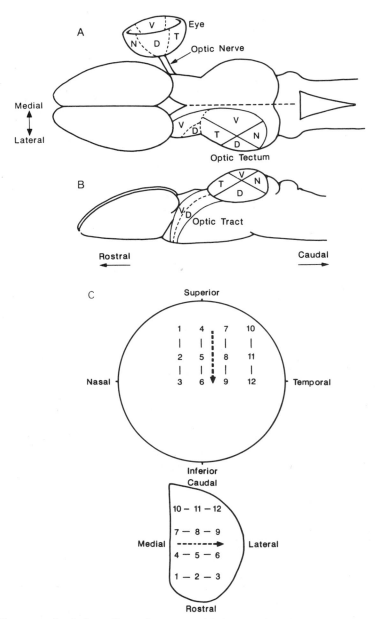

Fig. 1. A) The axons of retinal ganglion cells connect with the contralateral optic tectum in a precise order, which is illustrated in this dorsal view of a frog brain. Using HRP to label specific populations of ganglion cells, the organization of both the axons and their terminals can be revealed. Axons from temporal retina (**T**) connect with rostral tectum, and those from nasal retina (**N**) with the caudal part, whilst the dorsal axons (**D**) connect laterally and ventral axons (**V**) medially. B) The segregation of dorsal and ventral axons in the optic tract leads axons to the appropriate part of the tectum for termination. C) The precision and orientation of the retinotectal projection can be demonstrated electrophysiologically by recording from the tectum responses to stimulation in the visual field. Rostral tectum (**1, 2, 3**) receives visual information from the nasal visual field (i.e. from temporal retinal cells) and there is an orderly progression of the responses from medial (**1**) to lateral (**3**) tectum as the stimulus moves from superior to inferior visual field.

the retina continues by annular increments, for approximately one to two years. Therefore, the newest retinal cells lie in the peripheral retina, whilst the oldest cells are in central retina.

The growth of the tectum starts at a somewhat later stage of development (see below) and continues during larval life, culminating shortly after metamorphosis (Straznicky and Gaze, 1972). Tectal growth occurs by the addition of cells in a progressive wave starting in the laterorostral part and continuing in a caudal and medial direction. The incongruous growth of the retina and tectum means that, for the internal order of the projection to be preserved, the entire array of connections must gradually move over the tectal surface during development (Gaze et al., 1979). (The details of this shift in connections will not be discussed here, but this phenomenon should be borne in mind as counter-evidence for existence of specific affinities between ganglion cells and target cells in the tectum). To preserve function, which starts early in the development of the system, each new generation of ganglion cell axons must add to the existing array of connections in proper order. This is achieved by an orderly sequence of ingrowth, together with the previously mentioned shift in connections. For the first generated ganglion cells this problem does not arise. They must simply navigate to, and form retinotopic connections with, the uninnervated tectal primordium.

The early development of the *Xenopus* retinotectal projection is described in detail by Ross and Easter (1990, this volume). Some observations are also important to note here: The earliest retinal axons grow into the diencephalon at stage 33/34 (early on the second day), where they form the optic tract, and reach their initial target region at stage 38/39 (approximately 10 hours later). In the optic tract they grow in a position adjacent to the fibres of the post-optic commissure and in the immediately subpial part of the developing diencephalon (Easter and Taylor, 1989).

THE PATHWAY OF GROWING RETINAL GANGLION CELL AXONS

In post-embryonic *Xenopus*, the optic tract extends from the deepest part of the diencephalon, adjacent to the ventricle, to the pial margin. The relative depth of a fiber in the optic tract reveals the time at which it grew into the system, indicative of an orderly sequence of ingrowth; deepest fibres are the oldest, whilst those at the pia are the most recent (Fig.2). The original suggestion that new growing retinal axons all grew peripherally arose from the observation that after a lesion of the tadpole optic nerve, regenerating fibres grew in the immediately subpial region of the optic tract (Gaze and Grant, 1978). As has been mentioned, we now know that the earliest retinal axons grow superficially and that new growing axons at later stages of development are found in similar positions. Why growing retinal axons prefer the subpial region is unclear. We know from regeneration experiments that fibres can grow in the deeper parts of the pathway if they are given access; however, they normally prefer the tract margin. This may reflect a concentration of some substrate factor around the subpial glial end feet, (Silver and Rutishauser, 1984), or, the presence of the immediately preceding generation of fibres which form a growth substrate (Wilson et al., 1988).

To look in detail exclusively at growing axons in the subpial region of the pathways, one can exploit the regenerative ability of the retinal axons. When an optic nerve is lesioned, the severed axons regrow through the subpial region where a profusion of growth cone profiles can be identified. One problem encountered in such regeneration experiments is the abnormality of the pathway. It is filled with degenerating debris and reactive glia. Although this may add complexity to the interpretation of observations, the similar behavior of regenerating axons and those growing *de novo*, and even the possible enhanced expression of extracellular matrix components by the reactive glia, make this a promising approach.

So, we know that each generation of axons normally grows in an orderly fashion through the subpial region of the optic tracts which leads them to the tectal periphery where they terminate. The central question is how do the fibres recognize the correct relative position in the periphery in which to form connections?

THE TOPOGRAPHIC ORGANIZATION OF CONNECTIONS

The hypothesis of neuronal specificity was proposed by Sperry after his observations of specific regeneration and functional recovery of the retinotectal projection, and the maladaptive regeneration which arose after the rotation of an eye (Sperry, 1963). He suggested that complementary labels

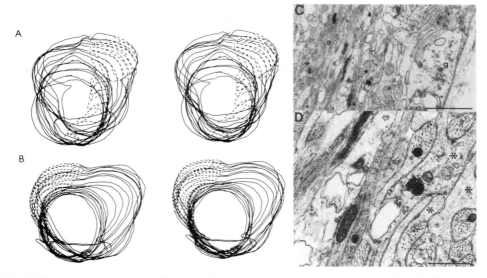

Fig. 2. Computer-generated three-dimensional reconstructions of transverse sections through A) the normal and B) the regenerated retinotectal projection labeled with HRP. In the normal projection the optic tract extends from deep in the diencephalon to the pial margin. In the regenerate, the entire projection is superficial. C) Electron micrograph of the subpial region of the optic tract showing the position of growth cone profiles which lie beneath the end feet of radial glia (**g**) and amidst other growing and recently grown axons (**a**). Scale bar 5μm.D) A higher magnification of the subpial region in C) showing growth cone profiles (*****). Scale bar 1 μm. (Reprinted with permission from Wilson et al., 1988).

existed in each array of neurons. A retinal ganglion cell, which bore a distinct "label", sent out its axon which responded to complementary "labels" expressed both along the route to its target (navigation cues) and in its target region (as a means of recognizing the correct cells with which to terminate). In absolute terms of a one-to-one specificity this theory is improbable, but it is plausible if gradients of labels exist in the retina and tectum and connections are formed in relative terms. In the chick visual system a graded distribution of an inhibitory factor has been found in caudal tectum, which may restrict temporal axon termination to rostral tectum (Allsopp and Bonhoeffer, 1990, this volume; Walter et al., 1987).

In *Xenopus*, although we have no similar candidate molecules for neuronal specificity, we have a wealth of evidence for the existence of such specific labeling of the ganglion cells. This evidence has come from a series of experiments involving manipulation of the embryonic eye. Parts of the eye cup can be removed and grafted, to construct eyes in which identified complements of ganglion cells are deleted, duplicated or relatively disarranged. The projections which later develop from operated eyes demonstrate that the original embryonic position of the ganglion cells faithfully predicts their relative sites of termination in the tectum. The best evidence for such stable positional labels in the retina comes from disarranged eyes in which half eyes are substituted for similar half eyes of opposite handedness (Fig.3). This operation results in a maximal discontinuity in polarity at the graft border which is detected in an abrupt change in orientation in the electrophysiologically recorded map as the stimulus passes from the host half eye to the graft (Gaze and Straznicky, 1980).

When is positional information established in the developing eye cup, and how are results of similar discontinuous eye graft experiments, apparently showing regulation of positional labels in the retina, reconciled with those described above?

In the late 1960s and early 1970s a series of experiments, performed by Jacobson and Hunt (1973), led to the claim that the developing eye cup had two distinct axes of polarity (naso-temporal and dorso-ventral), which were specified independently at different stages of development (stage 28 and stage 32). Similar experiments did not yield the same results in the hands of other investigators, who found evidence of retinal polarity from the earliest stages of differentiation of the eye cup (stage 21/22). This conflict has been attributed to differences in operative technique, especially in the ionic concentration of the operating solutions used. The *Xenopus* eye cup has a remarkable ability to regenerate missing or damaged tissue, and this process can give rise to duplication or the replacement of eye tissue depending upon the nature of the deficit and the mode of healing (Ide et al., 1984).

Recently, experiments by O'Rourke and Fraser (1986b;1989), showed that cells generated at the periphery of the graft during late tadpole life connected to the tectum according to their position in the eye, rather than to the expected position assuming their derivation from the embryonic tissue of the graft. In agreement with the results of Gaze and Straznicky (1980), the initial projection from the grafted cells was according to their embryonic origins, so there is no controversy about the existence of retinal labels. It is only at later stages of development that the different result emerges. It is unclear whether this is a result of true "respecification" of cells in the graft germinal epithelium, or some degenerative phenomena in the graft germinal epithelium with replacement or regeneration by cells derived from the host tissue.

The initial projections from "compound" eyes are also relevant to the question of whether or not the early tectum carries cellular labels. Such compound eyes are made by substitution of one half of an embryonic eye by the opposite half of an eye of opposite handedness. This results in the deletion of half of the normal population of ganglion cells and a duplication of the other half. Later, when fibres grow from the eye to the brain, the initial projections from double-ventral and double-temporal eyes show that the part of the tectum which normally receives axons from the deleted half-retina is vacant, but the part of the tectum appropriate for the nature of the compound eye, is innervated (Straznicky et al., 1981). For double-nasal compound eyes, on the other hand, the fiber projection covers the greater part of the tectum from the start. With the exception of these double nasal projections, the findings can be interpreted as evidence in favour of early regional tectal labeling. It is also possible, however, to argue that these compound eye results would fit the idea that the main determinant of the initial projection is the distribution of fibres in the pathway; and such an interpretation would fit the results from all three classes of compound eye, not just two.

RETINOTOPICITY IN THE OPTIC PATHWAYS

In the normal tadpole or metamorphosed frog, ganglion cell axons are arranged in the optic tract according to their position of retinal origin. Dorsal and ventral axons are segregated into the lateral and medial parts of the tract, temporal axons show relative cohesion in the center of the tract, whilst nasal axons are dispersed across its entire width (Fawcett and Gaze, 1982). This distribution leads them to the appropriate region of the tectum for termination (see Fig.1). Within the optic nerve, axons are not retinotopically ordered but in the region of the chiasm axons select a tract trajectory which has been shown experimentally to depend upon an embryonically specified identity (Taylor, 1987). For example, axons arising from a double-ventral "compound-eye" all make their appropriate selection for medial tract, leaving the lateral part of the tract devoid of axons (Fawcett and Gaze, 1982; Fig.4). All ventral axons therefore enter the tectum from its rostro-medial edge and none from its rostro-lateral edge. If similar pathway choices are made by the first retinal axons in the optic tracts, then a rough retinotopicity will exist in the projection, generated by pathway-choices rather than by target-recognition.

So far, the evidence for retinotopic organization during the initial outgrowth through the optic tract is positive, but limited to dorsal and ventral axons, which occupy the lateral and medial parts of the optic tract (Holt, 1984; Holt and Harris, 1986). Appropriately, the initial terminal arbors also show a retinotopic dorsal/ventral segregation. Intriguingly, the initial distributions of nasal and temporal arbors overlap completely (O'Rourke and Fraser, 1986a). It seems likely that this lack of a

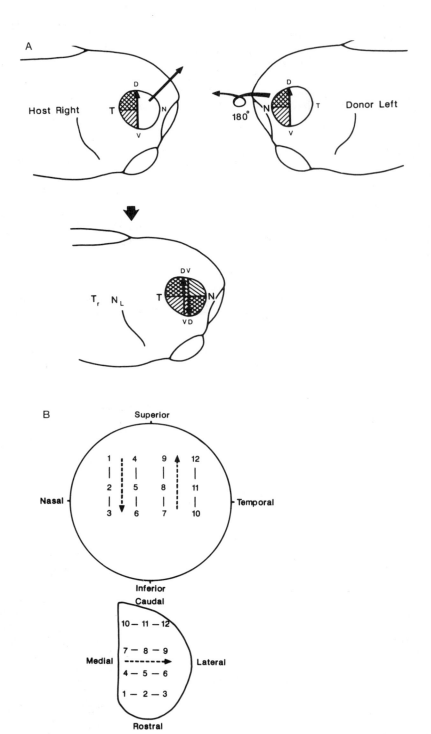

Fig. 3. A) The operation to form a discontinuous temporal-right/nasal-left eye. The nasal retina from the right eye of the host is replaced by the nasal part of a left eye. The graft must be inverted by 180 degrees to be accommodated into the orbit. This creates a radical disjunction in the positional inter-relationships of cells at the graft border, where dorsal and ventral cells are abutted. B) Electrophysiological recording of the projections from such eyes show a corresponding reversal of polarity at the graft border, indicating that the ganglion cells of each half of the eye have connected to the tectum according to their original embryonic position in the eye. (Figure on facing page.)

demonstrable naso-temporal difference is related to the cellular identity of the initial target region, as described below. Later, around stage 47, the characteristic nasotemporal differences emerge and may be demonstrated with fiber-tracing methods (O'Rourke and Fraser, 1986a) and also electrophysiologically (Gaze et al., 1974). The initial crude topography of the retinotectal map may therefore simply reflect this orderly ingrowth, rather than specific connectivity. However, the crude order of the initial projection may also establish the pattern of tectal "cues" underlying the precise topography of the subsequently developing projection.

DEATH AMONG THE RETINAL GANGLION CELLS

Studies of the early stages of visual system development have mainly concentrated upon the axons and their arbors, but recent investigations of both the ganglion cells and their target cells have revealed that some assumptions are surprisingly off the mark. For example, it has long been assumed that there is no significant cell death in the frog retina, during the formation of the retinotectal projection. This contrasts with the known massive cell loss in developing mammalian and chick retinae. To examine this issue, advantage has been taken of the annular growth of the frog retina (Fig.5A). Counting cells within central retina, as delineated by labeling mitotic cells at a specified stage of development, has produced some striking results showing extensive cell death.

Using this method, Jenkins and Straznicky (1986), have shown some 20% of the retinal ganglion cells present at stage 53 have died by metamorphosis, whilst Gaze and Grant (unpublished), have estimated that 45% of the ganglion cells at stage 45 have been lost by metamorphosis. Between stages 39 and 45 the results are more intriguing. At these early stages the cell counts are difficult, since the total number of cells is small, but one can derive a general impression of a peak in the relative level of cell death, somewhere in the region of 66%. This means that at least two thirds of the cells which initially send axons to the tectum are dying.

What evidence is there that the first growing retinal axons are a "pioneer" population?

The concept of "pioneer" axons has been best illuminated in studies of the development of the invertebrate nervous system. By definition a "pioneer" is one of the first axons to grow along a pathway and its implied role is one of pathfinding. Other axons may then use the pioneer as a substrate to form a nerve or tract. Once the pioneer has established the route, its function may be complete and it may then be eliminated. In the developing retinotectal system of *Xenopus*, the first born ganglion cells partially fulfil these criteria; they are the first to grow to the tectum, forming the optic nerve and the optic tract and 66% of them die. The initial projection is formed by many axons, so in this case there is not one pioneer axon, but a whole population of pioneers. An interesting speculation is that the early fibres may form the "template" for the segregation of dorsal from ventral axons in the tract. Subsequent generations of retinal axons could then make their pathway choice by fasciculating with their appropriate predecessors. The first axons may also play a role in inducing specific labels among the tectal cells, an idea which is discussed below.

THE ORIGIN OF THE TECTUM

Shortly after stage 45 two events which relate to the formation of the projection occur: the segregation of nasal from temporal arbors, and the coincident emergence of relatively precise retinotopography, as demonstrated electrophysiologically. A third fact also stands out; in studies of tectal cell genesis the first post-mitotic cells are generated at about stage 45 (Straznicky and Gaze, 1972) (Fig.5B). If there is no tectum when the first retinal axons arrive, at stage 38/39, then it becomes relevant to ask what is the nature of the initial target, in relation to which the fibres arborize? To address this issue, tectal cell genesis has been re-examined. Administration of labels which mark mitotic cells before stage 45 does **not** reveal a population of unlabeled cells in the most rostral part of the tectum at metamorphosis (Gaze and Grant, unpublished). Thus tectal cells present at metamorphosis were formed at or around stage 45. (The possibility that cells may become postmitotic earlier than this, and then die before metamorphosis, cannot be ruled out because it has so far not

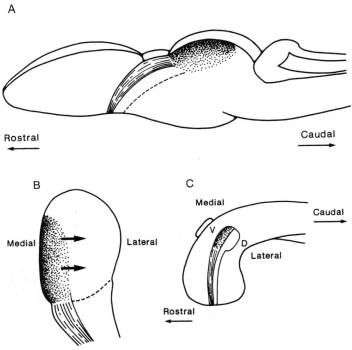

Fig. 4. A) The retinotectal projection from a double-ventral compound eye as demonstrated by HRP labeling. In the optic tract all the axons have selected the medial part of the tract, reflecting their ventral retinal origin, and enter the tectum from its rostro-medial pole. B) During development the projection from a double-ventral eye initially terminates medially on the tectum, which may reflect the pattern of ingrowth of the axons or could suggest some form of target affinity between ventral retinal axons and medial tectal cells. As the projection increases in size, the terminals shift progressively more lateral. C) At stage 39, when the first axons arrive at their first target region, near to the tectal precursor region, those from ventral and dorsal retina are segregated within the optic tracts producing an initial segregation of the terminal arbors.

been feasible to identify such cells.)   So, the region where the first optic axons arborize is close to where the tectum will later develop, but is not the tectum. What significance does this delayed tectal development have for the formation of connections?

After administration of label for mitotic cells before stage 45, the bulk of neuronal cells that are heavily labeled at metamorphosis are found in the pretectal nucleus and in the posterior thalamic nucleus. These are retino-recipient centers at the diencephalic-mesencephalic junction, and could form the initial targets for retinal axons. The di-mesencephalic junction is the first part of this region of the brain to form, and thereafter tectal development proceeds caudally, while the development of the diencephalon proceeds rostrally (Tay and Straznicky, 1982). In relation to these differences in the polarity of their development, it is interesting that the projections to the diencephalic nuclei have a rostro-caudal orientation which is the reverse of that to the tectum (Scalia and Fite, 1974).

Could the first retinal axons to arrive in the vicinity of the tectum play a role in its genesis or in the establishment of positional labels?

It has been shown by Raymond and Easter, that retinal axons have a modulatory effect on cell division in the goldfish tectum (Raymond et al., 1983). After de-afferentation, the level of mitosis in the caudal tectum declines, but is restored upon reinnervation, initially at a higher than normal (compensatory?) level. In the frog, the onset of cell genesis in the tectum is preceded by retinal axon ingrowth and arborisation, so there is the potential, as yet not demonstrated, for a stimulatory effect. However, if an eye is removed in embryo, the tectum still develops (although it is smaller than normal), suggesting that the retinal input is not essential. We don't know if such a de-afferented tectum develops with a normal time course, or whether the diminished size of the tectum results from cell death or reduced mitosis. So, retinal axons could have a modulatory role in tectal development.

Retinal axons have been shown to induce positional labels in the goldfish tectum, recognized by regenerating axons which terminate accordingly (Schmidt, 1978). It is therefore plausible that the initial population of retinal axons, arranged in crude retinotopic order, could induce a corresponding array of regional labels in the emerging tectal cell population.

PROPOSALS FOR THE FORMATION OF THE INITIAL RETINOTECTAL PROJECTION

In summary, the ideas proposed in this chapter can be restated as a hypothesis for the initial formation of a retinotopically organized pattern of connections. Ganglion cells in the retina, each bearing some form of embryonically-derived cell label, send out axons through the optic pathways. They grow in the subpial region of the pathway, either because of their association with fibres in the post-optic commissure, or because of some favored substrate associated with the glial end feet. In the optic tract, axons actively sort according to their retinal positional labels and occupy different regions of the pathway. At the dorsal midbrain they recognize a cue, possibly the early developing pretectal neurons, and arborize. Because of the retinotopic organization of the axons from dorsal and ventral retina, the initial terminal arbors are correspondingly retinotopically arranged. Subsequently, tectal cell genesis commences, possibly involving stimulatory interaction by the retinal axons, and connections are formed. Tectal cells receiving synaptic input from a particular population of ganglion cells become "specified" through these contacts. As more tectal cells develop, the arbors of temporal and nasal axons segregate, exhibiting their differential affinities for rostral and caudal tectum. A large proportion of ganglion cells formed during this period of tectal development will later die for reasons which are as yet unknown. Ensuing generations of axons use the preceding generations of axons to guide them through the appropriate part of the subpial tract to the tectum, where they arrive at an appropriate site for termination. Target cells which received input from ganglion cells of a similar retinal origin, are more attractive to the followers of those inputs, so relative order is preserved as the projection enlarges.

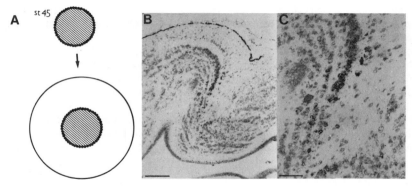

Fig. 5. A) If a label for mitotic cells is administered at stage 45, an annulus of cells will be labeled in the retinal margin (black), identifying the population of cells born at this stage. This marked annulus also conveniently defines the population of ganglion cells which existed in central retina at stage 45 (hatched) and these can be counted. If a similarly labeled eye is allowed to continue to grow, the defining annulus of cells persists, allowing the number of cells in central retina to be counted at a later stage. Cell death accounts for the fall in cell numbers within the defined region of central retina during the interval between the two counts. B) A low and (C) a higher power micrograph of a horizontal section through the tectum of a postmetamorphic frog, showing that the first tectal cells to be labeled after administration of tritiated thymidine at stage 45 form the most rostral part of the tectum. Scale bars: B) 100 μm, C) 50 μm.

Does retinal ganglion cell activity have a role in the establishment of ordered connections?

In the frog the formation of specific intertectal connections between regions of the tectum receiving inputs from ganglion cells viewing the same part of visual space is probably directed by correlated visual activity. Similarly, activity has been suggested to underlie the linkage between the auditory and visual projections to the mammalian colliculus. There is also a wealth of evidence for activity based refinement of regenerated projections in the frog retinotectal system and in the formation of discontinuous striped projections in double innervation experiments, where a single tectum receives a duplicated retinal input. In the later case, the stripes may be formed by an interplay between mechanisms leading similarly labeled axons to terminate in a particular tectal position and a repulsive segregating force generated by their dissimilar activity. It is known that once the initial population of retinal ganglion cell axons has formed a crude retinotopic array over the tectal surface, either by orderly ingrowth or by target cell recognition, there is a refinement of connections generating a precise retinotopicity. This refinement process could be driven by ganglion cell activity.

ACKNOWLEDGEMENTS

We thank Mr. Terry Richards for preparing the figures.

REFERENCES

Easter, S. S., and Taylor, J. S. H., 1989, The development of the *Xenopus* retinotectal pathway: selective fasciculation guides growing axons to their targets, *Development,* (in press).

Fawcett, J. W., and Gaze, R. M., 1982, The retinotectal fiber pathways from normal and compound eyes in *Xenopus, J. Embryol. Exp. Morphol.*, 72:19.

Gaze, R. M., Feldman, J. D., Cooke, J., and Chung, S. H., 1979, The orientation of the visuotectal map in *Xenopus*; developmental aspects, *J. Embryol. Exp. Morphol.*, 53:39.

Gaze, R. M., and Grant, P., 1978, The diencephalic course of regenerating retinotectal fibres in *Xenopus* tadpoles, *J. Embryol. Exp. Morphol.*, 44:201.

Gaze, R. M., Keating, M. J., and Chung, S. H., 1974, The evolution of the retinotectal map during development in *Xenopus, Proc. R. Soc. Lond. [Biol.], 185*:301.

Gaze, R. M., and Straznicky, C., 1980, Stable programming for map orientation in disarranged embryonic eyes in *Xenopus, J. Embryol. Exp. Morphol.*, 55:143.

Holt, C. E., 1984, Does timing of axon outgrowth influence retinotectal topography in *Xenopus*?, *J. Neurosci.*, 4:1130.

Holt, C. E., and Harris, W. A., 1986, Order in the initial retinotectal map in *Xenopus*: a new technique for labelling growing nerve fibres, *Nature,* 301:50.

Ide, C. F., Reynolds, P., and Tompkins, R., 1984, Two healing patterns correlate with different neural connectivity patterns in regenerating embryonic *Xenopus* retinae, *J. Exp. Zool.,* 230:71.

Jacobson, M., and Hunt, R. K., 1973, Origins of neuronal specificity, *Sci. Am.,* 228:26.

Jenkins, S., and Straznicky, C., 1986, Naturally occurring and induced cell death: a retinal whole mount autoradiographic study in *Xenopus, Anat. Embryol.*, 174:59.

O'Rourke, N. A., and Fraser, S. E., 1986a, Dynamic aspects of retinotectal map formation revealed by a vital-dye fiber-tracing technique, *Dev. Biol.*, 114:265.

O'Rourke, N. A., and Fraser, S. E., 1986b, Pattern regulation in the eye bud of *Xenopus* studies with a vital-dye fiber-tracing technique, *Dev. Biol.*, 114:277.

O'Rourke, N. A., and Fraser, S. E., 1989, Gradual appearance of a regulated retinotectal projection pattern in *Xenopus laevis, Dev. Biol.*, 132:251.

Raymond, P. A., Easter, S. S. jnr., Burnham, J. A., and Powers, M.K., 1983, Postembryonic growth of the optic tectum in goldfish; II modulation of cell proliferation by retinal fiber input, *J. Neurosci.*, 5:1092.

Scalia, F., and Fite, K., 1974, A retinotopic analysis of the central connections of the optic nerve of the frog, *J. Comp. Neurol.,* 158:455.

Schmidt, J. T., 1978, Retinal fibres alter tectal positional markers during the expansion of the half retinal projection in goldfish, *J. Comp. Neurol.*, 177:279.

Silver, J., and Rutishauser, U., 1984, Guidance of optic axons *in vivo* by a preformed adhesive pathway on neuroepithelial endfeet, *Dev. Biol.*, 106:485.

Sperry, R. W., 1963, Chemoaffinity in the orderly growth of nerve fiber patterns and connections, *Proc. Natl. Acad. Sci., USA*, 50:703.

Straznicky, C., and Gaze, R. M., 1971, The growth of the retina in *Xenopus laevis*; an autoradiographic study, *J. Embryol. Exp. Morphol.*, 26:67.

Straznicky, C., and Gaze, R. M., 1972, The development of the tectum in *Xenopus laevis*:: an autoradiographic study, *J. Embryol. Exp. Morphol.,* 28:87.

Straznicky, C., Gaze, R. M., and Keating, M.J., 1981, The development of retinotectal projections from compound eyes in *Xenopus, J. Embryol. Exp. Morphol.*, 62:13.

Tay, D., and Straznicky, C., 1982, The development of the diencephalon in *Xenopus, Anat. Embryol.*, 163:371.

Taylor, J. S. H., 1987, Fibre organization and reorganization in the retinotectal projection of *Xenopus, Development*, 99:393.

Walter, J., Henke-Fahle, S., and Bonhoeffer, F., 1987, Avoidance of posterior tectal membranes by temporal retinal axons, *Development*, 101:909.

Wilson, M. A., Taylor, J .S .H., and Gaze, R. M., 1988, A developmental and ultrastructural study of the optic chiasma in *Xenopus, Development*, 102:537.

IN VIVO CORRELATES OF *IN VITRO* STUDIES OF AXONAL GUIDANCE:

RETINAL TRANSPLANTATION IN THE MAMMALIAN RETINOTECTAL SYSTEM [*]

Mark Hankin (scribe), Raymond Lund (lecturer)

Department of Neurobiology Anatomy and Cell Science
University of Pittsburgh
Pittsburgh, Pennsylvania, USA

INTRODUCTION

It is nearly 100 years since Ramón y Cajal first described the bulbous ends of immature axons (see Ramón y Cajal, 1937), and 80 years since Harrison (1910) provided convincing evidence that these structures were, indeed, growth cones. In the intervening time, a great deal of interest has been directed towards elucidating the mechanisms by which axons are first guided along their pathway of outgrowth to their target regions, and then are matched with appropriate sets of neurons to form functional synaptic circuits.

Investigations of these issues have utilized several approaches. Many descriptions of axonal pathfinding *in vivo* have been generated by studying the normal development of specific projections, and experimental manipulations have been studied to determine which factors during development affect the normal maturational events. Such studies have led to inferences about the mechanisms underlying the normal developmental events. As cell and molecular biology have matured, the endeavor to define the cues which guide axons has been transferred into the tissue culture dish. Numerous studies of this type have consequently identified specific substrates which promote neurite outgrowth *in vitro*, and it has been suggested that appropriate distributions of these components in the developing animal might play a role in guiding axons to their correct targets.

Furthermore, configurational changes in substrate molecules may provide polarity information which axons could use to guide them towards an appropriate target. Finally, diffusible molecules could function to sustain cells so that they are able to survive and emit processes ("trophic maintenance"): they could also, if released by a localized source, serve to direct axons along a diffusion gradient towards the source ("tropic guidance"). It should be noted that, depending on the circumstances, a diffusible molecule could function both as a trophic or tropic factor.

Each experimental approach to studying development, however, carries important caveats. Studies of normal development, for example, usually do not take into account the dynamic nature of the living animal, and may be limited by the difficulty of not knowing whether individual changes are causative or simply correlative. Another point of concern is whether mechanisms deduced from investigations on one species transfer directly to other species and phyla. One issue, which is relevant to the studies described in this paper, concerns the effect of increasing the size of the developing brain

---

[*] This chapter to be cited as: Hankin, M., and Lund, R.,1990, *In vivo* correlates of *in vitro* studies of axonal guidance: retinal transplantation in the mammalian retinotectal system, in: "Systems Approaches to Developmental Neurobiology," P. A. Raymond, S. S. Easter, Jr., and G. M. Innocenti, eds., Plenum Press, New York.

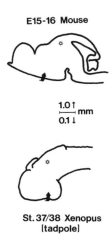

E15-16 Mouse

1.0 ↑
———— mm
0.1 ↓

St. 37/38 Xenopus
[tadpole]

Fig. 1. Schematic sagittal views illustrating the relative scale of the brains of embryonic mouse (E15-16) compared to the *Xenopus* tadpole. The stages shown are when retinal axons (arrow) first approach their target, the tectal primordium (asterisk). While both brains are drawn to the same size, the *Xenopus* brain is actually approximately an order of magnitude smaller (note scale bar).

on the effective range of distance-dependent phenomena, such as diffusible molecules. While there are many factors which could limit the absolute range of diffusible molecules in the developing brain (e.g., the physical arrangement and chemical composition of the extracellular space, the physicochemical properties of the diffusing molecule, and the concentration of the substance), it is possible that their effective range is relatively greater in smaller brains than in larger brains (Fig. 1). Thus, it is necessary to consider potential guidance mechanisms not only as they relate to other factors which influence outgrowth, but also in the context of the spatial relationships in the developing brain of the species in question.

Likewise, *in vitro* investigations, while allowing the problem to be approached at the cell and molecular levels, cannot replicate either the complex *in vivo* microenvironment or the gross tissue relationships in which axonal outgrowth takes place. Another question is whether properties ascribed to neurons in a culture dish reflect the *in vivo* condition. For example, the cell surface antigen Thy-1, usually only found on retinal ganglion cells and their processes (Barnstable and Drager, 1984; Perry et al., 1984), under some conditions can be expressed on astrocytes in culture (Pruss, 1979; Perry et al., 1984). Another striking example of the intricate controls regulating cell surface molecules *in vivo* may be seen in the expression on optic axons of the cell surface glycoprotein M6 (Lund et al., 1986), antibodies to which block neurite outgrowth and cell migration *in vitro* (Lagenaur et al., 1984). While this cell surface molecule is initially distributed over the entire primary optic pathway during early development, over the first 3 postnatal weeks it is lost from the optic nerve and, by maturity it becomes restricted to intraretinal and terminal domains of optic axons. Thus, a single axon may regulate its cell surface constituents depending on the local environment.

It is essential therefore to consider axonal outgrowth and target innervation in the context of the complex regulatory events that occur *in vivo* during the period of normal development. The developmental events responsible for the formation of connections seem to depend not only on programs intrinsic to the neurons, but also on a variety of extrinsic factors. Modulation of such factors during development substantially alters anatomical connections and associated physiology and behavior. How far neural development can proceed without particular extrinsic cues, and exactly how such cues modulate the development of specific neural elements are central problems in our understanding of how functional assemblages of neurons are formed.

RETINAL TRANSPLANTATION

Several years ago Lund and co-workers (Lund and Haushka, 1976; McLoon and Lund, 1980; Hankin and Lund, 1987; Sefton and Lund, 1988), examined the possibility of transplanting embryonic neural tissue to the neonatal rodent brain in the hope of providing an *in vivo* preparation which might complement ongoing *in vitro* studies of axonal guidance. The goal of these studies has been to confront growing axons in an experimental setting with the microenvironment of the developing rodent brain, and subsequently to analyze the abilities and patterns of axonal outgrowth with respect to normal and abnormal substrates, pathways and target fields.

Attention has been focused on the development of the mammalian retinotectal projection because it is well studied anatomically in developing and adult animals, and because it has clearly defined functional properties. In developing this transplantation preparation there were several important considerations. First, it was important to define the normal maturation of the system (including transient events which occur during development) so that the stage of development at the time of transplantation could be specified for both the donor and recipient tissues. Second, it was important to know whether the transplantation procedure itself significantly interfered with the developmental process. Was there massive cell death shortly after transplantation? Did particular cell types die as a normal sequence? Were the transplants rejected by the host or did they suffer other effects of being recognized as "non-self"? Third, there should be features significant to the organization and function of the visual system which were relatively easy to assay after experimental manipulation. Fourth, once established, the system should be available for manipulation to permit examination of plasticity of mature patterns of neural organization. Finally, in keeping with the stated overall goal, the transplantation studies should have parallels with *in vivo* and *in vitro* experiments.

Embryonic mouse CD-1 (E12-13) retinae were placed into the brainstem of neonatal Sprague-Dawley rats (P1). In most cases, one or both eyes were removed at the time of transplantation to increase the density of innervation of host nuclei by transplant-derived axons. At selected times after transplantation, animals were fixed and sections of the brain were processed to show transplant projections. For xenogeneic transplants (mouse-to-rat), sections were stained to demonstrate transplant-derived projections either with (1) mouse neuron-specific antibodies (Lund et al., 1985), (2) the Fink-Heimer stain for degenerating fibers following a "immune lesion" of the transplant (for a description of this technique, see Lund et al., 1987), or (3) normal silver stains (Lund and Westrum, 1966; Rager et al., 1979). As a result of these cross-correlative staining methods, it was possible to identify transplant-derived projections with confidence using any one staining method.

Transplanted retinae developed laminae characteristic of retinae *in situ* according to a normal timetable (Hankin and Lund, 1987). The emergence of specific cell classes and their distinctive morphologies remained faithful to the normal patterns. Retinae generally integrated quickly into the host neuropil, and exhibited projections which participated in functional pathways of the host visual system. Transplanted retinae exhibit electroretinograms similar to those recorded from a normal, intact eye and can mediate electrically-derived tectal responses (Simons and Lund, 1985), mediate light-evoked responses in cortical area 18a (Craner et al., 1989), are capable of driving a pupillary response in an intact host eye (Klassen and Lund, 1987) and are able to channel sensory information that alters complex behaviors of the host (Coffey et al., in press).

SELECTIVITY OF CONNECTIONS

In order to provide a baseline for studies of the interactions between transplanted retinae and host brains, Radel, Hankin and Lund (1989) examined the connections made with the host brain and how they are modified by transplant location. The most extensive connections with host visual nuclei were made by transplants located on the dorsal midbrain. These showed projections to the superior colliculus (mammalian homologue of the optic tectum), the pretectum (including the nucleus of the optic tract and olivary pretectal nucleus), the outer shell of the dorsal lateral geniculate nucleus (dLGN) and the accessory optic nuclei. All of these are normal targets of optic axons. No projections were seen to other potential targets, including the inner core of the dLGN, the ventral LGN, the intergeniculate leaflet or to the suprachiasmatic nucleus even when transplants were placed in the region of the optic chiasm, or on the adjacent optic tract. The same selectivity was found for grafts in other locations, although some regions were less predictably innervated.

It appears, therefore, that retinal transplants exhibit a selectivity of innervation that is not dictated simply by proximity to the target nucleus. There are a number of possible explanations for the selectivity of innervation patterns. It may be the result of a timing mismatch between the graft and host tissues, or perhaps it might reflect the absence of a specific ganglion cell type(s) that fails to survive the transplantation procedure. Although the ganglion cells in the transplant show a relatively normal cell size histogram (Perry et al., 1985), it should be noted that there are many fewer cells than normal.

Do axons from specific populations, or classes, of retinal ganglion cells each express different types of outgrowth behavior, perhaps responding selectively to guidance cues depending on the origin of those signals?

The patterns of outgrowth and the selectivity of innervation by transplant-derived axons must be interpreted with caution on this point. It does seem clear that certain classes of ganglion cells will innervate different regions, for example W- and Y-cells go to the superior colliculus, X-cells to the lateral geniculate nucleus, and perhaps another class to the suprachiasmatic nucleus. This sort of selectivity of innervation may also play a role in determining the outgrowth from transplanted retinae, and in the end, which target regions will get innervated. Additionally, such phenomena may also depend on second order events, such as whether the outputs from those regions have connected, or whether afferents from other regions are present. Perhaps another related question is whether axons derived from transplants originating from specific retinal quadrants (for example, nasal versus temporal) show projections to different tectal regions.

DEVELOPMENT OF TRANSPLANT-DERIVED PROJECTIONS

The earliest outgrowth of axons from retinal transplants can be detected 1-2 days after transplantation. Retinae placed close to the surface of the brainstem send axons towards the superior colliculus, and these course in a band within 20 μm of the *glia limitans*. Transplants placed deep in the midbrain show outgrowth towards the superior colliculus as long as these transplants are within a little more than 1mm from the tectal surface. More ventrally located tegmental transplants show no outgrowth unless they come in close proximity to the ventral brainstem surface, in which case they follow a surface course to the superior colliculus.

These observations led us to suggest that there may be two components to optic axon growth that had been artificially segregated by the transplantation procedure (Fig. 2A). One pattern of outgrowth follows substrates localized to the subpial margin of the brainstem. Although this component of outgrowth appears to be oriented towards the tectum, this might be in response to substrate cues rather than diffusible factors, since the distances over which this growth occurs (as much as 5mm) far exceeds the distance over which freely diffusible substances might be effective. There are several potential substrates for growth of the graft-derived axons, including laminin, which is transiently expressed along the developing optic pathway (Cohen et al., 1987; Liesi and Silver, 1988), and N-CAM, which is present on glial end feet in the region of growing axons (Silver and Rutishauser, 1984). It has been shown that sialic acid residues on N-CAM molecules along the optic pathway of developing chicks changes with proximity to the tectum (Schlosshauer et al., 1984), providing a possible physical basis for the oriented growth.

The second pattern of optic axon outgrowth, exemplified by transplants embedded in the brainstem, shows little evidence of substrate specificity and instead suggests a target-directed neurotropic response. Thus, retinae located in the midbrain parenchyma (up to approximately 1mm from the surface of the superior colliculus) project axons which are oriented towards the tectum, even from the earliest time they can be detected (Fig. 2A). These axons may be seen to associate with a number of different substrates in the midbrain (radial glia, blood vessels, as well as other neurons and their processes), but they do not appear to receive directional cues simply from the geometric alignment of these elements. Therefore, the highly stereotyped orientation of these projections suggests that optic axons are responding to a long-distance cue emanating from the target region.

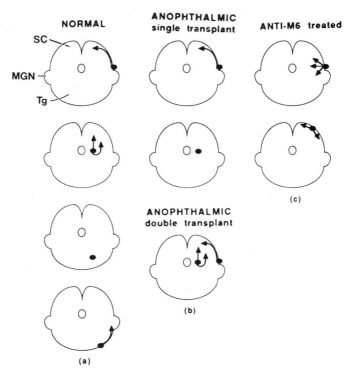

Fig. 2. Schematic coronal sections through the midbrain showing the axonal outgrowth patterns from retinal transplants placed in different postions in normal rats (column a), in *ocular retardation* mice (column b), and in normal rats after pretreatment of donor mouse retinae with mouse-specific antibody (anti-M6) that *in vitro* blocks neurite outgrowth on certain substrates (column c). Abbreviations: **MGN**, medial geniculate nucleus; **SC**, superior colliculus; **Tg**, tegmentum. The *glia limitans*, composed of glial endfoot processes aligned beneath the pial surface, is represented by the outline of the midbrain. Reprinted from Lund et al., in press.

In vivo studies in the retinotectal system of the *Xenopus* tadpole (Harris, 1986) support a similar conclusion for optic axons originating 200-300 μm from the tectal neuropil. However, recent work (Harris, 1989) also implicates substrate-bound cues in directional growth towards the target, and it is not yet clear in this system how such cues might modify the effects of the long-distance signals. Chemotropic guidance has also been suggested in several other systems (Lumsden and Davies, 1983; Tessier-Lavigne et al., 1988). *In vitro* studies have shown brain- or tectum-derived neurotrophic factors that maintain retinal ganglion cells (Nurcombe and Bennett, 1981; McCaffery et al., 1982; Turner et al., 1983). Similar factors could operate over a concentration gradient to produce the effects seen here.

Additional studies have dissociated these modes of growth further. The *ocular retardation* mutant mouse (*or^J*) is characterized by a failure of optic axon outgrowth from a rudimentary eye that undergoes degeneration (Theiler et al., 1976; Robb et al., 1978; Silver and Robb, 1979). Thus, unlike the rats used in the preceding transplant studies, the *or^J* tectum never receives optic axon innervation, and a retinal transplant placed in the midbrain is, therefore, confronted with a "virgin" tectum. Transplants placed on the surface of the midbrain as in the previous studies rapidly innervate the superior colliculus (Fig. 2B). By contrast, transplants placed in the tegmentum, less than 1mm from the superior colliculus, fail to show evidence of more than rudimentary axon outgrowth. In order to test whether optic input to the tectum is necessary before the tectum will exert its chemotropic influence, optic input was provided to the superior colliculus through a surface transplant. When a second retina was simultaneously co-transplanted into the tegmentum, the deep tegmental graft showed directed outgrowth towards the tectum. Therefore, it appears that tectal cells can only exert a neurotropic influence once they have received an optic innervation.

The identity of the cells in the superior colliculus that might produce diffusible chemotropic molecules is unknown, but they could be either neuronal or nonneuronal. It is interesting to note that the first neurons in the optic tectum of rodents and chicken are born prior to the arrival of the first optic axons (LaVail and Cowan, 1971; Mustari et al., 1979; Altman and Bayer, 1981; Edwards et al., 1986), whereas the situation appears to be reversed in *Xenopus* (Straznicky and Gaze, 1972). Thus, it is somewhat difficult to postulate a common mechanism for diffusible chemoattractants of neuronal origin across all species.

Another way in which it has been possible to dissect further the guidance cues in the rodent retinotectal projection has been through the use of monoclonal antibodies which perturb the system. Lund and colleagues (Hankin, Lund and Lagenaur, unpublished) have recently used a mouse-specific antibody to the neuronal cell surface glycoprotein M6 to interfere with axonal outgrowth (Fig. 2C). In culture, anti-M6 blocks neurite outgrowth from cerebellar neurons (Lagenaur et al., 1984); the efficacy appears to be substrate-dependent (Lagenaur, personal communication). Retinae transplanted to the midbrain surface after incubation in anti-M6 still projected axons into the host brain. However, instead of following the subpial pathway used by untreated retinal axons, axons from the treated retinae projected directly across the subpial region into the underlying midbrain neuropil. This suggests that M6 plays a critical role in recognition of subpial pathway guidance cues. Whether the antibody specifically blocks a receptor on the growth cone, or interferes with non-specific processes that have more to do with the physiology of the cell (i.e., osmotic or ionic regulation) is not yet clear. Correlative studies *in vitro* may help to address this intriguing issue.

CONCLUSION

The studies described in this paper use retinal transplantation as a tool to address the issue of axonal guidance and connectivity in an *in vivo* experimental setting. Although the main focus of this presentation has been to emphasize aspects of the preparation relevant to development, it is important to note that transplanted retinae are also capable of utilizing light input in a physiologically significant manner to modulate specific functional reflexes and complex behaviors in the host (Simons and Lund, 1985; Klassen and Lund, 1987; Craner et al., 1989; Coffey et al., in press). However, since it does not seem that retinae transplanted to the midbrain surface project in a topographically organized fashion onto the host tectum (Galli et al., 1989), it remains an open question as to whether it will be possible for transplanted retinae to mediate visual behaviors which depend on topographic mapping of visual input.

The expression of different, experimentally separable patterns of optic axon outgrowth suggests that guidance results from an elaborate interaction between substrate dependence, polarity cues and tropic guidance. During normal development, it may be suggested that growing optic axons on reaching the brainstem follow substrate cues close to the brainstem surface, being directed by polar cues towards the dorsolateral midbrain and the tectum. Once there, they quickly form the first synapses, and this process may stimulate neurons or associated glia in the tectum to produce a diffusible factor. This may serve several purposes: it could divert axons from the surface substrate; it could improve the efficiency of tectopetal growth by late growing axons; or it could serve to change the growth process from one of extension to one of terminal ramification.

How far will an axon grow in the CNS before it goes into its "arborization mode?"

This is one area which we have not yet addressed. It seems fair to say that this may relate to properties of the host as much as to intrinsic properties of the axon. In addition to specific molecular event(s) which may play a role in signaling an end to growth, myelination also begins at about the same time that many growth processes in the CNS cease. It is not known, however, whether such events are a cause for growth to stop, or whether they are the result of growth coming to an end. It might be interesting to explore this issue as it relates to the situation in the frog, where growth can continue throughout the life of the animal.

The existence of multiple cues for axonal guidance suggested by these, and other studies, raises the question of how growth cones determine which cue to follow if two or more cues overlap either spatially or temporally. The outgrowth from retinal transplants suggests that axonal guidance cues may be hierarchically ranked. This would allow a growth cone, depending upon its the past history of interactions, to respond preferentially to one cue amongst several according to a cellular algorithm. Thus, axons in the optic nerve would be guided by cues expressed in that region (e.g., axon-axon and/or axon-glia), but not (at least in animals such as mice and rats) to long-range cues emanating from the target region. At each subsequent point in the optic pathway, new cues would be expressed, and the growth cone would respond to each appropriate one depending on intrinsic, as well as extrinsic factors. Only when within range of a target-derived diffusible cue, would the growth cone respond. It should be noted that multiple cues may also regulate different properties of the growth cone and elongating axon (e.g., adhesion, outgrowth promotion, directionality), so that spatially overlapping cues may act on the growth cone at the same time.

It would appear, therefore, that the quite artificial circumstances presented by intracerebral transplantation may be useful for dissociating biological processes that would be hard to recognize by studying normal development, and furthermore such studies may also provide a perspective of developmental events which can be correlated with *in vitro* studies.

ACKNOWLEDGEMENTS

The authors would like to acknowledge past and present colleagues whose work on various aspects of retinal transplants has been mentioned in this paper: Fen-Lei Chang, Peter Coffey, Sandra Craner, Lucia Galli, Ling-Sun Jen, Henry Klassen, Carl Lagenaur, Steve McLoon, Hugh Perry, Jeff Radel, Kanchan Rao, Nick Rawlins, Ann Sefton and Dan Simons.

REFERENCES

Altman, J., and Bayer, S.A., 1981, Time origins of neurons of the rat superior colliculus in relation to other components of the visual and visuomotor pathways, *Exp. Brain Res.,* 42:424.

Barnstable, C.J., and Drager, U.C., 1984, Thy-1 antigen: a ganglion cell specific marker in rodent retina, *Neuroscience,* 11:847.

Coffey, P.J., Lund, R.D., and Rawlins, J.N.P., Retinal transplant-mediated learning on a conditioned suppression task in rats, *Proc. Natl. Acad. Sci. USA,* 18:7248.

Cohen, J., Burne, J.F., McKinlay, C., and Winter, J., 1987, The role of laminin and the laminin/fibronectin receptor complex in the outgrowth of retinal ganglion cell axons, *Dev. Biol.,* 122:407.

Craner, S.L., Radel, J.D., Jen, L.S., and Lund, R.D., 1989, Light-evoked cortical activity produced by illumination of intracranial retinal transplants: experimental studies in rats, *Exp. Neurol.,* 104:93.

Edwards, M.A., Caviness, V.S.Jr., and Schneider, G.E., 1986, Development of cell and fiber lamination in the mouse superior colliculus, *J. Comp. Neurol.,* 248:395.

Galli, L., Rao, K.R., and Lund, R.D., 1989, Transplanted rat retinae do not project on a topographic fashion on the host tectum, *Exp. Brain Res.,* 74:427.

Hankin, M.H., and Lund, R.D., 1987, Role of the target in directing the outgrowth of retinal axons: ransplants reveal surface-related and surface-independent cues, *J. Comp. Neurol.,* 263:455.

Harris, W.A., 1986, Homing behavior of axons in the vertebrate brain, *Nature,* 320:266.

Harris, W.A., 1989, Local positional cues in the neuroepithelium guide retinal axons in embryonic Xenopus brain, *Nature,* 339:218.

Harrison, R.G., 1910, The outgrowth of the nerve fiber as a mode of protoplasmic movement, *J. Exp. Zool.,* 9:787.

Klassen, H., and Lund, R.D., 1987, Retinal transplants can drive a pupillary reflex in host rat brains, *Proc. Natl. Acad. Sci. USA,* 84:6958.

Klassen, H., and Lund, R.D., 1988, Anatomical and behavioral correlates of xenograft-mediated pupillary reflex, *Exp. Neurol.,* 102:102.

Lagenaur, C.F., Fushiki, S., and Schachner, M., 1984, Monoclonal antibody M6 blocks neurite extension in cultured mouse cerebellar neurons, *Soc. Neurosci. Abstr.,* 10:759.

LaVail, J.H., and Cowan, W.M., 1971, The development of the chick optic tectum. II. Autoradiographic studies, *Brain Res.,* 28:421.

Liesi, P., and Silver, J., 1988, Is astrocyte laminin involved in axon guidance in the mammalian CNS?, *Dev. Biol.,* 130:774.

Lumsden, A.G.S., and Davies, A.M., 1983, Earliest sensory nerve fibers are guided to peripheral targets by attractants other than nerve growth factor, *Nature,* 306:786.

Lund, R.D., and L.E. Westrum, 1966, Neurofibrils and the Nauta method, *Science,* 153:1397.

Lund, R.D., and Hauschka, S.D., 1976, Transplanted neural tissue develops connections with host rat brain, *Science,* 193:583.

Lund, R.D., Chang, F.-L.F., Hankin, M.H., and Lagenaur, C.F., 1985, Use of a species-specific antibody for demonstrating mouse neurons transplanted to rat brains, *Neurosci. Lett.,* 61:221.

Lund, R.D., Perry, V.H., and Lagenaur, C.F., 1986, Cell surface changes in the developing optic nerve of mice, *J. Comp. Neurol.,* 247:439.

Lund, R.D., K.R. Rao, M.H. Hankin, H.W. Kunz, and T.J. Gill Jr, 1987, Transplantation of retina and visual cortex to rat brains of different ages; maturation, connection patterns, and immunological consequences, *Ann. N.Y. Acad. Sci.,* 495:227.

Lund, R.D., Radel., J.D., Hankin, M.H., Klassen, H., Coffey, P.J., and Rawlins, J.N.P., in press, Development and functional integration of retinal transplants with host rat brains, in: "Brain Repair," A. Bjorklund, A. Aguayo, and D. Ottoson, eds., Macmillan Press, London.

McCaffery, C.A., Bennett, M.R., and Dreher, B., 1982, The survival of neonatal ganglion cells in vitro is enhanced in the presence of appropriate parts of the brain, *Exp. Brain Res.,* 48:377.

McLoon, S.C., and Lund, R.D., 1980, Specific projections of retina transplanted to rat brain, *Exp. Brain Res.,* 40:273.

Mustari, M.J., Lund, R.D., and Graubard, K., 1979, Histogenesis of the superior colliculus of the albino rat: a tritiated thymidine study, *Brain Res.,* 164:39.

Nurcombe, V., and Bennett, M.R., 1981, Embryonic chick retinal ganglion cells identified in vitro: their survival is dependent on a factor from the Res., 44:249.

Perry, V.H., Morris, R.J., and Raisman, G., 1984, Is Thy-1 expressed only by ganglion cells and their axons in the retina and optic nerve?, *J. Neurocytol.,* 13:809.

Perry, V.H., Lund, R.D., and McLoon, S.C., 1985, Ganglion cells in retinae transplanted to newborn rats, *J. Comp. Neurol.,* 231:353.

Pruss, R.M., 1979, Thy-1 antigen on long-term cultures of rat central nervous system, *Nature,* 280:688.

Radel, J.D., Hankin, M.H., and Lund, R.D., 1989, Selectivity of connections made by retinal transplants, *Soc. Neurosci. Abstr.,* 15:1367.

Rager, G., S. Lausmann, and F. Gallyas, 1979, An improved silver stain for developing nervous tissue, *Stain Technol.,* 54:193.

Ramón y Cajal, S., 1937, "Recollections of My Life," American Philosophical Society, Philadelphia.

Robb, M., Silver, J. and Sullivan, R., 1978, *Ocular retardation (or) in the mouse. Invest. Ophthalmol. Vis. Sci.,* 17:468.

Schlosshauer, B., Schwarz, U., and Rutishauser, U., 1984, Topological distribution of different forms of neural cell adhesion molecule in the developing chick visual system, *Nature,* 310:141.

Sefton, A.J., and Lund, R.D., 1988, Cotransplantation of embryonic mouse retinal with tectum, diencephalon, or cortex to neonatal rat cortex, *J. Comp. Neurol.,* 269:548.

Silver, J. and Robb, R.M., 1979, Studies on the development of the eye cup and optic nerve in normal mice and in mutants with congenital optic nerve aplasia, *Dev. Biol.,* 68:175.

Silver, J., and Rutishauser, U., 1984, Guidance of optic axons in vivo by a preformed adhesive pathway on neuroepithelial end-feet, *Dev. Biol.,* 106:485.

Simons, D.J., and Lund, R.D., 1985, Fetal retinae transplanted over tecta of neonatal rats respond to light and evoke patterned neuronal discharges in the superior colliculus, *Dev. Brain Res.,* 21:156.

Straznicky, K., and Gaze, R.M., 1972, The development of the tectum in Xenopus laevis: an autoradiographic study, *J. Embryol. Exp. Morphol.*, 28:87.

Tessier-Lavigne, M., Placzek, M., Lumsden, A.G.S., Dodd, J., and Jessell, T.M., 1988, Chemotropic guidance of developing axons in the mammalian central nervous system, *Nature,* 336:775.

Theiler, K., Varnum, D.S., Nadeau, J.H., Stevens, L.C. and Cagianut, B., 1976, A new allele of *ocular retardation*: early development and morphogenetic cell death, *Anat. Embryol. (Berlin),* 150:85.

Turner, J.E., Barde, Y.-A., Schwab, M.E., and Thoenen, H., 1983, Extract from brain stimulates neurite outgrowth from fetal rat retinal explants, *Dev. Brain Res.*, 6:77.

EMBRYONIC-ADULT INTERACTIONS: CELLULAR MECHANISMS INVOLVED IN

PURKINJE CELL REPLACEMENT BY NEURONAL GRAFTING *

Patricia Gaspar (scribe), Constantino Sotelo (lecturer)

INSERM U 106
Bâtiment de Pédiatrie, Hôpital Salpêtrière
Paris, FRANCE

INTRODUCTION

Because of the relative simplicity and orderliness of its circuitry, the cerebellum is an attractive model to study the development of the mammalian central nervous system. We will discuss two approaches which have been used in the laboratory of C. Sotelo to study the developing cerebellum. The first is the attempted replacement of missing parts of the adult cerebellar circuitry by embryonic grafts. This approach, mainly developed with Cuca Alvarado-Mallart (Gardette et al., 1988, Sotelo and Alvarado-Mallart, 1986, 1987a, b) was envisaged as a way of asking whether or not the timing of cell to cell interactions was necessary for the building up of the cerebellar circuitry. The second approach, largely a result of the work of Marion Wassef (Wassef et al., 1985, 1987, 1989a,b) and other collaborators has been directed at finding cues or patterns which might guide the organization of precise projectional maps in the cerebellum. This approach led to the investigation of zonal organization within the cerebellum.

BRIEF ANATOMICAL REVIEW

The relative simplicity of the cortical cerebellar structure is due to the small number of cell types, five in all, each connected to the others in a stereotyped manner. The basic circuitry was established by Cajal (1889) at the turn of the century and is summarized in Figure. 1. The cerebellar cortex appears as a 3-layered structure: the single cell layer of Purkinje cells (PC) is sandwiched between an upper molecular layer and a lower granular layer. The PC is the only output cell of this system, sending its efferents mainly to the deep nuclei. Two types of excitatory inputs converge directly or indirectly on PCs: the climbing fibers and the mossy fibers. The climbing fibers (CF) arise from the contralateral inferior olive and establish direct synaptic contacts on the proximal dendritic arbor of PCs in a unique one-to-one relationship, i.e. 1 CF contacts 1 and only 1 PC. Mossy fibers arise from several brainstem nuclei and from the spinal cord and contact PCs indirectly through relay neurons, the granule cells. The latter send out their axons in the molecular layer in the form of parallel fibers (PF) which synapse on the distal part of PC dendritic arbors. Besides the granule cells, there are three other types of interneurons, all inhibitory: the basket cells, which send out terminals around the cell body of PCs, the stellate cells, with terminals synapsing on PC dendrites, and the Golgi cells, which contact the granule cells.

---

* This chapter to be cited as: Gaspar, P. and Sotelo, C., 1990, Embryonic-adult interactions: cellular mechanisms involved in Purkinje cell replacement by neuronal grafting, in: "Systems Approaches to Developmental Neurobiology," P. A. Raymond, S. S. Easter, Jr., and G. M. Innocenti, eds., Plenum Press, New York.

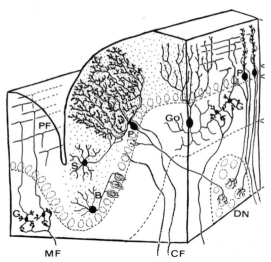

Fig.1. Schematic representation of the cerebellar circuitry in perspective. The front plane is sagittal and the vanishing plane is frontal (see text for comment). **B**, basket cells; **CF**, climbing fibers; **DN**, deep nuclei; **G**, granule cells; **Go**, golgi cell; **P**, Purkinje cell; **PF**, parallel fibers; **S**, stellate cell.

CEREBELLAR GRAFTS

The Model

By placing embryonic tissue in an adult host cerebellum, we can investigate the way in which these two tissues interact. Will the embryonic neurons mature at their normal pace or will they be influenced by the contact with an adult environment? Will the adult host react to the presence of embryonic tissue by reexpressing some of its transient developmental features? Ultimately the question is whether the grafted neurons will become integrated into the wiring diagram of the adult cerebellum, that is, will they form the proper connections with the appropriate partner cells?

This issue was examined using as hosts animals with lesions of the cerebellum. Most of our work has been done with a spontaneous cerebellar lesion, the Purkinje cell degeneration (PCD) mutation in mice. In these mutants, the PCs start to die by the second postnatal week, after having established all their connections. Eventually, they completely disappear by the 45th postnatal day, while the other neuronal elements of the cerebellar circuit are basically unchanged. Embryonic cerebellar tissue was taken from the cerebellar anlage of E12 normal mice, that is, at the peak of the proliferative period for PCs. Tissue fragments or cell suspensions were grafted into the PC-free cerebellar cortex of 2-months-old PCD mice. The fate of the grafted PCs could be followed with calbindin immunostaining (and other cell specific markers of PCs). Calbindin antibodies stain the entire extent of the PC, and the staining is quite selective for PCs within the cerebellar cortex.

Long-Term Replacement of the Missing Circuitry

In order to replace the missing PCs of the host, the grafted cells would need to meet three requirements: 1) migrate out of the graft into the the host tissue; 2) grow adequate dendritic arbors, thereby allowing the principal afferences to sprout and re-establish synaptic connections at the right places; and 3) grow an efferent axon to re-establish the cerebellar output. These issues were examined in animals that survived 2 months after grafting (Sotelo and Alvarado-Mallart, 1986, 1987).

Neuronal migration of the grafted PC does occur. Grafted neurons could be seen at distances as far as 700 μm away from the graft in the molecular layer of the host cerebellum (Fig. 2). However, the spatial organization differed from that of normal adults: the PCs did not form a typical monolayer, but instead invaded the entire width of the molecular layer in abnormal positions. PCs never intruded into the granular layer, however, which is therefore presumably a less permissive environment.

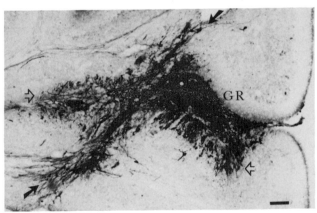

Fig. 2. Cerebellum of a PCD mouse 2 months after transplantation of embryonic cerebellar fragments. PCs are immunolabeled with calbindin antibody. Note the absence of labeled cells from the host. From the labeled remnant graft (**GR**) the principal migratory streams can be noted: along the pipette track (filled arrows); laterally spreading away from the graft remnant, and radially within the host's molecular layer (open arrows). Bar: 66 µm.

When compared to other grafting systems that have been described in the adult mammalian CNS, this migration of PCs is a quite unusual feature. Furthermore, the apparent specificity of the migration, which only involved PCs, raises a number of unresolved questions. What force could specifically drive these cells and no others out of the graft? Are there any trophic factors provided by the host? Another possibility is that because the mutant host cerebellum lacks PCs, only PCs in the graft are free of competitive interactions with host neurons of like class, and thereby move out to colonize the empty territory. In support of this notion is the observation that similar grafts made into normal mice hosts resulted in almost no observable migration of the PCs, except in places where the host tissue had been destroyed by the pipette track or by kainic acid lesion (Armengol et al., 1989).

The dendritic outgrowth of the grafted PCs follows a normal pattern. By 2 months after grafting, the PCs had a fairly normal dendritic tree in which both proximal and distal segments could be identified. Furthermore, despite their rather abnormal positions, their dendritic arbors tended to remain constrained within the sagittal plane, as would be the case normally. This arrangement may be important for the connections between PC dendrites and their afferents to become properly established.

The question then arises as to whether these PCs receive any synaptic input from the host, either direct olivo-cerebellar climbing fibers or indirect spino-cerebellar fibers. This question was approached with electrophysiological methods in a collaborative study with Francis Crepel et al. in Orsay (Gardette et al., 1988). Using an *in vitro* slice preparation and intracellular recordings of the grafted PCs, it was demonstrated that the large majority of the impaled cells were responsive to electrical stimulation of the underlying white matter. The response properties recorded in PCs allow one to distinguish between simple spikes (corresponding to the monosynaptic input of CF), complex spikes (corresponding to the disynaptic input of mossy fibers), as well as later inhibitory responses (due to a postsynaptic inhibition by stellate and basket cells). All of these responses were recorded from the grafted PCs. Therefore, one can assume that synapses have been established between the host and the graft. This has been further corroborated in ultrastructural studies (Sotelo et al., 1984, 1986).

Grafted PC axons sometimes grow out of the cerebellar cortex to reach their principal target, the host's deep cerebellar nuclei. This last connection is apparently the most difficult for the grafted neurons to achieve. We observed it in only a limited number of cases, and only when the graft was close enough to the deep nulcei (the critical distance was 600 µm). Even then, the density of PC terminal arborization was much lower than in a normal cerebellum.

There are several reasons why we might expect the output connections to be difficult to make. One reason is that oriented axonal outgrowth must occur in a cellular context which is intermediate between a developing and a regenerating system. The growing axons will encounter many of the obstacles of the latter situation, namely the absence of guiding cues and perhaps the presence of a non-permissive substratum formed by adult CNS myelin. Another limiting factor may be a competition for PC axons between the deep nuclei of the host and residual neurons in the deep nuclei of the graft which are often present. The latter, being at a developmental stage parallel to that of the grafted PCs, may be a more favorable target. Indeed, the majority of grafted PC axons are directed toward the deep nuclear neurons of the graft remnant, and only a small minority find their way to the host's deep nuclei.

The scarcity of this output connection is obviously a limiting factor for a complete integration of the grafted PC in the mutant cerebellar circuitries. Does this mean that recovery of function, that is reduction of the motor deficits presented by these mutant mice, would therefore be expected to be minor?

We have not examined this issue specifically with any behavioral tasks. Furthermore, the possibility that some aberrant connections may be formed by the grafted PCs cannot be discarded. For example, the PC axons form aberrant plexuses in the host's molecular layer, which could mediate the direct inhibitory interconnections between PCs. Another example is the absence of pericellular basket fibers around the grafted cells; the empty baskets of the host seem to be unreactive to the presence of embryonic tissue. There are also a few ectopic synapses, that is, afferents improperly segregated on the PC dendritic tree, but there are never any heterologous synapses, that is, synapses between cell categories which would not normally be connected to each other (e.g. mossy fibers and PC).

Maturation of Cerebellar Grafts-Comparison with Normal Development

The relatively coherent integration of the grafted PCs into the cerebellum of adult mutant mice led Sotelo and co-workers to suggest that the grafted neurons may recapitulate all their normal ontogenic steps, even though they are placed in an abnormal adult environment. To examine this, the principal developmental events in grafts and during normal development were compared (Sotelo et al., 1987b). In doing this comparison one must bear in mind that the first day post-graft (DPG) corresponds to the 13th embryonic day. The period of 3 to 21 DPG which was examined therefore corresponds to the E16-P14 period in normal development.

The time window of PC cell proliferation, which is normally 90 hours, is not modified by the grafting procedure even though the cell manipulations involved are done at the peak of the proliferative period and may, *a priori*, have disrupted this timing.

Two migratory streams from graft to host were observed, one tangential and the other radial (Fig. 2). Only the latter axis is reminiscent of migration occurring during normal cerebellar development. The tangential axis of migration is unique to the graft. Migrating cells originate from the main body of the graft, at the graft-host interface. At 4 to 5 days after grafting, immature cells stream tangentially from the periphery of the graft into the host's cerebellar cortex, between the pial surface and the parenchyma. They extend up to 700 μm, forming a multiple layer proximally , and thinning down to a single row of cells distally. The second, radial migratory pathway originates either from the lateral extensions which form around the graft or from the subpial location, where the first migratory route had brought them. In the first case, the PCs move down into the host's molecular layer through broken patches of the basal lamina. A tentative interpretation for this is that the PC growth cones release some proteolytic enzyme, as has been shown in other systems *in vitro* (Krystosek and Seeds, 1981). Then, whatever their previous route, PCs invade the molecular layer by sending inwardly oriented processes. In both cases, the cells are radially polarized, with a long leading process which reaches down to the granular layer, where it stops.

A potential radial substrate in the molecular layer could be provided by the Bergmann glial fibers, which are present in the adult cerebellar cortex and are particularly abundant in the mutant. Indeed, direct appositions of migrating PC and glial fibers were occasionally observed. This migratory path is rather similar to that which is observed during development, where the immature PC migrate radially, probably along the radial glia. However, the direction of migration is inverted (upwards in normal development).

The 3 phases of dendritic maturation described for PCs during development can also be observed in the grafts: i) fusiform cell phase (when PCs are migrating); ii) stellate cell phase with disoriented dendrites; iii) flattening of the dendritic arbor with profuse branching. The timing of these developmental features does not seem to be modified for the embryonic PCs placed in an adult environment.

In normal development, the synaptic investment of the PC cell body and dendritic tree with axon terminals is time-locked with the maturation of its dendritic tree. Climbing fibers (CF) arrive first, moving up from the cell body (PC phase 2) to the primary dendrites, which are then invested with parallel fibers (PC phase 3), and finally the formation of contacts with the basket and stellate cells occurs (Larramendi, 1968).

What happens in the graft? During the migratory phase of fusiform cells, hardly any synapses are observed, as would be the case in normal development. Synaptogenesis starts 10 to 11 DPG (PC cell phase 2), following the normal developmental timing. However, the pattern is different for the grafted cells in that synaptogenesis for CF occurs now almost simultaneously with synaptogenesis from basket cells and from parallel fibers. An explanation for this discrepancy would be that, at similar developmental stages, the normal developing PCs will find only the CF, whereas the grafted PCs will find all the different categories of axons already present in the adult molecular layer. Nevertheless , after a phase of very active synaptogenesis, the typical segregation of these synapses on the different segments of the PC ultimately occurs also in the grafts.

The refinement of the climbing fiber projection is thought to occur through a selective elimination of some of the CF synapses. The evidence here is mainly electrophysiological (Crepel et al., 1976). Analysis of PC cell responses after stimulation of the underlying white matter have led to the suggestion that there is a transient multiple innervation by CF during development. Indeed, the excitatory postsynaptic potentials of PC are not all-or-none, as in the adult cerebellum, but fluctuate, in a stepwise manner, with the intensity of the stimulation. The progression of this multiple innervation is very characteristic: it starts at P3 with the synaptogenesis of CF, peaks at P5 , and decreases sharply from P6 to P12 when all PCs become monoinnervated.

Electrophysiological analysis on the grafted cells, similarly revealed a phase of transient multiple innervation 10 to 13 days after grafting. However, the time window of this phenomenon was much reduced when compared to normal development. All PCs were singly innervated by 14 days after transplantation. This may be related to the considerations raised previously, that CF and PF are established together and that the competition between these 2 inputs plays a role in the regression of this multiple innervation.

Direct anatomical demonstration of the transient multi-innervation is still lacking, but its persistence in adults has been shown in experimental situations where the granular cells are destroyed early, thereby eliminating the competition of CF with parallel fibers (Sotelo et al., 1981).

These observations suggest that the transplanted embryonic cells have recapitulated their normal phases of development with approximately normal timing. The fact that these cells were able to form many of the appropriate connections with the host suggests that the embryonic transplant has recreated a favorable microenvironment for synaptogenesis.

FORMATION OF PROJECTION MAPS

Despite its rather monotonous, uniform appearance in classical histological preparations, the cerebellum is characterized by a functional heterogeneity which becomes obvious when one examines more closely its connections and microchemical structure. There is a zonal organization mainly related to the distribution of inputs and outputs. For example, the two principal cerebellar afferents, the olivo-cerebellar and the spino-cerebellar systems, are both characterized by a very specific regional pattern of termination, organized as discrete longitudinal bands. Inside these bands, the projections are further organized with a precise somatotopic order and in a point-to-point manner, at least for the olivo-cerebellar system (Sotelo et al., 1984). How is this topographic organization assembled ? What parameters could guide the formation of these maps? One suggestion supported by some evidence is that the chemical heterogeneity of the PCs themselves provides recognition cues for the different afferent inputs.

Formation of Topographical Projections to the Cerebellar Cortex does not Require Synaptogenesis

A converse notion would be that synaptogenesis could in some way determine the formation of a patterned cerebellar projection. For example, a widespread, nonspecific projection could later be refined by a selective process of regression of some connections and validation of others. However,

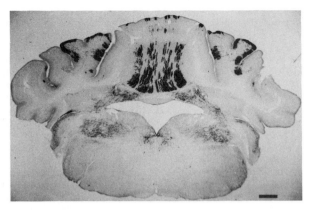

Fig. 3. Calbindin immunostaining of a cerebellum of a *nervous* mutant mouse: the remaining PCs appear as darkly staining bands. Their distribution delimits a radial zonation, symmetrically distributed with respect to the midline. Bar: 500 μm

this view is not supported by observations in the rat, since the topographical pattern of the main projections is already formed during the perinatal period (Arsenio-Nunes and Sotelo, 1984, Sotelo et al., 1984), although the cerebellar cortex is quite immature at that stage and contains few synapses. Thus the olivo-cerebellar projectional map is organized in its definitive pattern with a clear banding organization at birth, 2 days before the beginning of synaptogenesis (Sotelo et al., 1984).

The development of the spino-cerebellar projection occurs with a slower time course, however (Arsenio-Nunes and Sotelo, 1984). During the first stage (P1) the afferent fibers underlie the grey matter, waiting below their proper field of termination (in the anterior vermis); later on (P3) they penetrate the cerebellar cortex, and they form a protocolumnar arrangement of fibers; and finally, they achieve their definitive adult columnar pattern of termination, simultaneously with the onset of mossy fiber synaptogenesis. To evaluate the possible role of their targets, the granule cells, Leonor Arsenio-Nunes investigated different agranular cerebellar mutants (Arsenio-Nunes et al., 1988). In the *weaver* mutation, where granular cells are affected primarily, no modification of this projection was observed. Similar observations were made after early destruction of the granular cells with X-ray irradiation. On the other hand, in the *staggerer* mutation, where the lesion of granular cells is secondary to a primary defect of PCs, the spinocerebellar map was never properly established (Arsenio-Nunes et al. 1988). These observations indicate that the target of the spinocerebellar projection, the granule cell, is not an essential element for the establishment of its topographical organization. PCs instead could be the organizing elements of this projection.

Transient PC Heterogeneity During Perinatal Development

Among the many antigens (proteins such as calbindin or Purkinje cell specific glycoproteins) which can be used as markers of PC, several have been noticed to have peculiar developmental patterns. That is, although they are expressed in all adult PCs they do do not appear simultaneously in all PCs during development (Wassef et al., 1985, 1989a). This heterogeneity becomes visible soon after PC migration. Furthermore the cell clusters delimited with the markers are usually non-overlapping (Wassef et al., 1985). This observation carries two implications. First, the heterogeneous expression of these antigens does not reflect different maturational stages among PCs. Second, the number of functional compartments which may thus be defined is considerably increased. Indeed a PC compartment could be tagged by the combination of several antigens (e.g. for 3 hypothetical markers A, B, C there would be 8 possible combinations, A+B+C+,A+B-C+, etc...).

These basic PC compartments, as defined by the expression of different antigens, appear in definite topographical locations at a given age. Therefore they provide a reproducible map for the incoming projections. In addition, the boundary between PC compartments could be used in the generation of gradients of positional information, according to the scheme proposed by Meinhardt (1983) (see Wassef et al., 1989a,b, for more ample discussion of this point).

What is the relationship between the PC -clusters and PC birth dates?

This is an important issue. Preliminary data (M.Wassef) indicate that such a relationship exists. However one PC cluster is not derived from a single cell clone, as indicated by the work of Mullen (Mullen, 1977) on PCD chimaeric mice.

Purkinje cell heterogeneity in the adult cerebellum. Can one find any remnants of this primitive compartmentation in adults? Two sets of data suggest that one can. First, in cerebellar mutations of the mouse, with various degrees of PC loss (*nervous*, PCD, *tambaleante*), the pattern of cell loss is characteristic : PCs are lost by clusters, in precise, reproducible topographical locations, outlining a zonal organization of surviving cells (Wassef et al., 1987) (Fig.3). Second, a few monoclonal antibodies, such as SAC1 (obtained by P.Streit) or Q113 (obtained by R.Hawkes) (Hawkes and Leclerc, 1987), both of which seem to label cell surface glycoproteins, stain only particular subpopulations of adult PCs, and delimit antero-posterior bands.

This chemical compartmentation does not seem to be determined by the arrival of afferent fibers since it is still visible in heterotopic transplantations of the cerebellum where none of the afferences are made (Wassef et al., 1989b). On the other hand, some recent tracing studies in the adult rat indicate that the projection fields of individual sectors of the olivo-cerebellar pathway, may conform to the histochemically distinct compartments (Wassef et al., 1989a, b).

This set of observations suggests that the chemical heterogeneity of PCs (whether transient or permanent) is expressed as part of an intrinsic developmental program. This heterogeneity could be sufficient to build a topographic map and could be utilized by the incoming afferences to organize their precise projectional map. The latter proposition must be explored in further experiments.

ACKNOWLEDGEMENTS

R.M. Alvarado-Mallart and Marion Wassef contributed substantially to the work described here.

REFERENCES

Arsenio-Nunes, M.L., and Sotelo, C., 1985, Development of the spinocerebellar system in the postnatal rat, *J.Comp. Neurol.*, 237::291.

Arsenio-Nunes, M.L., Sotelo, C., and Wehrle, R., 1988, Organization of spinocerebellar projection map in three types of agranular cerebellum: Purkinje cell Vs. granule cell as the organizer element, *J.Comp. Neurol.*, 273:120.

Armengol, J. A., Sotelo, C., Angaut, P., and Alvarado-Mallart, R. M., 1989, Organization of host afferents to cerebellar grafts implanted into kainate lesioned cerebellum in adult rats. Hodological evidence for the specificity of host-graft interactions, *Eur. J. Neurosci.*, 1:75.

Cajal, S.R., 1889, Sur l'origine et la direction des prolongations nerveuses de la couche moléculaire du cervelet, *Aus der Int. Monatsschrift. Anat. Phys. VI, Heft.*, 4:1.

Crepel, F., Mariani, J., and Delhaye-Bouchaüd, N., 1976, Evidence for a multiple innervation of Purkinje cells by climbing fibers in the immature rat cerebellum, *J.Neurobiol.*, 7:567.

Gardette, R., Alvarado-Mallart, R.M., Crepel, F., and Sotelo, C., 1988, Electrophysiological demonstration of a synaptic integration of transplanted Purkinje cells into the cerebellum of the adult Purkinje Cell Degeneration mutant mouse, *Neuroscience*, 24:777.

Hawkes, R., and Leclerc, N., 1987, Antigenic map of the rat cerebellar cortex: the distribution of parasagittal bands as revealed by a monoclonal anti-Purkinje cell antibody mab Q113, *J.Comp.Neurol.*, 256:29.

Krystosek, A., and Seeds, W., 1981, Plasminogen activator secretion by granule neurons in cultures of developing cerebellum, *Proc. Natl. Acad. Sci. USA*, 78:7810.

Larramendi, L.M.H., 1969, Analysis of synaptogenesis in the cerebellum of the mouse, in: "Neurobiology of Cerebellar Evolution and Development," R.Llinas, ed., American Medical Association, Chicago, pp.803.

Meinhardt, H., 1983, Cell determination boundaries as organizing regions for secondary embryonic fields, *Dev. Biol.*, 96:375.

Mullen, R.J., 1977, Site of *pcd* gene action and Purkinje cell mosaicism in cerebella of chimaeric mice, *Nature,* 270:245.

Sotelo, C., 1981, Development of synaptic connections in genetic and experimentally induced cerebellar malformations, in: "Development in the Central Nervous System", D.R. Garrod and J.D. Feldman, eds., Cambridge University Press, Cambridge, pp.61.

Sotelo, C., Bourrat, F., and Triller, A., 1984, Postnatal development of the inferior olivary complex in the rat. II. Topographic organization of the immature olivocerebellar projection, *J.Comp. Neurol.,* 222:177.

Sotelo, C., and Alvarado-Mallart, R.M., 1986, Growth and differentiation of cerebellar suspensions transplanted into the adult cerebellum of mice with heredo-degenerative ataxia, *Proc.Natl.Acad.Sci. USA,* 83:1135.

Sotelo, C., and Alvarado-Mallart, R.M., 1987a, Reconstruction of the defective cerebellar circuitry in adult Purkinje cell degeneration mutant mice by Purkinje cell replacement through transplantation of solid embryonic grafts, *Neuroscience,* 20:1.

Sotelo, C., and Alvarado-Mallart, R.M., 1987b, Embryonic and adult neurons interact to allow Purkinje cell replacement in mutant cerebellum, *Nature,* 327:421.

Wassef, M., Zanetta, J.P., Brehier, A., and Sotelo, C., 1985, Transient biochemical compartmentalization of Purkinje cells during early cerebellar development, *Dev. Biol.,*111:129.

Wassef, M., Sotelo, C., Cholley, B., Brehier, A., and Thomasset, M., 1987, Cerebellar mutations affecting the postnatal survival of Purkinje cells in the mouse disclose a longitudinal pattern of differentially sensitive cells, *Dev. Biol.,* 124 :379.

Wassef, M., Angaut, P., Arsenio-Nunes, L., Bourrat, F., and Sotelo, C., 1989a, Purkinje cell heterogeneity: its role in organizing the topography of the cerebellar cortex connections, in: "Neurobiology of the cerebellar systems," R.Llinas and C.Sotelo, eds., Oxford University Press, New York (in press).

Wassef, M., Sotelo, C , Thomasset, M., Granholm, A. C., Leclerc, N., Rafrafi, J., and Hawkes, R., 1989b, Expression of compartmentation antigens in cerebellar transplants, *J. Comp. Neurol.* (in press).

THE REGULATION OF NEURONAL MORPHOLOGY AND INNERVATION IN DEVELOPING AND ADULT ANIMALS: ANATOMICAL, PHYSIOLOGICAL AND *IN VIVO* OBSERVATIONS [*]

Anthony-Samuel LaMantia (scribe), Dale Purves (lecturer)

Department of Anatomy and Neurobiology
Washington University School of Medicine
St. Louis, MO, USA

INTRODUCTION

This chapter summarizes two related but distinct lines of investigation carried out by Dale Purves and his colleagues over the past several years: the first deals with the ways in which a neuron's morphology and innervation are regulated by the neuron's target, and the second deals with the development of methods by which neuronal morphology and connectivity can be monitored in living animals.

Studies of the influence of targets on neuronal morphology and connectivity both during development and in adulthood, provide insight into the ways in which the structural and functional demands of an individual animal's body regulate the organization of the nervous system. The experiments summarized here address these issues in the mammalian sympathetic pathway, a relatively simple and accessible part of the peripheral nervous system. The results indicate that trophic interactions between neurons and their targets play an important role in the determination of convergence and divergence in neural pathways by modulating the complexity of postsynaptic dendrites and the numbers of axons that innervate them.

This modulation of neuronal morphology and innervation may continue over an animal's entire lifetime. Ongoing adjustments in neural organization require that individual neurons possess some capacity for modifying their shape and connections. Visualization of neurons in living animals over weeks or months enables one to assess directly the amount of change that individual neurons or groups of neurons undergo during the course of a lifetime. These techniques have been applied to both the peripheral and central nervous systems to show that individual elements in the living nervous system can change throughout life.

THE REGULATION OF NEURONAL MORPHOLOGY AND CONNECTIVITY IN THE AUTONOMIC NERVOUS SYSTEM

The Relationship Between Neuronal Morphology and Animal Size

For years neurobiologists have noted a correlation between the size of an animal and the size and complexity of its nervous system; however, the potential significance of this relationship has been

---

[*] This chapter is to be cited as: LaMantia, A.-S., 1990, The regulation of neuronal morphology and innervation in developing and adult animals: anatomical, physiological and *in vivo* observations, in: "Systems Approaches to Developmental Neurobiology," P. A. Raymond, S.S. Easter, Jr., and G.M. Innocenti, eds., Plenum Press, New York.

largely ignored (for review see Purves, 1988). It seems sensible to ask whether or not this relationship reflects interactions between neurons and the targets they serve, and what are anatomical and physiological consequences of these interactions? One important consequence may be the modulation of convergence and divergence in neuronal pathways. Convergence and divergence represent, respectively, the number of axons which innervate a particular target neuron, and the number of targets which any particular neuron innervates. These two properties influence the ways in which neural systems relay and process information.

The regulation of neuronal complexity and innervation appears to depend upon competition for trophic support from the target (Purves and Lichtman, 1980; Purves et al.,1988). These trophic interactions reflect the interdependent relationships between neurons and the cells that they innervate, which may be either other neurons or non-neuronal cells such as muscles or glands. Trophic effects may be evident over days, weeks, months or an entire lifetime. These sorts of interactions were originally proposed to regulate the numbers of neurons innervating a particular target; however, they may also play a role in regulating the pattern and arrangement of individual dendritic and axonal arbors as well as the synaptic connections they make (for review, see Purves et al., 1988).

The relationship between neuronal size and complexity and target size is evident in comparisons of the dendritic complexity, afferent innervation and tonic activity of homologous autonomic neurons from different species which vary widely in size. These comparisons have been made primarily between neurons of the superior cervical ganglion, a collection of sympathetic autonomic neurons which are innervated by preganglionic axons from intermediolateral motor column of the spinal cord. The superior cervical ganglion cells in turn innervate a variety of peripheral targets. If one compares cell size, dendritic complexity and the number of axons of superior cervical ganglion neurons from mammalian species of different sizes, a systematic relationship can be seen (Fig. 1). In a small mammal like the mouse, each superior cervical ganglion cell has only a few primary dendrites (Purves and Lichtman, 1985), is innervated by relatively few preganglionic axons (Purves et al., 1986) and has a low rate of ongoing synaptically driven spontaneous activity (Ivanov and Purves, 1989). In contrast, in rabbits, which are approximately 100 times larger than mice, individual superior cervical ganglion cells are larger, have many more primary and secondary dendrites, are innervated by more preganglionic axons, and have a higher rate of activity. In animals of intermediate size--for example the hamster, the rat, and the guinea pig--the size, morphology and tonic activity of superior cervical ganglion cells also vary according to this general rule (Purves et al., 1986). Thus morphological complexity, synaptic organization and physiological function all vary with animal size. This correlation implies that neurons can adapt to the targets they innervate, and that the adaptation is reflected in both the anatomy and physiology of the system. It is likely that the ability of the system to process information varies as well, since one result of the relationship between animal size and neuronal complexity is a change in the amount of convergence and divergence. These adaptations occur primarily during development; however ongoing adjustments may also be made throughout an animal's lifetime. The adjustments may provide a means by which the organization of the nervous system is matched to the changing size and functional demands of an animal's body.

Studies of the development of parasympathetic autonomic ganglion cells that have no dendrites, either at birth or in maturity, show that these neurons are multiply innervated early in postnatal development and subsequently come to be singly innervated by a process of input elimination (Lichtman,1977; Hume and Purves, 1981). This phenomenon suggests that preganglionic axons compete with each other and that one outcome of this process determines the number of afferent axons that innervate each target neuron. The object of this competition may be trophic factors provided by the target neurons. The relatively small size of these cells without dendrites may limit the amount of trophic support available, thus limiting the number of axons which are eventually related to each cell.

In contrast, in the rabbit ciliary ganglion (a sympathetic autonomic ganglion that innervates the iris of the eye) the ganglion cells have from one to ten primary dendrites at birth (Fig. 2). Initially, ciliary neurons with few or no primary dendrites are innervated by as many as 7 different axons, as are those with several primary dendrites. In adults, however, the innervation of ciliary ganglion cells is correlated with the number of primary dendrites and the overall degree of dendritic complexity (Hume and Purves,1981; Purves and Hume, 1981): neurons with few or no dendrites are innervated by one or two axons, while those with several primary dendrites and multiple second order branches are innervated by up to 7 axons. Apparently the number of axons that finally innervate an individual neuron over the course of postnatal development depends largely on the dendritic complexity of the neuron.   During development in the ciliary ganglion,   cells with more dendrites can be considered a larger target, capable of providing sufficient trophic support for multiple preganglionic axons. The size of these targets, the ciliary ganglion cells, is controlled in turn by the size of their peripheral targets and the ability of these targets to provide trophic support. These observations suggest that

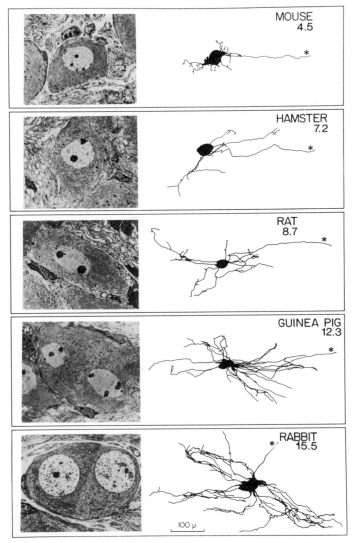

Fig. 1. Systematic variation of cell size and dendritic complexity in superior cervical ganglion (SCG) cells from five different mammalian species. The cell have been labeled by intracellular injection of horseradish peroxidase following intracellular recording to determine the number of inputs. The correlation between cell soma size, number and complexity of primary and secondary dendrites and animal size is readily apparent in the series of electron micrographs and camera lucida drawings of representative superior cervical ganglion cells examined in mice, hamsters, rats, guinea pigs and rabbits. The number in the lower right hand corner of each panel is the mean number of preganglionic axons which innervate SCG cells in each species. This number is determined by measuring the stepwise increments in postsynaptic response elicited by increasing stimulation of the preganglionic nerve. (Adapted from Purves et al., 1986.)

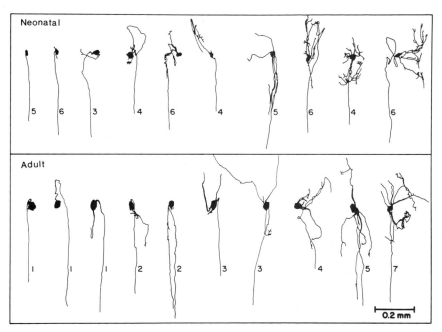

Fig. 2. Dendritic complexity and preganglionic innervation in neonatal and adult rabbit ciliary ganglia. A) Ciliary ganglion cells appear immature at birth, however, a full range of dendritic complexities can be distinguished. In contrast, the number of innervating axons(numbers to the right of each axon) is approximately 5 at birth regardless of dendritic complexity. B) In the adult, the extent of dendritic complexity still varies widely; however, the number of innervating axons varies in register with the dendritic complexity. (Adapted from Hume and Purves, 1981; Purves and Hume, 1981.)

neurons are sensitive to the amount of target derived trophic support available at several levels in the autonomic pathway--thus the direction of trophic interactions from target to innervating neuron may be reiterated at several levels of the autonomic motor pathway.

The nature of trophic interactions in the autonomic pathhways can be assessed in greater detail by performing four different types of experiments. First, the influence of preganglionic axons on the elaboration of dendritic morphology of autonomic neurons can be examined by cutting the axons early in development (Voyvodic, 1987): ganglion cells that develop in the absence of preganglionic innervation are similar in size to normal cells, and have similar numbers of primary dendrites. Second, the importance of the target for the maintenance of normal ganglion cell morphology can be demonstrated by cutting the post ganglionic axons in order to deprive the neurons of their trophic support (Yawo, 1987): the dendritic complexity of axotomized ganglion cells is greatly reduced. Apparently the targets, rather than innervating axons, play a primary role in the determination and maintenance of dendritic morphology and connectivity in this system. Third, the size of the peripheral target of developing autonomic neurons can be manipulated at birth (Voyvodic,1989). These studies demonstrate that there is a robust correspondence between target size and dendritic complexity (Fig. 3A): larger targets result in larger and more extensive dendritic arborizations while smaller targets result in smaller dendritic arborizations. These effects are not influenced by preganglionic axons since similar results are seen after denervation of the ganglion (Voyvodic, 1989). Finally, nerve growth factor (NGF), a trophic factor known to be supplied to autonomic neurons by their targets, can be administered systemically during postnatal development, presumably increasing the amount of this factor available to the autonomic neurons (Snider, 1988). In animals treated with NGF, the size and complexity of autonomic ganglion cell dendritic arborizations is greatly enhanced during the course of postnatal development (Fig. 3B), implying that the amount of this trophic factor available influences neuronal morphology in addition to neuronal survival. Together, these four experiments demonstrate that target-mediated trophic interactions have a profound influence on the size and complexity of sympathetic neurons.

All of these observations are consistent with the conclusion that trophic interactions between a neuron and its target play a primary role in determining the number and distribution of connections that neuron will eventually make over the course of development. These factors, which influence the amount of convergence and divergence in the pathway, will necessarily influence the way in which information is relayed and processed, thus modulating the functional capacity of the system. Positive evidence for target control of dendritic morphology in the autonomic nervous system, along with negative evidence for the lack of a role for innervating axons, suggests that in this motor pathway

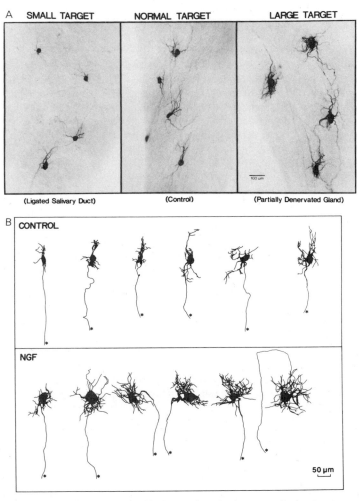

Fig 3. Experimental demonstrations of trophic interactions in the sympathetic nervous system. A) The effect of manipulating target size on the dendritic morphology of SCG cells. In animals in which relative target size was increased by eliminating all but one of the post-ganglionic nerves innervating the salivary gland, dendritic complexity is dramatically increased. In animals where the target is decreased in size by ligating the salivary duct, dendritic complexity is dramatically decreased (adapted from Voyvodic, 1989). B) The effect of systemic administration of NGF on dendritic morphology of SCG cells. NGF was administered to newborn rats by subcutaneous injection, and this procedure was repeated daily in the same rats for two weeks. The soma size, number of primary dendrites, and extent of dendritic arborization were all dramatically increased in the NGF-treated animals. (Adapted from Snider, 1988.)

103

trophic regulation of neuronal connections may be polarized from periphery to target. This polarity would provide an animal with an effective way of matching the neuronal apparatus to move its body with the size and form of the body to be moved. An opposite polarity might be expected for sensory systems, where the influence of afferents from peripheral sensory receptors might modulate the complexity of central neuronal targets in order to accommodate expanding sensory surfaces or changing functional demands.

The observations in the ciliary ganglion suggest that the range of dendritic complexity at birth is great enough to account for varying degrees of convergence. What then is the significance of the trophic and competitive interactions which happen after birth? Are they at all responsible for controlling the number of primary dendrites?

The interpretation of the data from the ciliary ganglion depends in part on the definition of dendritic complexity. While there is a full range of primary dendrites at birth, the numbers and complexity of secondary dendrites continues to increase systematically. This target-controlled aspect of dendritic complexity may influence the establishment of adult numbers of synapses made by innervating axons. The number of primary dendrites is important in determining the amount of convergence; however, the elaboration of secondary dendrites may provide increased trophic support for additional synapses made by the innervating axons. The processes which determine the numbers of primary dendrites on sympathetic neurons are not known: this aspect of the initial differentiation of sympathetic neurons may depend equally upon intrinsic properties of the cells and early trophic influence from the diverse targets that they innervate.

Are similar trophic effects on dendritic morphology or numbers of innervating axons seen in the spinal motor neurons which innervate the autonomic ganglia, and to what extent can the propagation of trophic interactions account for the development of neuronal morphology and synaptic organization in other peripheral and central pathways?

At present, there is little available information which addresses these questions directly. For example, the number and complexity of innervation of spinal motor neurons versus autonomic neurons makes comparisons between the first and second level of the sympathetic motor pathway difficult. Within the spinal cord, target-mediated trophic interactions may not be the only influence on neuronal morphology. Innervating axons may also play a role, raising the possibility of axonally released trophic factors as well as target-derived trophic factors. The balance between these two forms of trophic influence may be shifted in favor of the target in motor systems where sensitivity to the size and state of the periphery is important, and in favor of innervating axons in sensory systems, where the number, complexity, and activity of inputs from the sensory receptors require adjustments within the target.

To summarize up to this point, correlations between target size and neuronal complexity reflect trophic interactions between neurons and their targets. These interactions operate both during development and in adulthood to coordinate neural architecture with changes in the size and function of an animal. One important aspect of these interactions is the modulation of convergence and divergence, which has important functional consequences. The correlation of neuronal size, complexity and innervation with animal size provides initial evidence in support of this conclusion. Studies of the development of preganglionic innervation of autonomic neurons with varying degrees of dendritic complexity indicate that the final correspondence between the number of innervating axons and the number of dendritic branches may be accomplished by eliminating inputs in accord with the size and structure of the target. In contrast, neither the initial nor the final dendritic complexity seems to depend on the presence of innervating axons throughout development. These observations suggest that in motor systems trophic interactions from target to innervating neuron may be reiterated at several levels of the pathway so that at each level the dendritic complexity of the relevant neurons is controlled by the amount of trophic support available in the target. In the autonomic nervous system, the target-mediated trophic interactions that result in the modulation of dendritic complexity during development are related to the absolute size of the target, which presumably reflects the amount of target derived trophic factors available. When neurons are confronted with a larger target, cell size and dendritic complexity increases, regardless of the presence or absence of innervating axons. These effects can be reproduced in part by increased circulating levels of NGF, a trophic substance released by the targets of sympathetic neurons. These observations are consistent with the conclusion that neurons compete with one another for finite amounts of target-derived trophic support and that their competition influences their structure and connectivity.

There seem to be several different meanings for the term "competition," is it possible to define this term more precisely?

In defining neuronal competition it is important to identify an object for that competition. Simple geometric notions such as "target space" are certainly insufficient for a detailed understanding of the phenomenon. For cell survival, competition can be defined as cells competing for a limited resource such as NGF or some other nutritive or survival factor. Similarly, for axonal competition, axons may compete for a limited resource like target derived trophic factors, specific postsynaptic receptors, or cell adhesion and other cell surface recognition molecules. In either case, the essential feature is a well defined object of competition, presumably molecular, that is available in limited quantities. The acquisition of this object of competition in turn provides feedback to the competitors.

OBSERVING NEURAL ARCHITECTURE IN INDIVIDUAL LIVING ANIMALS OVER TIME

Dendritic and Synaptic Remodelling in the Peripheral Nervous System

Over the past five years it has become possible to observe neural architecture over time in living animals using a combination of vital fluorescent dyes, low-light-level video microscopy and digital image processing (for review see Purves and Voyvodic, 1987; Purves, 1989). The vital fluorescent dyes enable one to add enough contrast to individual neural elements so that they may be distinguished from the surrounding, uncontrasted neuropil. In this way, individual elements can be seen with sufficient resolution. Low-light-level video microscopy allows one to detect and amplify low intensity light signals. This is essential to minimize light-induced damage caused by exposing fluorescently stained living cells to light. Digital image processing facilitates the acquisition and storage of video images by converting them to an array of computer encoded intensities. Images stored in this way may be further enhanced using computational methods which accentuate contrast, emphasize edges, or subtract background information.

Using these techniques one can begin to determine whether or not individual neurons change their dendritic morphology or pattern of innervation during adulthood. When a superior cervical ganglion cell is injected intracellularly with the vital dye 6-carboxyfluorescein (Purves and Hadley, 1985), it is possible to resolve the cell's dendritic arbor using the microscopic imaging techniques described above (see also Fig. 4A). Intracellular recordings show no detectable alterations in the synaptic functions of these cells. After the initial imaging experiment, the animal is allowed to recover and after periods of a few days to several months, the appropriate cell is located using morphological landmarks in the ganglion, reinjected with dye and imaged once again (Purves and Hadley, 1985, Purves et al., 1986). Comparisons of images obtained in this way show that the pattern and size of the smaller dendritic branches of an individual neuron change substantially over time, while the primary dendrites are more stable (Fig. 4B). The net change is toward increasing complexity, although both extension and retraction of dendrites occurs.

The existence of ongoing progressive changes in the postsynaptic dendrites of adult sympathetic ganglion cells suggests that the innervation of these cells might also change. *In vivo* imaging techniques also prove to be useful in addressing this issue, and the results of this line of investigation indicate that synapses are capable of turnover and rearrangement in adult animals (for review see Purves, 1989). This issue was first explored at the mammalian neuromuscular junction. Motor neuron endplates undergo varying degrees of change from minimal (Lichtman et al., 1987) to substantial (Herrera and Banner, 1987; Wigston, 1989), depending on the species and the type of muscle examined. In contrast, mammalian sensory endings appear to undergo rapid remodeling: the pattern of sensory endings in the cornea changes appreciably over periods as short as one day (Harris and Purves, 1989). Thus the arrangement of synapses on non- neuronal targets in the periphery can change over time in adult animals. Experiments to address this issue for synapses on neuronal targets were carried out on neurons of the submandibular salivary duct ganglion. The neurons of this ganglion lack dendrites, and this feature greatly simplifies the mapping and comparison of fluorescently labeled synaptic boutons over time. After an intravenous injection of the vital fluorescent dye 4-Di-1-Asp, one of a family of mitochondrial specific probes which permit the preferential visualization of synaptic endings (Magrassi et al., 1987), the complete pattern of synaptic boutons on identified ganglion cells can be seen. Control experiments using methylene blue, a histological dye which stains preganglionic axon terminals, confirm the anatomical completeness of the *in vivo* imaging method, and intracellular recordings confirm the functional integrity of the synapses. When this procedure is repeated in the same animal after intervals of up to three weeks, significant, but apparently gradual, rearrangement of boutons can be seen (Fig. 4C). The direct observations of dendritic and synaptic remodeling described above indicate that ongoing modulation of neuronal connections can occur after what is usually considered to be the period of "development" has come to an end. This ongoing change may reflect the subtle operation of trophic interactions between neurons and their targets to accommodate the less dramatic, but nonetheless important changes that an adult animal undergoes over days, weeks, months or years. These include changes in size and shape, adaptations to new environments, the acquisition of new behaviors, and learning and memory.

Development of Neuronal Groups in the Central Nervous System

In general, the mammalian brain is thought to be anatomically stable once the process of development ends, even though most animals continue to grow, and their brains continue to increase in size long after the fetal and early postnatal period. One reason for this impression of eventual stability may be the limitation of traditional anatomical techniques employed in individuals of differing ages. The ability to observe changes in individual neural elements over time in the central nervous system may permit new insights into the question of anatomical stability in the mammalian brain. The larger numbers of neurons and increased diversity of connections in the brain, however, make changes in individual neuronal morphology even more difficult to examine than in the peripheral nervous system. In addition, it is not clear that individual dendrites and synaptic boutons are the appropriate units for analyzing changes in neural architecture in the central nervous system. An equally important feature of the mammalian brain is the accumulation of subsets of neurons and the axons that innervate them into neuronal groups or processing units like columns in the visual cortex, whisker barrels in the somatosensory cortex or glomeruli in the olfactory bulb. These neuronal processing units constitute yet another aspect of neural organization whose size, shape, numbers or distribution might change either during development or in adulthood. The prevalence of these units, and their distinct anatomical and functional characteristics, suggests that they may be the currency by which the most important business of the brain is transacted. Surprisingly, little information is

---

Fig 4. A) Diagram of experimental set-up used for in vivo imaging of neural architecture in living animals (see Purves and Voyvodic, 1987; Purves, 1989). B) Dendritic remodeling over periods of three months in SCG cells in the mouse. In these tracings of video images, there are instances of dendritic extension (open arrows) as well as dendritic retraction (closed arrows). The general direction of the changes is toward increased dendritic complexity. C) Synapse rearrangement on the surface of parasympathetic ganglion cells from the submandibular ganglion of the mouse. After a period of three weeks the distribution of synaptic boutons (black dots) has changed dramatically (adapted from Purves et al, 1988). (Adapted from Purves et al., 1986.)

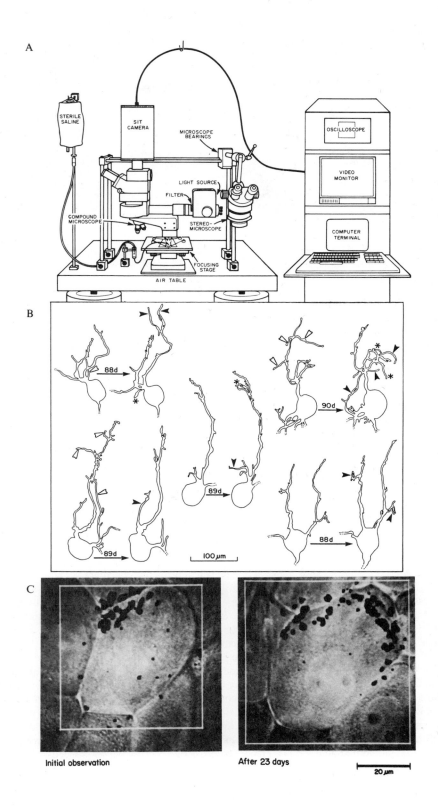

A

STERILE SALINE

SIT CAMERA

MICROSCOPE BEARINGS

LIGHT SOURCE

FILTER

COMPOUND MICROSCOPE

STEREO-MICROSCOPE

FOCUSING STAGE

AIR TABLE

OSCILLOSCOPE

VIDEO MONITOR

COMPUTER TERMINAL

B

88d

*

90d

*

*

89d

89d

100 μm

88d

C

Initial observation

After 23 days

20 μm

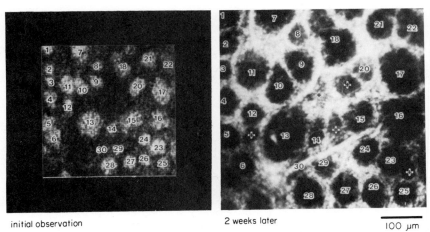

initial observation

2 weeks later

100 µm

Fig. 5. Progressive addition of glomeruli in the olfactory bulb of the developing mouse. The initial image was obtained in an anesthetized three day old mouse pup by exposing the olfactory bulb with the dura intact, staining the bulb with the vital fluorescent dye RH414, and imaging the bulb with a scanning confocal microscope. The final image was obtained when the animal was approximately 3 weeks old, by staining the surface of the bulb with Sudan black after perfusion with aldehyde fixatives. Corresponding glomeruli in the initial and final images are numbered, newly added glomeruli are indicated with "+" signs. Notice that the new glomeruli are intercalated into an existing, stable pattern which persists in spite of addition and growth of glomeruli. (Adapted from LaMantia and Purves, 1989.)

currently available which addresses the ways in which the number and pattern of these processing units is established during development and is maintained in maturity.

A number of observations of central nervous system development suggest that many essential features of central neural architecture arise from primarily regressive processes. Thus adult patterns of connectivity are thought to be sculpted from a surplus of cells, axons, dendrites and synapses (Cowan et al., 1984), and functionally relevant circuits are thought to be selected from redundant or excessive connections both during development and in adulthood (Changeux and Danchin, 1976; Edelman, 1987). There is little to suggest that entirely new neuronal circuits are added progressively as an animal matures, at least for birds and mammals. One difficulty encountered in assessing the addition or elimination of neuronal elements during development is that one can never be entirely sure that the changes detected by comparing different animals at distinct ages represent purely regressive or progressive processes. Conceivably, addition of new neural elements--whether they are dendrites or synapses, or perhaps entire processing units--might continue as an overwhelmingly regressive process was occurring. Following the size, shape and neighbor relations of identified neuronal processing units in a living animal over time might allow one to assess the contribution of progressive and regressive phenomena to the development of the mammalian brain.

The results of *in vivo* observations of the developing olfactory bulb in individual mice (LaMantia and Purves, 1989) demonstrate that glomeruli--the primary neuronal processing units of the bulb--are added progressively throughout a prolonged period of postnatal development. In these experiments the glomeruli were stained through the intact dura with the fluorescent dye RH414 (Grinvald et al., 1984), and imaged with an MRC 500 laser confocal microscope. Histological and electron microscopical examination of olfactory bulbs stained and imaged in this way show no detectable short-or long-term damage to the tissue. Using this technique to observe the same population of glomeruli at two different occasions in the same animal (Fig. 5), LaMantia and Purves have determined that glomerular addition is a gradual, constructive process which proceeds without the elimination of existing units. Thus the net addition of glomeruli, whose rate and magnitude can be estimated by counting in standard histological sections (Pomeroy et al., 1989), is a purely progressive process; there is no hidden regressive component. The construction of new units continues for at least

2 months postnatally. The *in vivo* observations of glomerular development in the olfactory bulb suggest that changes in central neural architecture can continue for prolonged periods after birth, and that neural development may include both regressive/selective and progressive/constructive components.

SUMMARY

It is possible to observe directly changes in neuronal architecture in both the peripheral nervous system and the central nervous system using vital fluorescent dyes, video microscopy, and digital image processing. In vivo imaging techniques give one the ability to distinguish changes in neuronal morphology and the distribution of neuronal elements; these changes have been undetected until now. Physiological, histological and electron microscopical controls indicate that these observations may be made without seriously compromising the integrity of the system. The observation of synaptic remodeling at the neuromuscular junction, in the cornea, and in autonomic ganglia, and of dendritic changes in autonomic ganglia and suggests that subtle changes in synaptic organization may occur continually throughout an animal's lifetime, perhaps in register with subtle changes in the size, form and function of the animal, or even with experience. The gradual addition of new processing units in the central nervous system indicates that new neuronal circuitry may also be added to the brain over a significant portion of the animal's life. The lack of elimination of glomeruli indicates that regressive or selective processes do not operate upon entire neuronal processing units in this system. These changes in neural architecture observed *in vivo* may underlie the adaptive capabilities of the nervous system that operate long past the developmental period perhaps throughout an animal's entire lifetime.

The olfactory system may be unique in that the receptor population in the olfactory mucosa continues to increase during much of postnatal development; furthermore, there is some evidence for postnatal neurogenesis in the bulb itself.

There is evidence that in rodents a significant number of olfactory receptor cells are added during postnatal development (Meisami and Safari, 1989) and in the adult (Graziadei and Monti- Graziadei, 1979). While this constant addition and turnover distinguishes the peripheral component of the olfactory system from other sensory systems, the rate of postnatal growth of the olfactory bulb is identical to that for the rest of the rodent brain. It is possible that the central targets of various sensory projections share some basic mechanisms to adjust to this growth. There is postnatal neurogenesis within the bulb, but it is limited primarily to periglomerular and granule cells(Hinds, 1967; Bayer, 1983). Although the periglomerular cells contribute to the glomerular neuropil it is important to point out that the major olfactory bulb component of the glomeruli, the mitral cells, are postmitotic at least three days before birth. Thus the progressive addition and growth of glomeruli probably does not depend primarily upon the addition of new neurons in the bulb.

What sorts of controls are possible for distinguishing between potential effects of the in vivo imaging procedures themselves and the biological phenomena one wishes to study?

At present, physiological, histological, and electron microscopical methods have been used to assess the effects of the imaging procedures on the integrity of the tissue studied. Although the imaging procedures are invasive, the controls indicate that there is little long-term effect of the techniques used to observe neural architecture over time. In addition, the results of the *in vivo* experiments provide a different sort of internal control. The gradual, progressive changes observed over weeks or even months in most systems are difficult to dismiss as artefacts arising from initial damage caused by the imaging techniques.

REFERENCES

Bayer, S. A., 1983, ^{3}H-Thymidine-radiographic studies of neurogenesis in the rat olfactory bulb, *Exp. Brain Res.*, 50:320

Changeux, J.P. and Danchin A., 1976, Selective stabilization of developing synapes as a mechanism for the specification of neuronal networks, *Nature*, 264:705.

Cowan, W. M., J. W. Fawcett, D. D. M. O'Leary, and B. B. Stanfield, 1984, Regressive events in neurogenesis, *Science*, 225:1258.

Edelman G.M., 1987, "Neuronal Darwinism: The Theory of Neronal Group Selection," Basic Books, New York.

Graziadei, P. P. C. and G. A. Monti-Graziadei., 1979, Neurogenesis and neuron regeneration in the olfactory system of mammals. I.Morphological aspects of differentiation and structural organization of the olfactory sensory neurons, *J Neurocytol.*, 8:1.

Grinvald, A., L. Anglister, J.A. Freeman, R. Hildesheim, and A. Manker, 1984, Real time optical imaging of naturally evoked electrical activity in intact frog brain, *Nature*, 308:848.

Harris, L. and D. Purves. 1989 Rapid remodeling of sensory endings in the corneas of living mice, *J. Neurosci.*, 9:2210.

Herrera, A. A. and Banner, L. R., 1987, Direct observation of motor nerve terminal remodelling in living frogs, *Soc. Neurosci. Abstr.*, 13:1665.

Hinds, J. W., 1968, Autoradiographic study of histogenesis in the mouse olfactory bulb. I. Time of origin of neurons and neuroglia, *J. Comp. Neurol.*, 134:287.

Hume, R. I. and Purves, D., 1981, Geometry of neonatal neurones and the regulation of synapse elimination, *Nature*, 293:469.

Ivanov, A. and Purves, D., 1989, Ongoing electrical activity of superior cervical ganglion cells in mammals of different sizes, *J. Comp. Neurol.*, 284:398.

LaMantia, A.-S. and Purves, D., 1989, Development of glomerular pattern visualized in the olfactory bulbs of living mice, *Nature*, (in press).

Lichtman, J. W., Magrassi, L. and Purves, D., 1987, Visualization of neuromuscular junctions over periods of several months in living mice, *J. Neurosci.*, 7:1215.

Magrassi, L., Purves, D. and Lichtman, J. W., 1987, Fluorescent probes that stain living nerve terminals, *J. Neurosci.*, 7:1207.

Pomeroy, S. L., LaMantia, A.-S. and Purves, D., 1989, Evidence that postnatal development of the mouse olfactory bulb occurs by gradual addition of newly constructed neural ensembles, *Soc. Neurosci. Abstr.*, 15:809.

Purves, D., Voyvodic, J. T., Magrassi, L. and Yawo, H., 1988, Nerve terminal remodeling visualized in living mice by repeated examination of the same neuron, *Science*, 238:1122.

Purves, D., 1988, "Body and Brain: A Trophic Theory of Neural Connections," Harvard University Press, Cambridge, MA.

Purves, D., 1989, Watching synaptic connections change in the living nervous system, *Sci. Amer.*, (in press).

Purves, D., Snider, W. D. and Voyvodic, J. T., 1988, Trophic regulation of nerve cell morphology and innervation in the autonomic nervous system, *Nature*, 336:123.

Purves, D. and Voyvodic, J. T., 1987, Imaging mammalian nerve cells and their connections over time in living animals, *Trends Neurosci.*, 10:398.

Purves, D. and Lichtman, J. W., 1980, Elimination of synaptic connections in the developing nervous system, *Science*, 210:153.

Purves, D. and Hume, R. I., 1981, The relation of postsynaptic geometry to the number of presynaptic axons that innervate autonomic ganglion cells, *J. Neurosci.*, 1:441.

Purves, D. and Lichtman, J. W., 1985, Geometrical differences among homologous neurons in mammals, *Science*, 228:298.

Purves, D., Hadley, R. D. and Voyvodic, J., 1986, Dynamic changes in the dendritic geometry of individual neurons visualized over periods of up to three months in the superior cervical ganglion of living mice, *J. Neurosci.*, 6:1051.

Purves, D., Rubin, E., Snider, W. D. and Lichtman, J. W., 1986, Relation of animal size to convergence, divergence and neuronal number in peripheral sympathetic pathways, *J. Neurosci.*, 6:158.

Snider, W. D., 1988, Nerve growth factor promotes dendritic arborization of sympathetic ganglion cells in developing mammals, *J. Neurosci.* 8:2628.

Voyvodic, J. T., 1989, Regulation of dendritic geometry in the rat superior cervical ganglion by peripheral targets, *J. Neurosci.*, (in press).

Voyvodic, J., 1987, Development and regulation of dendrites in the rat superior cervical ganglion: influence of preganglionic innervation, *J. Neurosci.*, 7:904.

Wigston, D. J., 1989, Remodelling of neuromuscular junctions in adult mouse soleus, *J. Neurosci.*, 9:639.

THE DEVELOPMENT OF CORTICAL PROJECTIONS [*]

Peter Kind (scribe)

Psychology Department
Dalhousie University
Halifax, Nova Scotia
CANADA

Giorgio Innocenti (lecturer)

Institute of Anatomy
Faculty of Medicine
University of Lausanne
SWITZERLAND

INTRODUCTION

The adult central nervous system can be thought of as a device for the 'adaptive structuration' of an animal's environment. The pattern of neuronal connectivity, which develops through genetic and experience-dependent processes, is one of the factors that determines an animal's perception of the surrounding world. It is not surprising, therefore, that the connectivity pattern of the mammalian brain as well as the developmental mechanisms that give rise to this pattern are among the most studied areas of neurobiology.

An interesting feature of the developing mammalian cortex is the overproduction of axons, followed by their subsequent removal. The development of the cerebral cortex, therefore, is a biphasic process whereby the transient, juvenile connectivity is replaced by the stabile, adult organization. In fact, the transition in architectural style from "Romanesque" to "Gothic" may be the best analogy for the changes in the "style" of cortical axonal projections from juvenile to adult mammals. In addition, these developmental changes share several features with the metamorphic development of holometabolous insects. The significance of the transient axonal population is unclear; however, the possibility that it represents a type of developmental error seems unlikely for two reasons. Firstly, it is improbable that the mechanisms of development are so imprecise as to result in the massive axonal elimination that is observed and, secondly, the transient projections are highly stereotyped within, and in some cases, between species. For these reasons, random developmental error appears to be an insufficient explanation for the formation of transient projections. It seems much more likely that the transient projections serve some function during development, presumably a morphogenetic function (Innocenti, 1988).

This lecture reviews the present knowledge of these transient projections with a focus on the development of the corpus callosum. For further elaboration of some of the concepts and a more complete review see Innocenti (1990).

ADULT ORGANIZATION OF THE CORTEX

The mammalian cortex is organized along radial and tangential directions. Radially, it can be divided into six layers, although boundaries between layers are not always distinct and some layers

---

[*] This chapter to be cited as: Kind, P., and Innocenti, G. M., The development of cortical projections, in: "Systems Approaches to Developmental Neurobiology," P. A. Raymond, S. S. Easter, Jr., and G. M. Innocenti, eds., Plenum Press, New York.

can be further subdivided. Layer IV receives the main thalamic input although thalamic projections of lesser magnitude have been found in other layers. Layers I-III, the supragranular layers, generally project to other cortical areas and the infragranular layers project to subcortical nuclei. In the visual system, callosally projecting neurons at the area 17/18 border are found mainly in layers III and IV, with a few in layer VI (Caminiti and Innocenti, 1981; Innocenti,1980). On the other hand, those neurons in the posteromedial lateral suprasylvian area (PMLS) and posterolateral lateral suprasylvian area (PLLS) which project across the callosum to areas 17 and 18 are found mainly in layer VI (Segraves and Innocenti, 1985) with a few in layer III (Innocenti and Clarke, 1984a,b).

Tangentially, the cortex is organized into discrete cytoarchitectonic areas. Each area is believed to serve specific functions and receives input from a distinct group of thalamic nuclei (Caviness and Frost, 1980). Within a sensory system, the areas and their interconnections define distinct lines of sensory processing as well as defining the hierarchies which exist within each line (Hubel and Livingstone, 1987; Livingstone and Hubel, 1987a,b; and Van Essen, 1985). A characteristic projection originates from neurons near the area 17/18 border and, through the callosum, terminates in the contralateral 17/18 border and retinotopically corresponding regions of other visual areas (Innocenti, 1986). The border between areas 17 and 18 is also the retinotopic location of the vertical meridian, and it is believed that the callosal connections are responsible for 'stitching' together the cortical representations of the two visual hemifields (Berlucchi et al., 1967; Choudhury et al., 1965; and Hubel and Wiesel, 1967). The callosal projection from PMLS conforms to the same retinotopic rules as those for areas 17 and 18. Although this area sends a minor projection to contralateral areas 17 and 18, its main callosal output goes to the homotopic regions of PMLS (Innocenti, 1986).

THE ORGANIZATION OF THE JUVENILE CORTEX

One of the most salient features of the juvenile cortex which distinguishes it from the adult cortex is the presence of numerous transient projections. These include cortical to subcortical (Adams et al., 1983; D'Amato and Hicks, 1978; Distel & Hollander, 1980; Stanfield et al., 1982; and Tsumoto et al., 1983), thalamo-cortical (Hubel et al., 1977; Kato et al., 1984, 1986; and Rakic, 1976), local and distant intrahemispheric (Clarke and Innocenti, 1986; Dehay et al., 1984; Innocenti and Clarke, 1984a; Katz and Wiesel,1987; Price and Blakemore, 1985a,b; and Price and Zumbroich, 1989) as well as in interhemispheric projections (Dehay et al., 1988; Innocenti et al., 1977; Innocenti and Caminiti, 1980; Ivy and Killackey,1981; and Olivarria and Van Sluyters, 1985). The interhemispheric projections were the first (Innocenti et al., 1977), and are to date, the most completely described. In the cat, transient callosal axons originate from most of areas 17 and 18 and reach homotopic regions in the contralateral hemisphere as well as numerous other visual areas (Fig. 1; Innocenti, 1981; and Innocenti and Clarke, 1984a,b) . From these studies and others in different sensory areas (Feng and Brugge, 1983; and Innocenti and Caminiti, 1980) and species (Chow et al., 1981; Ivy et al., 1979; Miller and Vogt, 1984; and Mooney et al., 1984), it appears that, unlike in adult animals, where neurons which project across the callosum are organized in discrete columns or clusters, in newborns there is a continuous band of cells projecting across the callosum. Additionally, in the cat, neurons in the auditory cortex were found extending axons to either ipsilateral or contralateral visual areas (Innocenti and Clarke, 1984a). Interestingly, when injections with retrograde labels were restricted to the grey matter of newborn cortex, the projection pattern was very similar to that of the adult. Only when the injection involved the white matter (and deep layer VI) were transient projections labelled (Innocenti and Clarke, 1984b; and Innocenti and Clarke, 1986). Whether these transient projections form synapses in the white matter remains unclear; however, a transient population of subplate neurons (Chun et al., 1987) and the dendrites of layer VI neurons extending into the white matter (Marin Padilla, 1977) could provide the targets for these transient axons.

Transient projections are characteristically patterned: 1) they originate specifically from certain cortical layers; 2) they have a rough tangential organization (ie. are topographically arranged); 3) they follow very stereotyped routes in the white matter and 4) they show characteristic behaviors at their sites of termination. It should also be mentioned that some projections never form. For example, a reciprocal transient projection from visual cortex to auditory cortex may be expected if transient axon development was not a selective process, but such a projection has never been demonstrated.

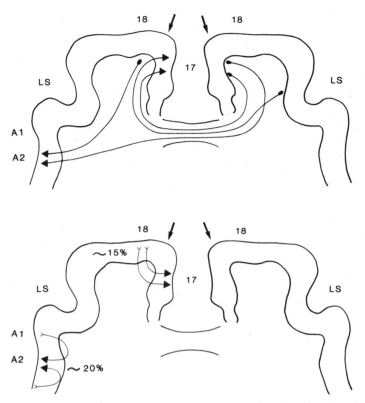

Fig. 1. Top: schematic representation of four types of neurons, characterized by different locations and the site of their transient projection. Two of these neurons are in the medial part of area 17 and their axons reach the white matter under the contralateral area 17, or the lateral suprasylvian areas (**LS**). Two other neurons are in auditory areas A1 and A2 and their axons reach the white matter under the ipsi- or contralateral areas 17 and 18. Bottom: schematic representation of the presumed final projection of the same neurons shown above, after elimination of the transient projections. Notice that they all form relatively short projections. Percent values refer to the fraction of areas 17 and A1, A2 neurons with transient projections for which the local, final projection could be documented.

RADIAL DISTRIBUTION OF TRANSIENT PROJECTIONS

In general, the radial distribution of callosally projecting neurons is similar in both adult and juvenile animals (Caminiti and Innocenti, 1980; Innocenti, 1980; and Segraves and Innocenti, 1985). Both white and grey matter injections retrogradely label many neurons in layers III and upper IV, but few cells in layer VI. A similar distribution was also found for the auditory to visual projection which disappears in the adult, although fewer neurons were found in layer IV (Innocenti and Clarke, 1984a). The radial origin of certain projections, however, does change. For example, the callosal projection from PMLS contralateral to area 17/18 originates from layers III and VI in the kitten, but the majority of the layer III projection is removed by adulthood leaving only layer VI neurons (Innocenti and Clarke, 1984b). Radial specificity has also been shown for cortical-subcortical projections (Stanfield et al., 1982).

The mechanisms that determine where a neuron will send its axon are still unclear. The laminar specificity of both transient and permanent neurons could mean that positional cues play a major role in determining axonal destination. Several lines of evidence, however, make such a simple hypothesis unlikely. For example, certain cortical neurons extend their axons along their 'chosen' pathways prior to acquiring their final radial position (Schwartz and Goldman-Rakic, 1986). In addition, neurons with the same radial position extend their axons along separate pathways and have different target regions (Innocenti et al., 1986 and Segraves and Innocenti, 1985). Lastly, the radial position of neurons can be severely altered by X-irradiation or treatment with cytotoxic drugs (Innocenti and Berbel, 1989a,b; Jones et al, 1982; and Jensen and Killackey, 1984), or by a genetic mutation, as in the *reeler* mouse (Caviness, 1977). This change in radial position, however, does not alter the neuron's choice of target.

Other possible determinants of axonal destination include birth date, clonal affiliation and serial position in a clone. The first seems unlikely because neurons of different layers often follow similar pathways and share a common target despite probable differences in birth date (Innocenti, 1986; Luskin and Shatz, 1985). In addition, neurons with similar birth dates can have completely different target regions. The role of clonal affiliation and position in determining axonal projection patterns is unknown in vertebrates; however, they have been shown to be important in invertebrates (Sulston and Horvitz, 1977).

TANGENTIAL ORGANIZATION OF JUVENILE PROJECTIONS

As previously mentioned, injections of retrograde tracer restricted to the grey matter of newborn kittens show a callosal projection pattern similar to that of adults (Clarke and Innocenti, 1986; and Innocenti and Clarke, 1984a,b). For example, axons of the callosum are labelled from injections into areas 17 and 18, only if the 17/18 border is involved. In addition, only neurons lying near the 17/18 border of the contralateral hemisphere are labelled. Injections which extend into the white matter, however, label a much larger, crescent-shaped zone in the contralateral hemisphere with its long axis oriented roughly mediolaterally (Innocenti and Clarke, 1984a,b). The crescent-shaped zone includes a continuous labelling through areas 17 and 18 and other visual areas, but also involves auditory areas. It is known that the callosal projections are topographically ordered because as the injection sites are moved in the anteroposterior direction, the labelled zone in the contralateral cortex moves accordingly. Interestingly, in a study performed by Nakamura and Kaneseki (1989), small injections into the adult cat presplenium labelled a zone of cortex very similar to that resulting from neonatal injection into areas 17 and 18. It appears, therefore, that the topography of the juvenile callosal projections may be related to that of axons in the corpus callosum; however, it is not known if the rudimentary topography of the juvenile callosum is necessary for the formation of the adult topographic projection.

TRANSITION FROM JUVENILE TO ADULT CONNECTIVITY

Despite the fact that the juvenile architecture is very different from that of the adult, it appears that the axons that do invade the cortex **can** become permanent, and those that remain confined to the white matter are eliminated. The cortical terminations, therefore, have an adult-like pattern at the time they are formed. When the visual callosal axons reach the contralateral cortex they enter a "waiting" phase in a region known as the cortical subplate (Feng and Brugge, 1983; Innocenti et al., 1981; Olavarria and Van Sluyters, 1985; and Rakic, 1977), and then a select group enter the cortex at the 17/18 border (Innocenti and Clarke, 1984b). The signal that mediates cortical invasion is still unknown, but maturation of the target tissue has been implicated, in particular in the geniculocortical projection where this "waiting" phase has also been observed (Shatz and Luskin, 1986).

Subsequent to the "waiting" phase, the transient projections are eliminated. Although cell death probably occurs during the development of the mammalian cortex, axonal elimination may be a more likely mechanism for explaining the loss of callosal projections (Innocenti et al., 1986). In order to distinguish between neuronal death and axon elimination, neurons with transient callosal axons projecting to area 17 of the kitten were retrogradely labelled with a long lasting tracer during the first postnatal week (Innocenti et al., 1986). The kittens were allowed to survive until the second postnatal month (after their transient callosal axons had been eliminated), at which time certain ipsilateral visual areas were injected with another tracer. The result was double-labelling of 15-20 % of area 17 neurons only when the late injections involved area 17 or 18. Late injection into other visual areas did not result in double-labelled neurons. It appears therefore that cell death was not involved in the removal of transient callosal axons. Instead, the long transient axon was probably liminated and the neuron

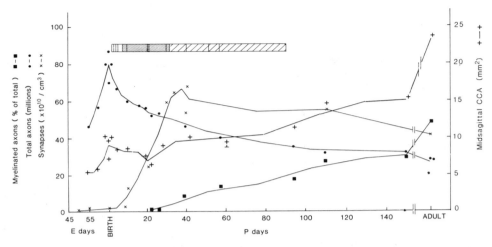

Fig. 2. Temporal relations of different aspects of cortical and callosal development in the cat, i.e., number of axons in the corpus callosum (dots), midsagittal cross-sectional area (CCA; +), myelination of callosal axons (squares), density of synapses in the visual cortex (x; Cragg, 1975). The horizontal rectangle represents the period of elimination of callosal projections from area 17, demonstrated with retrograde transport by Innocenti and Caminiti (1980). Vertical lines in the rectangle indicate the age of one kitten at the time of HRP injection. Stippling indicates the period of elimination of the projection, considered to extend from the age of the oldest kitten in which the injection was still fully exuberant to that of the youngest kitten in which the projection seemed to be as in the adult. Two phases are distinguished, the first (heavy stippling) corresponds to the bulk of the elimination, from most of area 17, the second (light stippling), corresponds to the elimination of projections close to the 17/18 border. Notice that most of the callosal axons and projections are eliminated before the onset of myelination. This massive elimination coincides with a pause in the growth of the CCA and occurs during the fast increase in the synaptic density. The peak in synaptic density is probably reached around PD70, not around PD37 as indicated here (Winfield, 1981). Thus the elimination of callosal axons and projections is most conspicuous during the initial quarter to third of synaptogenesis in area 17. (Modified from Berbel and Innocenti, 1988).

established a permanent local or association projection. Research completed by Katz and Wiesel (1987) and O'Leary and Terashima (1988) indicates that, in the case of interareal and corticofugal projections, the permanent axon is actually a side branch of the transient axon as opposed to a separate axon. The elimination of the transient projection, therefore, results in the normal axonal morphology of adult neurons.

In the cat, the loss of transient projections temporally coincides with a 70% reduction of the total callosal axons (Berbel and Innocenti, 1988; and Koppel and Innocenti, 1983). This relationship is important because it suggests that the elimination of transient projections actually causes a decrease in the number of callosal axons; however, in the monkey, the loss of transient axons does not occur at the same time as axon loss in the callosum (LaMantia and Rakic, 1984). It is unclear why this species difference occurs; however, several explanations seem plausible. In the monkey, there may be a significant time lag between the loss of dye-transporting abilities of the axon, and the loss of the axon from the corpus callosum seen through electron microscopy. Furthermore, it is quite likely that the early phase of axon loss in the monkey is being masked by a simultaneous addition of axons to the corpus callosum. Finally, more detailed tracer studies on the development of interhemispheric connections in the monkey seem to be needed.

The transition between juvenile and adult cortical connectivity occurs simultaneously with several other cortical processes (Fig. 2); and, while correlations are often not indicative of causal relationships, they may provide useful clues into some of the mechanisms which lead to the stabilization or elimination of axons. Firstly, axon elimination is closely timed to the onset of the fast

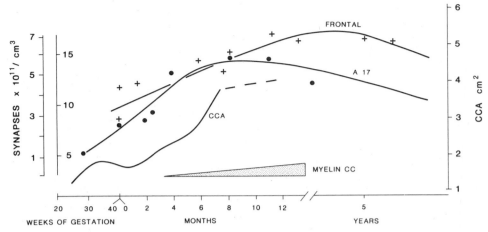

Fig. 3. Temporal relations of different aspects of cortical and callosal development in man, ie. midsaggital CCA (Clarke et al., 1989), synaptogenesis in area 17 (dots; curve fitted by eye; Huttenlocher et al., 1982) and in frontal cortex (crosses, curve fitted by eye; Huttenlocher, 1979), and myelination of callosal axons (light microscopic observation of Yakovlev and Lecours, 1969). Notice that CCA appears to decrease between the end of gestation and the first postnatal month. This period may correspond to the massive elimination of transient callosal projections and axons in man: as in the cat the suspected elimination occurs before myelination and during the initial phase of fast synaptogenesis in the cortex.

phase of synaptogenesis (Berbel and Innocenti, 1988). Therefore, either the two events are independent, or a causal relationship exists between them, or they are both dependent on a common developmental occurrence. Second, the elimination of callosal axons occurs prior to the onset of myelination (Berbel and Innocenti, 1988). This is important because it implies that the fate of a given axon may be determined before myelination.

In the cat, the massive loss of callosal axons is correlated with, and is probably responsible for, a decrease in the cross-sectional area (CCA) of the corpus callosum (Berbel and Innocenti, 1988). In humans, a decrease in cross-sectional callosal area occurs during the final two gestational, and the subsequent two postnatal months (Clarke et al., 1989). The temporal relation between the decrease in CCA, the fast-phase of synaptogenesis and myelination is very similar to that of cats (Figure 3). Therefore, the decrease in CCA in humans may be a reliable indicator of at least part of the loss of transient callosal axons.

During the period of axonal stabilization and elimination, a massive molecular reshuffling must be occurring within the axons. Indeed, Figlewicz et al. (1988) showed that the levels of the three neurofilament subunits increased in the kitten corpus callosum over the first postnatal month. The low (L) and medium (M) molecular weight subunits were present at birth and steadily increased over the first postnatal month. When an antibody directed against a phosphorylated epitope of the high (H) molecular weight subunit was used, staining appeared on postnatal day (PD) 11 and continued to increase until PD 18. A separate antibody directed against an unphosphorylated epitope of H subunit, and possibly the M subunit, however, did not label the corpus callosum until PD 25, and staining increased steadily until PD 39 (Innocenti et al., in progress). The L and M subunits form the core of the neurofilaments, while the H subunit crosslinks and may stabilize the neurofilaments (Berbel and Innocenti, 1988; and Hirokawa, 1986). The increase in the H subunit occurs during the massive axon elimination and stabilization (Fig. 4). One feature which may distinguish the permanent from the transient axons, therefore, may be the formation of a mature cytoskeleton. It is still impossible to discern, however, whether the maturation of the axonal cytoskeleton is the primary mechanism in determining an axon's fate, or whether it is a secondary phenomenon triggered by a prior molecular decision.

THE REGULATION OF AXONAL SURVIVAL IN THE CEREBRAL CORTEX

Despite the recent progress in understanding the role of the cytoskeleton in the development of the cortex, it seems unlikely that any unitary process will completely explain the elimination of transient axons during cortical development. Instead, the regulation of the juvenile to adult transition is probably controlled by a complex network of interacting factors, the net result of which may be the disassembly or stabilization of the cytoskeleton. The exact nature of these factors has been partially examined through perturbation experiments designed to examine the importance of 1) the nature of the animal's early visual experience, 2) the integrity of the afferent periphery and its projection and 3) the integrity of the target region, including its afferent projections, on the elimination and stabilization of callosal axons.

The role of visual experience and the afferent periphery in the development of the visual callosal pathways has been examined by altering the nature of the early visual experience through induced horizontal strabismus (Innocenti and Frost, 1979; and Lund et al., 1978), monocular (Innocenti and Frost, 1979) and binocular deprivation (Innocenti et al. 1985), monocular and binocular enucleation (Innocenti and Frost, 1979, 1980) and dark-rearing (Frost and Moy, 1989; and Lund and Mitchell, 1979). As mentioned above, the area 17/18 border is also the retinotopic location of the vertical meridian, and, the role of the callosally projecting neurons is to stitch together the two visual hemifields. A horizontal strabismus shifts the geometrical midline and, therefore, may alter the location of the callosally projecting neurons to a more temporal or nasal retinotopic area, depending on whether the strabismus is divergent or convergent, respectively. Interestingly, strabismus causes a modest expansion in the distribution of callosally projecting neurons in area 17, but the magnitude of the change seems unrelated to the angle of the strabismus. Similar results were found in cats that were monocularly deprived (MD) until three months of age from birth and in cats which had 10 days of normal vision prior to binocular deprivation (Innocenti et al., 1985). Binocular deprivation from birth until one month of age had no effect on the development of the callosal neurons when followed by normal vision. Finally, monocular and binocular enucleations resulted in a similar widespread distribution of callosally projecting neurons. It would appear, therefore, that these conditions of altered visual exposure result in the stabilization of normally transient axons. One should bear in mind, however, that very few axons were stabilized compared to the large number of transients which were still eliminated. In addition, for both the monkey (Dehay et al., 1989) and man (Clarke et al., 1989) callosal maturation may be a prenatal event. These findings necessitate the involvement of mechanisms independent of vision in the regulation of axonal elimination.

The complete removal of pattern vision through bilateral lid suture resulted in a 50% decrease in the number of visual callosal neurons in kittens (Innocenti et al., 1985) and reduced the density of callosal terminations in areas 17 and 18 (Innocenti and Frost, 1979, 1980). These results indicate that although visual experience may not be sufficient to rescue large numbers of normally transient axons, normal pattern vision is necessary in the maintenance of a normal visual callosal projection.

The role of the afferent periphery, though well studied, remains somewhat ambiguous. Shatz (1977) showed that Siamese cats had an expanded zone of callosally projecting neurons, and that the magnitude of the expansion varied proportionally with the degree of abnormal crossing at the chiasm. Since this study, however, attempts to systematically change the callosal projection through altering the afferent periphery have resulted in more modest effects which were often species specific. Monocular and binocular enucleation on embryonic monkeys (Dehay et al., 1989), kittens (Innocenti and Frost, 1979, 1980), and rat and hamster pups (Olavarria and Van Sluyters, 1984; Rhoades and Delacrose, 1980; and Rothblat and Hayes, 1982) led to a small expansion of the callosally projecting region; whereas, binocular enucleation resulted in a decrease in the total number of callosally projecting neurons in kittens but not in monkeys or rats (though no quantitative analysis was performed in the latter two species). It is possible that the fate of the callosal axons is already determined at birth, therefore, alteration of the periphery in newborns would have little effect. Such a scenario seems unlikely, however, because congenitally anophthalmic mice and rats show a very similar expansion in the callosal projecting region relative to that of neonatally enucleated animals (Olavarria and Van Sluyters, 1984; and Olavarria et al., 1987).

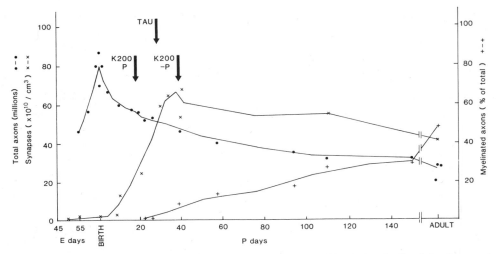

Fig. 4. Temporal relations of morphological and biochemical aspects of cortical and callosal development in the cat. The curves of number and myelination of callosal axons and synaptic density are the same as those shown in Fig. 2. Arrows point to the first, unequivocal appearance of three cytoskeletal proteins in callosal axons, the phosphorylated heavy subunit of neurofilaments (**K200 P**; Figlewicz et al., 1988), the adult forms of the juvenile microtubule associated proteins **Tau** (Riederer et al. in preparation), a partially dephosphorylated form of the heavy subunit of neurofilaments (**K200 -P**), or possibly of the medium neurofilament subunit.

Although enucleation experiments also alter the visual experience of the animals, it appears that the patterns observed following enucleation are not due to the changes in visual experience. Binocular enucleation (Innocenti and Frost, 1980) produced qualitatively and quantitatively different results from those of binocular lid suture (Innocenti et al., 1985; and Innocenti and Frost, 1985) and dark rearing (Frost and Moy, 1989). In conclusion, it appears that while both visual history and afferent integrity can alter the visual callosal projection, other, more primary factors must be determining the fate of callosal axons.

While the effects of visual experience and the afferent periphery on the visual callosal projections are becoming better understood, their mode of action still remains a mystery. For example, it is unclear whether the above mentioned experimental paradigms are directly affecting the callosally projecting neurons, or whether they are affecting the contralateral targets. It is possible that the target region is releasing a trophic factor for which the incoming fibres compete. Changes in the target secretion of this trophic factor could certainly alter the nature of the callosal projection. Experiments designed to test the competition hypothesis, however, are fraught with difficulty. For example, simply showing that one neuronal population is eliminated while another survives is not sufficient evidence of competition in the cortex. It may be impossible to completely rule out the effects of secondary inputs elsewhere in the network.

Recently, while examining the effects of target tissue lesions on the development of callosal projections, Innocenti and collaborators noted that neonatal injections of ibotenic acid (IBO) into areas 17 and 18 of newborn kittens completely eliminated the granular and infragranular layers (Assal et al., 1989; Innocenti et al., 1987; Innocenti and Berbel, 1989a,b). The result was a thinner cortex or "microcortex" which was very similar to microgyria - a human cortical dysplasia. The supragranular layers had not finished migrating at the time of the injections and appeared to be virtually unaltered by the IBO injection. The microcortex does exhibit several features of normal development: it receives a projection (though somewhat reduced) from the lateral geniculate nucleus and also exhibits orientation and direction selectivity. One interesting abnormality of the microcortex, however, is its ability to maintain the ipsilateral and contralateral auditory inputs but not the transient projection from area 17.

The white matter below the injured area becomes infiltrated with astrocytes indicating that a trophic factor may play a role in the stabilization of normally transient projections. The selectivity of the stabilization process (auditory but not area 17 axons), makes the idea of a general trophic factor unlikely. It does not, however, rule out the possibility of several trophic factors or possible differential effects of supra and infragranular layers on the incoming callosal axons.

While the regulation of survival of cortical axons is proving to be a very complicated process, recent clinical observations stress the potential relevance of the problem for human pathology. Lyon and collaborators (in press) have recently described an apparently new syndrome characterized by congenital necrotizing myopathy, cardiomyopathy, cataracts and atrophy of the white matter tracts such as the corpus callosum and the pyramidal tract. The atrophy of these tracts could result from an exaggeration of the normal axon elimination which occurs during development. It is possible that the mechanism necessary for the proper maintenance of cortical axons malfunctions and this leads to cytoskeletal deficits.

CONCLUSION

Although the presence of massive axonal exuberance in the juvenile mammalian cortex is a very well characterized developmental phenomenon, the function and regulation of this axon overproduction is still unclear. Even though the presence of transient connections may appear to contradict the idea that a neuron is prespecified for recognition of a given target, such a conclusion should be approached with caution. Some prespecification of axonal destination may be involved in the development of the visual callosal axons. For example, the transient axons are arranged in a topographic order and only those axons near the area 17/18 border extend into the grey matter. The latter suggests that only certain populations of axons possess the ability to recognize distinct target regions. In addition, certain connections, such as the visual to auditory cortex, never develop, even though they may be expected to if no prespecification occurs. For these reasons, the existence of a genetically determined recognition signal cannot be ruled out; however, the mechanisms which mediate this process must be different from those traditionally associated with the prespecification hypothesis.

Finally, the formation of the adult neural network is not regulated by any single developmental mechanism. Instead, the interaction of numerous higher order factors, seem to control the stabilization and elimination of juvenile neural connections.

The purpose of metamorphosis is to create a new body plan and, hence, a new nervous system in order to accomplish a completely different lifestyle. The transient axons, on the other hand, serve no obvious function. Therefore, is the analogy of the development of the mammalian cortex to metamorphosis an accurate one? Could the exuberance be better explained as a phylogenetic phenomenon rather than a developmental one?

The analogy to metamorphosis was used to emphasize the huge differences in the nervous systems of juvenile and adult animals. One consequence of metamorphosis is a completely new network of neuronal connections and perhaps this is how we should view the transition from the juvenile to adult neural network. The analogy may be even more substantial. Metamorphosis is initiated by a hormonal signal in both insects and amphibians. Recent findings by R. Hawkes and collaborators suggest that thyroid hormones may be necessary for the elimination of transient callosal projections and the cytoskeletal maturation of the remaining axons.

Of course it is possible that the transient projections are a direct result of phylogeny, though it is unlikely that the ancestor of the cat had a connectivity pattern resembling that of a newborn kitten. Instead, certain transformations may have occurred in phylogeny which have resulted in exuberancy. For example, during development axons must first choose a pathway and then choose a target. Therefore, these two choices must be closely related - presumably through phylogeny. It is possible that

121

during evolution, there was an increase in target areas without an increase in pathway choice. One possible result of such a scenario is an increase in the number of axons in a given pathway, which may eventually result in exuberancy.

During the development of the callosal projections many peripheral events occur such as the alignment of the two eyes. These events can be somewhat variable and occur completely independently of the CNS. Since the purpose of the callosal projection is to accurately amalgamate the two visual hemifields, is it not possible that the purpose of the exuberancy is to allow a certain degree of flexibility into these peripheral events? In fact, is some degree of flexibility not necessary in order to properly coordinate peripheral and central events in the nervous system?

It is possible that a certain sub-population of the transient visual callosal axons do play a role in the proper formation of binocular vision. This functional explanation, however, cannot explain the magnitude of the transient axonal population.

It may be that the projections close to the area 17/18 border serve this function and that the same sub-population of neurons are being stabilized in the strabismus and deprivation experiments. In addition, we must be very careful to distinguish between the cause and the function of the exuberancy. The cause, in our opinion, is probably a mismatch of cues along the pathways and cues at the target. The axons are initially only interested in the pathway and are ignorant of their destination. The function of the exuberancy of connections is a separate phenomenon. The overgrowth of axons may provide the system with a certain amount of flexibility and this may explain why exuberancy was preserved in evolution. In fact, some transient axons can be stabilized by performing certain experimental manipulations. Allowing for a certain degree of flexibility during the development of binocular vision may be one role for the exuberant projections.

REFERENCES

Adams, C.E., Mihailoff, G.A., and Woodward, D.J., 1983, A transient component of the developing corticospinal tract arises in visual cortex, *Neurosci. Lett.*, 36:243.

Assal, F., Melzer, P., and Innocenti, G.M., 1989, Functional analysis of a visual cortical circuit resembling human microgyria, *Eur. J. Neurosci.Suppl.* ,2:256.

Berbel, P., and Innocenti, G.M., 1988, The development of the corpus callosum in cats: a light- and electron-microscopic study, *J. Comp. Neurol.*, 276:132.

Berlucchi, G., Gazzaniga, M.S., and Rizzolatti, G., 1967, Microelectrode analysis of transfer of visual information by the corpus callosum, *Arch. Ital. Biol.*, 105:583.

Caminiti, R., and Innocenti, G.M., 1981, The postnatal development of somatosensory callosal connections after partial lesions of somatosensory areas, *Exp. Brain. Res.*, 42:53.

Caviness, V.S., 1977, Reeler mutant mouse: a genetic experiment in developing mammalian cortex, in: "Approaches to the Cell Biology of Neurons", Cowan, W.M. and Ferrendalli, J.A., eds., Society for Neuroscience, Bethesda, MD, p. 27.

Caviness, V.S., and Frost, D.O., 1980, Tangential organization of thalamic projections to the neocortex in the mouse, *J. Comp. Neurol.*, 194:335.

Choudhury, B.P., Whitteridge, D., and Wilson, M.E., 1965, The function of the callosal connections of the visual cortex, *Q. J. Exp. Physiol.*, L:214.

Chow, K.L., Baumbach, H.D., and Lawson, R., 1981, Callosal projections of the striate cortex in the neonatal rabbit, *Exp. Brain. Res.*, 42:122.

Chun, J.J.M., Nakamura, M.J., and Shatz, C.J., 1987, Transient cells of the developing mammalian telencephalon are peptide-immunoreactive neurons, *Nature*, 325:617.

Clarke, S., and Innocenti, G.M., 1986, Organization of immature intrahemispheric connections, *J. Comp. Neurol.*, 251:1.

Clarke, S., Kraftsik, R., Van der Loos, H., and Innocenti, G.M., 1989, Forms and measures of adult and developing human corpus callosum: is there sexual dimorphism?, *J. Comp. Neurol.*, 280:213.

Cragg, B.G., 1975, The development of synapses in the visual system of the cat, *J. Comp. Neurol.*, 160:147.

D'Amato, C.J., and Hicks, S.P., 1978, Normal development and post-traumatic plasticity of corticospinal neurons in rats, *Exp. Neurol.*, 60:557.

Dehay, C., Bullier, J., and Kennedy, H., 1984, Transient projections from the frontoparietal and temporal cortex to areas 17, 18 and 19 in the kitten, *Exp. Brain Res.*, 57:208.

Dehay, C., Horsburgh, G., Berland, M., Killackey, H., and Kennedy, H., 1989, Maturation and connectivity of the visual cortex in monkey is altered by prenatal removal or retinal input, *Nature*, 337:265.

Dehay, C., Kennedy, H., and Bullier, J., 1988, Characterization of transient cortical projections from auditory, somatosensory, and motor cortices to visual areas 17, 18 and 19 in the kitten, *J. Comp. Neurol.*, 272:68.

Distel, H., and Hollander, H.,1980, Autoradiographic tracing of developing subcortical projections of the occipital region in fetal rabbits. *J. Comp. Neurol.*, 192:505.

Feng, J.Z., and Brugge, J.F., 1983, Postnatal development of auditory callosal connections in the kitten, *J. Comp. Neurol.*, 214:416.

Figlewicz, D.A., Gremo, F., and Innocenti, G.M., 1988, Differential expression of neurofilament subunits in the developing corpus callosum, *Dev. Brain Res.*, 42:181.

Frost, D.O., Moy, Y.P.,1989, Effects of dark rearing on the development of visual callosal connections, *Exp. Brain Res.*, (in press).

Hirokawa, N., 1986, Quick- freeze, deep-etch visualization of the axonal cytoskeleton, *Trends Neurosci.*, 9:67.

Hubel, D.H., and Livingstone, M.S., 1987, Segregation of form, color, and stereopsis in primate area 18, *J. Neurosci.*, 7:3378.

Hubel, D.H., and Wiesel, T.N., 1967, Cortical and callosal connections concerned with the vertical meridian of visual fields in the cat, *J. Neurophys.*, 30:1561.

Hubel, D.H., Wiesel, T.N., and LeVay, S., 1977, Plasticity of ocular dominance columns in monkey striate cortex, *Philos. Trans. R. Soc. Lond. [Biol.]*, 278:377.

Huttenlocher, P.R., 1979, Synaptic density in human frontal-cortex-developmental-changes and effects of aging, *Brain Res.*, 163:195.

Huttenlocher, P.R., Courten de C., Garey, L.J., and Van der Loos, H., 1982, Synaptogenesis in human visual cortex - evidence for synapse elimination during normal development, *Neurosci. Lett.*, 33:247.

Innocenti, G.M., 1990, The development of cortical connections, in: "Progress in Sensory Physiology", Springer-Verlag, (in press).

Innocenti, G.M., 1980, The primary visual pathway through the corpus callosum: morphological and functional aspects in the cat, *Arch. Ital. Biol.* 118:124.

Innocenti, G.M., 1986, General organization of callosal connections in the cerebral cortex. in: "Cerebral Cortex", vol. 5, Jones, E.G. and Peters, A.,eds., Plenum Press, New York, p. 291.

Innocenti, G.M., 1981, Transitory structures as substrate for developmental plasticity of the brain, *Dev. Neurosci.*, 13:305.

Innocenti, G.M., 1988, Loss of axonal projections in the development of the mammalian brain, in: "The Making of the Nervous System," Parnavelas, J.G., Stern, C.D., and Stirling, R.V., eds., Oxford University Press, Oxford, p. 319.

Innocenti, G.M., and Berbel, P., 1989a, Analysis of an experimental cortical network: i) architectonics of areas 17 and 18 after neonatal injections of ibotenic acid; similarities with human microgyria, *J. Neural Transplant* , (in press).

Innocenti, G.M., and Berbel, P., 1989b, Analysis of an experimental cortical network, ii) connections of areas 17 and 18 after neonatal injections of ibotenic acid, *J. Neural Transplant*, (in press).

Innocenti, G.M., Berbel, P., and Melzer, P., 1987, Stabilization of transitory corticocortical projections following lesions provoked by neonatal ibotenic injections, *Neurosci. Abstr. Suppl.*, 22:S227.

Innocenti, G.M., and Caminiti, R., 1980, Postnatal shaping of callosal connections from sensory areas, *Exp. Brain Res.*, 38:381.

Innocenti, G.M., and Clarke, S., 1984a, Bilateral transitory projection to visual areas from auditory cortex in kittens, *Dev. Brain Res.*, 14:143.

Innocenti, G.M., and Clarke, S., 1984b, The organization of immature callosal connections, *J. Comp. Neurol.*, 230:387.

Innocenti, G.M., Clarke, S., and Kraftsik, R., 1986, Interchange of callosal and association projections in the developing visual cortex, *J. Neurosci.*, 6:1384.

Innocenti, G.M., Fiore, L., and Caminiti, R., 1977, Exuberant projection into the corpus callosum from the visual cortex of newborn cats, *Neurosci. Lett.* 4:237.

Innocenti, G.M., and Frost, D.O., 1979, Effects of visual experience on the maturation of the efferent system to the corpus callosum, *Nature*, 280:231.

Innocenti, G.M., and Frost, D.O., 1980, The postnatal development of visual callosal connections in the absence of visual experience or of the eyes, *Exp. Brain Res.*, 39:365.

Innocenti, G.M., Frost, D.O., and Illes, J., 1985, Maturation of visual callosal connections in visually deprived kittens: A challenging critical period, *J. Neurosci.*, 5:255.

Innocenti, G.M., Koppel, H., and Clarke, S., 1981, Glial phagocytosis during the postnatal reshaping of visual callosal connections, *Neurosci. Lett. Suppl.*, 7:S160.

Ivy, G.O., Akers, R.M., and Killackey, H.P., 1979, Differential distribution of callosal projection neurons in the neonatal and adult rat, *Brain Res.*, 173:532.

Ivy, G.O., and Killackey, H.P., 1981, The ontogeny of the distribution of callosal projection neurons in the rat parietal cortex, *J. Comp. Neurol.*, 195:367.

Jensen, K.F., and Killackey, H.P., 1984, Subcortical projections from ectopic neocortical neurons, *Proc. Natl. Acad. Sci. USA*, 81:964.

Jones, E.G., Valentino, K.L., and Fleshman, J.W., 1982, Adjustment of connectivity in rat neocortex after prenatal destruction of precursor cells of layers II-IV, *Dev. Brain Res.*, 2:425.

Kato, N., Kawaguchi, S., and Miyata, H., 1984, Geniculocortical projection to layer I of area 17 in kittens: orthograde and retrograde HRP studies, *J. Comp. Neurol.*, 225:441.

Kato, N., Kawaguchi, S., and Miyata, H., 1986, Postnatal development of afferent projections to the lateral suprasylvian visual area in the cat: an HRP study, *J. Comp. Neurol.*, 252:543.

Katz, L.C., and Wiesel, T.N., 1987, Postnatal development of intrinsic axonal arbors of pyramidal neurons in cat striate cortex, *Soc. Neurosci. Abstr.* 13:1025.

Koppel, H. and Innocenti, G.M., 1983, Is there a genuine exuberancy of callosal projections in development? A quantitative electron microscope study in the cat, *Neurosci. Lett.*, 41:33.

LaMantia, A-S., and Rakic, P., 1984, The number, size, myelination, and regional variation of axons in the corpus callosum and anterior commissure of the developing rhesus monkey, *Soc. Neurosci. Abstr.*, 10:1081.

Livingstone, M.S., and Hubel, D.H., 1987a, Connections between layer 4B of area 17 and thick cytochrome oxidase stripes of area 18 in the squirrel monkey, *J. Neurosci.*, 7:3371.

Livingstone, M.S., and Hubel, D.H., 1987b, Psychophysical evidence for separate channels for the perception of form, color, movement, and depth, *J. Neurosci.*, 3416.

Lund, J.S., and Mitchell, D.E., 1979, The effects of dark-rearing on visual callosal connections of cats, *Brain Res.*, 167:172.

Lund, R.D., Mitchell, D.E., and Henry, G.H., 1978, Squint-induced modification of callosal connections in cats, *Brain Res.*, 144:169.

Luskin, M.B., and Shatz, C.J., 1985, Neurogenesis of the cat's primary visual cortex, *J. Comp. Neurol.*, 242:611.

Lyon, G., Arita, F., Le Galloudec, E., Vallee, L., Misson, J-P., and Ferriere, G., 1989, A disorder of axonal development, necrotizing myopathy, cardiomyopathy and cataracts: a new familial disease, *Ann. of Neurol.*, (in press).

Marin-Padilla, M., 1977, Dual origin of the mammalian neocortex and evolution of the cortical plate, *Anat. Embryol.*, 152:109.

Miller, M.W., and Vogt, B.A., 1984, The postnatal growth of the callosal connections of primary and secondary visual cortex in the rat, *Dev. Brain Res.*,14:304.

Mooney, R.D., Rhoades, R.W., and Fish, S.E., 1984, Neonatal superior collicular lesions alter visual callosal development in hamster, *Exp. Brain Res.*, 55:9.

Nakamura, H., and Kanaseki, T., 1989, Topography of the corpus callosum in the cat, *Brain Res.*, 485:171.

Olavarria, J., Bravo, H.., and Ruiz, G., 1988 The pattern of callosal connections in posterior neocortex of congenitally anophthalmic rats, *Anat. Embryol.*, 178:155.

Olavarria, J., Malach, R., and Van Sluyters, R.C., 1987, Development of visual callosal connections in neonatally enucleated rats, *J. Comp. Neurol.*, 260:321.

Olavarria, J., and Van Sluyters, R.C., 1984, Callosal connections of the posterior neocortex in normal-eyed, congenitally anophthalmic, and neonatally enucleated mice, *J. Comp. Neurol.*, 230:249.

Olavarria, J., and Van Sluyters, R.C., 1985, Organization and postnatal development of callosal connections in the visual cortex of the rat, *J. Comp. Neurol.*, 239:1.

O'Leary, D.D.M., and Terashima, T., 1988, Cortical axons branch to multiple subcortical targets by interstitial axon budding: implications for target recognition and "waiting periods", *Neuron*, 1:901.

Price, D.J., and Blakemore, C., 1985a, Regressive events in the postnatal development of association projections in the visual cortex, *Nature*, 316:721.

Price, D.J., and Blakemore, C., 1985b, The postnatal development of the association projection from visual cortical area 17 to area 18 in the cat, *J. Neurosci.*, 5:2443.

Price, D.J., and Zumbroich, T.J., 1989, Postnatal development of corticocortical efferents from area 17 in the cat's visual cortex, *J. Neurosci.*, 9:600.

Rakic, P., 1976, Prenatal genesis of connections subserving ocular dominance in the rhesus monkey, *Nature*, 261:467.

Rakic, P., 1977, Prenatal development of the visual system in rhesus monkey, *Philos. Trans. R. Soc. Lond. [Biol.]*, 278:245.

Rhoades, R.W., and Dellacroce, D.D., 1980, Neonatal enucleation induced an asymmetric pattern of visual callosal connections in hamsters, *Brain Res.*, 202:189.

Rothblat, L.A., and Hayes, L.L., 1982, Age-related changes in the distribution of visual callosal neurons following monocular enucleation in the rat, *Brain. Res.*, 246:146.

Schwartz, M.L., and Goldman-Rakic, P.S., 1986, Some callosal neurons of the fetal monkey frontal cortex have axons in the contralateral hemisphere prior to the completion of migration, *Soc. Neurosci. Abstr.*, 12:1211.

Segraves, M.A., and Innocenti, G.M., 1985, Comparison of the distributions of ipsilaterally and contralaterally projecting corticocortical neurons in cat visual cortex using two fluorescent tracers, *J. Neurosci.*, 5:2107.

Shatz, C.J., 1977, Anatomy of interhemispheric connections in the visual system of Boston Siamese and ordinary cats, *J. Comp. Neurol.*, 173:497.

Shatz, C.J., and Luskin, M.B., 1986, The relationship between the geniculocortical afferents and their cortical target cells during development of the cat's primary visual cortex, *J. Neurosci.*, 6:3655.

Stanfield, B.B., O'Leary, D.D.M., and Fricks, C., 1982, Selective collateralo elimination in early postnatal development restricts cortical distribution or rat pyramidal tract neurones, *Nature*, 198:371.

Sulston, J.E., and Horvitz, H.R., 1977, Post-embryonic cell lineage of the nematode *Caenorhabditis elegans*, *Dev. Biol.*, 56:110.

Tsumoto, T., Suda, K., and Sato, H., 1983, Postnatal development of corticotectal neurons in the kitten striate cortex: a quantitative study with the horseradish peroxidase technique, *J. Comp. Neurol.*, 219:88.

Van Essen, D.C., 1985, Functional organization of primate visual cortex, in: "Cerebral Cortex", vol. 3, Peters, A. and Jones, E.G., eds., Plenum Press, New York, p. 259.

Winfield, D.A., 1981, The postnatal-development of synapses in the visual-cortex of the cat and the effects of eyelid closure, *Brain Res.*, 206:166.

Yakovlev, P.I., and Lecours, A.-R., 1967, The myelogenetic cycles of regional maturation of the brain, in: "Regional development of the brain in early life," Minkowski, A., ed., Blackwell Scientific Publications, Oxford, p. 3.

THE VISUAL SYSTEM OF FLIES: ANALYSIS OF THE NUMBER, SPECIFICITY, PLASTICITY, AND PHYLOGENY OF IDENTIFIED SYNAPSES [*]

René Marois (scribe)   I. A. Meinertzhagen (lecturer)

Department of Psychology   Life Sciences Centre
Yale University   Dalhousie University
New Haven, CT, USA   Halifax, Nova Scotia, Canada

INTRODUCTION

The functional interactions of a neural circuit are established primarily by its pattern of synaptic connections. Understanding the process of synapse formation and its regulation is therefore paramount to an analysis of circuit organization. To formulate the rules for the assembly of synaptic microcircuits requires as a minimum a simple system that nonetheless possesses the major architectural principles of all nervous systems, and that is easily amenable to precise, detailed analysis. The first neuropil of the fly's optic lobe, the lamina, meets many of these requirements. As background, the structural organization and ontogeny of the defined circuits of this highly stereotyped neuropil have already been thoroughly investigated. This chapter presents recent studies that have exploited these advantages to decipher the operational steps in the formation of synaptic microcircuits and their regulation, plasticity, and evolution.

DESCRIPTION OF THE SYSTEM

The first neuropil in the insect's optic lobe is built on a modular principle (Strausfeld and Nässel, 1981) established by the projection from the innervating photoreceptors of the overlying ommatidia (Meyerowitz and Kankel, 1978). Each module, or cartridge, comprises a set of photoreceptor terminals innervating a fixed set of interneurons. The ensemble is ensheathed, and therefore structurally isolated, by sheets of glial cells. What makes this system so attractive and tractable is the high degree of structural stereotypy it exhibits. Each cell and its synaptic contributions in a cartridge can be individually identified from serial-section electron microscopy. Although most of the findings are based on studies using the housefly, *Musca* , cell number and identity are sufficiently conserved to allow generalizations to other Diptera (Shaw and Meinertzhagen, 1986), and the judicious inclusion in this review of findings on other species.

Of the ten or so cell classes and their more than dozen major synaptic classes found in every lamina cartridge in *Musca* (Strausfeld and Campos-Ortega, 1977), only those cells that participate in two of the synaptic classes are relevant to this chapter. In a typical cartridge, six photoreceptor term-

---

[*] This chapter to be cited as: Marois, R., and Meinertzhagen, I. A., 1990, The visual system of flies: analysis of the number, specificity, plasticity, and phylogeny of identified synapses, in: "Systems Approaches to Developmental Neurobiology," P. A. Raymond, S. S. Easter, Jr., and G. M. Innocenti, eds., Plenum Press, New York.

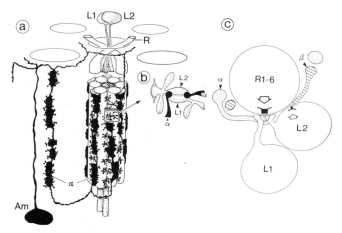

Fig. 1. Schematic diagram of a cartridge in the lamina of the housefly, *Musca*. Only the cellular elements relevant to this review are illustrated. (a) Six photoreceptor terminals (**R1-R6**) surround two central lamina monopolar neurons (**L1, L2**). Processes of amacrine cells (**Am**) are also synaptic participants. (b) Enlarged inset showing the postsynaptic sites of the photoreceptor tetrad synapse viewed in the plane of the presynaptic membrane. One process from each of the two monopolar neurons abuts the presynaptic site at the terminal. Typically, the polar positions of the synaptic tetrad are occupied by two a processes. (c) The synaptic circuit of the afferent tetrad and **L2** feedback synapses. T-shaped presynaptic ribbons are present in both the photoreceptor tetrad synapse (large open arrow), and in the dyad synapse of **L2** feeding back upon a photoreceptor and a ß process from **T1** (small open arrow). (Modified from Shaw and Meinertzhagen, 1986.)

inals (R1-R6) that each originate in a different overlying ommatidium provide the major synaptic input upon two monopolar cells, L1 and L2, at dendritic spines emitted at regular intervals along the longitudinal axis of the monopolar cells' axons. The input synapse is typically a tetrad, with the photoreceptor terminal presynaptic on processes of both L1 and L2, their dendrites or axons, and on two other postsynaptic elements which mostly comprise two alpha (a) processes from a lamina amacrine cell (Fig. 1). Abutting the presynaptic membrane of the terminal is the presynaptic ribbon, a table-shaped organelle comprising a pedestal surmounted by a platform, and forming a characteristic T in cross section (Trujillo-Cenóz, 1965). Postsynaptically, membranous cisternae are clearly recognizable underlying the synaptic membranes of L1 and L2. About 200 such sign-inverting tetrad synapses exist per photoreceptor terminal in *Musca,* constituting the preponderant synaptic class of the lamina neuropil. They are a model for the synapses with multiple postsynaptic elements found widespread in many other nervous systems, both invertebrate (Watson and Burrows, 1982) and vertebrate (Dowling and Boycott, 1966).

Another synaptic class important to this discussion is the feedback synapse from L2 back upon its photoreceptor inputs (Fig. 1). In *Musca,* this is a dyad synapse which, besides the photoreceptor, incorporates a process from the medullary basket cell, T1, as a second postsynaptic element to L2 (Kral and Meinertzhagen, 1989). In addition, many other synaptic classes exist in each cartridge, with populations of varied sizes, of which the more accessible tetrad synapse and its feedback partner are taken to be representative.

DEVELOPMENT

During pupal development the photoreceptors of the retina, which develops from the eye imaginal disc, innervate the growing optic lobe through a pathway already established by the axon bundle of a group of larval photoreceptors (Trujillo-Cenóz and Melamed, 1973). The photoreceptor axons of an individual ommatidium fasciculate together on their way to the lamina through the optic stalk between the eye disc and the brain, but at the lamina they later come to diverge from each other. Eventually each will innervate a different cartridge along with those other photoreceptors from neighboring ommatidia that share the same visual field. Photoreceptor development and axonal morphogenesis occur in four distinct waves (Meinertzhagen, 1973): (1) Commencing in the third instar larva, a rapid phase of fiber growth enables the slender growth cone of the photoreceptor axon to reach the outer surface of the lamina; (2) next, the growth cones expand and their filopodia explore adjacent growth cones in the outer surface of the lamina to generate a shallow plexus; (3) then the growth cones slowly migrate laterally towards the appropriate developing cartridge; (4) finally, the receptor terminals grow centripetally along the monopolar cell axons of the appropriate cartridge, leading to a deepening of the lamina plexus which is completed by about 50% of pupal development. In the crustacean *Daphnia,* at least, it is the incoming photoreceptor axons that cue the sequence of neurite outgrowth from the monopolar cells of the lamina (Macagno, 1984).

An essential feature of the system is that synaptogenesis occurs only after all the major kinetic features of growth in the developing lamina have ceased. By 50% of pupal development, both photoreceptor and monopolar axonal elongation have ceased, while neurites of L1 and L2 have insinuated themselves in the interstices of the surrounding photoreceptor terminals. Two important consequences of these events are that: 1) The axons of both the photoreceptor and monopolar cells are juxtaposed for a long time (20 hrs. or more for *Musca*) before they embark upon synaptogenesis; 2) it is the postsynaptic partners that initiate local growth prior to synapse formation, with dendritic processes from L2 or L1 contacting the presynaptic membrane of the photoreceptor terminal (Meinertzhagen and Fröhlich, 1983; see below). The rules of synapse formation in this system (Meinertzhagen, 1984) may as a result differ somewhat from those in operation at the neuromuscular junction (*c.f.* Bennett and Pettigrew, 1976), where it is the presynaptic nerve that approaches the postsynaptic muscle fiber to initiate synaptogenesis.

Synapse Formation

Adult *Musca* photoreceptor terminals each have about 200 tetrad synapses. By the time synaptogenesis begins at 60% of pupal development, however, very few newly formed synapses are tetrads; rather, they are almost exclusively monads and dyads (Fröhlich and Meinertzhagen, 1983). With further development the frequency of monads decreases while dyads and triads are more frequently encountered. These are finally outnumbered after emergence by tetrads. It is concluded that, during development, there is a progressive assembly of postsynaptic elements at sites destined to become tetrads, resulting in the transformation of a particular synaptic site from a monad to a dyad, then to a triad and finally a tetrad, as new postsynaptic elements are incorporated (Fig. 2). This increase in the number of tetrads formed occurs against the backdrop of a net elimination amongst the total number of synaptic sites during late pupal and early adult development (Fröhlich and Meinertzhagen, 1983).

Tetrad synapse formation not only occurs sequentially, but also obeys very strict combinatorial rules (Fig. 2). First, a postsynaptic element that would normally not be incorporated in the mature tetrad (such as the ß process of T1) is never encountered in a developing synapse. Second, of the range of synaptic combinations that are theoretically possible amongst the elements that do normally participate in normal tetrads, only a fraction actually exists. For instance, a tetrad with two postsynaptic L1 processes is never encountered. Third, the sequential order of adding of postsynaptic elements is constrained. For instance, the first postsynaptic element to be added is either L1 or L2 (with an equal chance for each), but not an amacrine cell process. Because this selectivity occurs in a dynamic system where numerous cell types have the opportunity to encounter each other, there must be active, mutual recognition between pre- and postsynaptic partners for each of the stages of tetrad formation, in a sequence that is unique for each of the possible combinations of the developing synapse. These recognition steps could be concatenated from the sequential feedback of signals proposed to occur in synapse formation elsewhere (Burry et al., 1984), resembling those postulated to explain the maturation of other aspects of synaptic interactions, such as synaptic potentiation (Stevens, 1989). Given the rare occurrence of an erroneous tetrad combination and the absence of any dyads or triads in the adult (Nicol and Meinertzhagen, 1982a), erroneous or incomplete tetrads must presumably be eliminated during development. It is only after tetrad formation is completed that the presynaptic ribbon finally develops and the tetrad enlarges (Meinertzhagen, 1984).

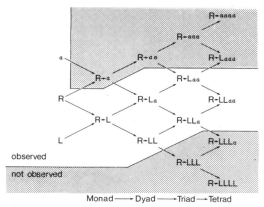

Fig. 2. Combinatorial rules during tetrad formation. Of all the theoretically possible combinations of normally occurring postsynaptic elements, only a fraction is observed (white area). Strict combinatorial rules ensure that other combinations never persist in the adult (stippled area). See text for further explanation. (Modified from Fröhlich and Meinertzhagen, 1983.)

NUMERICAL REGULATION OF SYNAPSES

In adults, the number of synaptic sites maintained by the photoreceptor terminal is highly regulated (Nicol and Meinertzhagen, 1982a). Interestingly, the slight variation ($\pm$ 2 SE are 10% of the mean number in *Musca*) strongly correlates with variations in photoreceptor terminal size. A similar relationship holds for the monopolar cells, L1 and L2, between the size of dendrites and the frequency of their postsynaptic sites (Nicol and Meinertzhagen, 1982b). But what regulates synaptic frequency? Does cell size depend on synaptic frequency, or does cell size dictate synaptic frequency?

This question can be addressed in the *Drosophila* mutant, *gigas* (ME 109; Ferrús and Garcia-Bellido, 1976), in which mutant patches generated by early somatic cross-over in the fly's eye have greatly enlarged corneal facets and ommatidial cells, relative to surrounding areas expressing the wild-type phenotype. Mutant photoreceptor terminals at these sites attain their increased size prior to synaptogenesis with their normal, wild-type interneuron partners in the lamina, and subsequently make significantly more synaptic contacts. Since the size of the synapses does not change in such mutants, it is concluded that receptor terminal size regulates synaptic frequency, but not synaptic size (Meinertzhagen, 1989). The causality of this relationship may be seen in the context of a need to minimize the metabolic cost of producing and maintaining synaptic sites, even if it does not reveal the functional strategy for how the particular number of tetrads itself has been selected.

Cell size may be just one of many factors that regulate synaptic frequency. Variations in the demand for synaptic partnership may also affect the number of synapses. That is, how does the cell's synaptic frequency respond to alterations in the density of presynaptic innervation? Is, for example, the control of synaptic frequency symmetrically distributed between the pre- and postsynaptic cells?

Fortunately, the eye of the fly presents us with a natural experiment to decide on this issue (Fröhlich and Meinertzhagen, 1987). Although a cartridge normally receives innervation from six photoreceptors, there are normally occurring areas of hypo- and hyperinnervated cartridges in the lamina (Meinertzhagen and Fröhlich, 1983; Fröhlich and Meinertzhagen, 1987). A zone of hyper-convergence of photoreceptor terminals occurs at the equator of the lamina - the region where the dorsal and ventral halves of the lamina meet - while fewer than six terminals converge upon cartridges at the lamina's edge.

Quantitative electron microscopic examination of these areas reveals that hyperinnervated cartridges do not have receptor terminals with greatly reduced synaptic frequencies, indicating that it is the postsynaptic neurons that have increased their synaptic inputs to accommodate the extra number of terminals (Fig. 3). On the other hand, cases of extreme hypoinnervation (two receptor terminals) led to an increase (1.5 times) in synaptic frequency of the presynaptic terminal, an increment that was still insufficient however to re-establish a normal number of synaptic sites for the postsynaptic cells

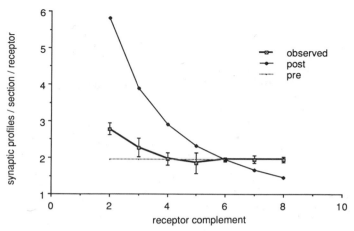

Fig. 3. Effect of different innervation ratios (number of photoreceptor cells contributing to each cartridge) on the synaptic frequencies of the receptor terminals. The frequency of synaptic profiles is expressed per photoreceptor terminal per EM section, as a function of the number of terminals innervating a cartridge (receptor complement). The receptor complement is normally six, but varies from two in the lamina's hypoinnervated circumference to eight in the hyperinnervated equatorial region. Normally innervated cartridges have, on average, two observed synaptic profiles per section per receptor terminal. The stippled horizontal line is the theoretical curve that would be obtained if synaptic frequency were completely determined by the presynaptic cell (i.e. two synaptic profiles per section per receptor terminal, regardless of their number innervating the cartridge). Filled circles indicate the theoretical curve that would be obtained if synaptic frequency were entirely regulated postsynaptically (i.e. the number of synaptic profiles decreases as their number of photoreceptor terminals increases, in order to maintain a constant number of postsynaptic sites). The observed values (open squares) are those expected from a presynaptic control of synaptic regulation, except under extreme cases of hypoinnervation, in which regulation appears to be under both pre- and postsynaptic control. (Redrawn from Fröhlich and Meinertzhagen, 1987.)

hyperinnervation, while both pre- and postsynaptic sites regulate their synaptic frequencies under conditions of extreme hypoinnervation. The differential effects of hypo- and hyperinnervation densities on synaptic frequency may be the reason for the inconsistency of conclusions based on other systems, where typically only one change in innervation ratio has been used (e.g. Constantine-Paton and Norden, 1986).

The changes in innervation ratio did not affect synaptic contact size, only synaptic frequency. Interestingly, the correlation between synaptic frequency and cell size also holds true in the hypo- and hyperinnervated cartridges for both the receptor terminals and the monopolar cell axons (Fröhlich and Meinertzhagen, 1987). Since Nature only varied receptor complement in her experiments, this must mean that synaptic input can affect cell size, which is the opposite conclusion from the previous experiments using *gigas*. The relationship between synaptic frequency and cell size may therefore be bilateral; larger cells may afford to pay for the metabolic cost of a greater number of synapses, but this cost might be partly offset by the formation of those synaptic sites, perhaps by providing a means of procuring more of some essential trophic factor, retrograde or anterograde as the case may be.

Relationship between Synaptic Frequency and Synaptic Size

The assertion that synaptic frequency varies directly with cell size holds only for a comparison between cells of a given age. This relationship is altered for a population of cells examined over a developmental period. Cell size increases during pupal development and peaks in adulthood. By contrast, the synaptic frequency of photoreceptor terminals peaks around 74% of pupal development

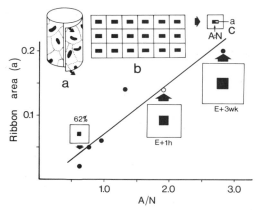

Fig. 4. Synaptic size increases proportionally as synaptic density decreases over the surface of the photoreceptor terminal. The ratio **A/N** is an inverse measure of synaptic density, derived as in b) and c), and illustrated in relation to the mean area of the synaptic ribbon for values obtained at 62% of pupal development, and at 1 hr and 3 wks. after emergence (**E**). Intervening values form a chronological series along the line of the graph, which the synaptic population ascends with increasing age. (a) Stylized representation of the cylindrical photoreceptor terminal with its synaptic sites represented by filled profiles. (b) Unrolled receptor membrane. The synaptic sites and their distributions are nowhere as regularly shaped and evenly spaced *in vivo* as represented here for sake of simplicity. (c) The receptor membrane area can be evenly divided amongst the synaptic sites to provide an imaginary patch of equal size to each. The area of this patch is the total membrane area, **A**, divided by the total number of synaptic sites, **N**. On average, each synaptic ribbon of area **a** presides over a membrane area A/N about ten times larger. Values of **a** and A/N represent population means. (From Meinertzhagen and Fröhlich, 1983.)

and decreases thereafter (Fröhlich and Meinertzhagen, 1983). A similar relationship also applies for the L2 feedback synapse (Kral and Meinertzhagen, 1989). As a result, synaptic density, the number of synapses per membrane area, decreases during development (Fig. 4). During the same period, however, there is a proportional increase in synaptic size, as measured by the area of the synaptic ribbon at the surviving sites (Fröhlich and Meinertzhagen, 1983; Kral and Meinertzhagen, 1989). The important implication is that throughout development the photoreceptor terminal conserves the fraction of its total membrane area (7-10%; Fröhlich and Meinertzhagen, 1983) devoted to synaptic sites (Fig. 4). Whether this holds true in perturbed cases, such as in the mutant *gigas,* is not known.

EFFECT OF ACTIVITY ON SYNAPTIC FREQUENCY

The evidence presented above argues for anatomical features such as cell size and innervation ratios as regulators of synaptic frequency. But the role of activity, or experience, as another factor influencing synaptic regulation has also to be considered. Although it has historically been seen as a driving force exclusively in vertebrate neural development (e.g. Easter et al., 1985), the importance of activity in forming neural circuits in insects has already been documented (Murphey, 1986). For instance, there are clear examples of the sensitivity of visual behavior of flies and bees to environmental conditions during early adult life (Hertel, 1982, 1983; Mimura, 1986, 1987).

In the adult fly's lamina, the strict numerical regulation of photoreceptor synapses does not necessarily imply their lack of plasticity, since animals are reared under standard conditions. Kral and Meinertzhagen (1989) have recently examined whether manipulation of the fly's visual environment could reveal a previously unconsidered plastic capacity in the lamina of the fly's optic lobe. They reared newly eclosed or young adult flies for one or two days in a flickering light and examined the frequency of L2 feedback synapses. The animals had one eye occluded with black paint, so as to

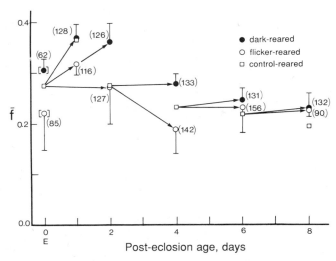

Fig. 5. The effect of rearing conditions on the mean frequencies *(f-bar)* of L2 feedback synapses in the lamina of the fly's optic lobe. Eyes of animals were exposed either to normal (control) light, to flickering light, or to dark, for one or two days at different times after emergence (**E**). The angular divergence between the arrows pointing to dark-reared and flicker-reared values reflects the magnitude of the differential effects of these lighting regimes on synaptic frequency. The arrows originate at the point values that synaptic frequencies in control animals would have attained prior to the commencement of differential rearing conditions, as based on frequencies obtained from normally reared animals of that age. Experimental values may also be compared with values of control animals sacrificed on the same day. Sample size is given by the number of cartridges (in brackets), usually from at least four eyes per sample point. (From Kral and Meinertzhagen, 1989.)

provide a comparison within animals between dark- and flicker-rearing conditions. They found that dark-rearing leads to a higher synaptic frequency than flicker-rearing (Fig. 5), and that maximal differences (30%) are reached by two to four days postemergence, after which the effects of differential rearing attenuate, disappearing by day 8. These results suggest that there is a critical period of plasticity similar to that reported for vertebrates (Rauschecker and Marler, 1987). Rearing for one day instead of two affected the synaptic frequency as well and, in fact, as little as six hours are sufficient to procure differential anatomical effects (Kral and Meinertzhagen, 1989). The effect is also reversible within the limits of the critical period; the consequences of rearing the animal in flicker light on day 1 are completely reversed by dark-rearing the animal on the following day. The size of synaptic contacts does not vary with rearing conditions, but the diameter of L2's axon increases with dark-rearing, providing additional evidence for plasticity.

How does the definition of your critical period as observed in the fly's lamina compare to the mammalian critical period?

The critical period could be defined as the time window during which experience may affect the circuitry of a maturing nervous system. The critical period observed here is in many ways similar to that detected in mammals (Rauschecker and Marler, 1987). It is observable after birth (emergence), when the animal is first exposed to the outside world; it has a finite duration - about 4 days, a fraction of which only is sufficient to alter the nervous system; and the effects are reversible, at least during this period of plasticity. Furthermore, behavioral correlates of a critical period in flies and bees have also been observed (Hertel, 1982; Mimura, 1986). The present study differs from the mammalian protocol insofar as dark-rearing was compared mainly with flicker-rearing conditions and not with normal rearing, because the normal group did not receive comparable visual exposure (see main text). It is also not known whether the differential effects created during the critical period persist well into adulthood, since experimental animals were always examined immediately after the end of the differential rearing condition, which lasted only one or two days. Nevertheless, a critical period for synaptic plasticity was clearly observed in the fly's lamina.

Why use flickering light as a comparison point for dark-rearing, instead of continuous light? And why measure the synaptic frequency of the L2 feedback synapses instead of that of the afferent tetrad synapse?

Flickering light was used because it was thought to be the most relevant visual feature for the lamina, the function of which appears to be to encode visual temporal contrasts (Laughlin, 1981; Shaw, 1984). Initially, we had intended to sample both afferent and feedback synaptic frequencies and, hence, the ratio between these. For technical reasons, the analysis of L2 feedback synaptic frequency was partially incompatible with the analysis of the tetrad frequency, mainly because the L2 synapses occur only at the most proximal lamina depth, where tetrad synapses, which are more evenly distributed throughout the lamina, are not reliably sampled.

Flies reared under normal environmental conditions and sacrificed at different periods after emergence reveal that normal L2 feedback synaptic frequencies vary with adult age (Fig. 5), peaking at day 1 postemergence. Dark-rearing appears to increase synaptic frequency over these normal conditions, but comparison between the normal and either experimental conditions is hampered by the fact that the time of the day at which normal animals were sacrificed for analysis was not controlled between groups. As a result, the normal groups experienced varied periods of daylight prior to sampling for EM, and this could account for at least part of the variability in synaptic frequency between normal and flicker - or dark - rearing, given the rapidity with which detectable synaptic change may occur (6 hrs).

Synaptic Turnover

A system with a fixed synaptic population size may nevertheless be in a dynamic state of regulation, with synapses turning over constantly, in a manner already widely canvassed (Cotman and Nieto-Sampedro, 1984). The fact that synaptic frequencies in the fly were observed both to decrease and increase under different conditions of age and activity, even as late as early adult life, suggests that synapses may break and form continually.

In the fly's lamina, the formation of new synapses has been observed during pupal and early adult development (Fröhlich and Meinertzhagen, 1983). In order to observe the loss of synapses, degeneration has recently been induced experimentally by photoablating photoreceptors (Brandstätter, Shaw, and Meinertzhagen, 1989). As the receptor terminal degenerates, the presynaptic ribbon of the L2 feedback synapse attached to a membrane vesicle internalizes into L2's axoplasm shortly before the synaptic partners disassemble. The recent observation (Brandstätter, unpublished observations) of such organelles in normal adult flies, albeit much less frequently, suggests that synapses may normally not be fixed, but may turn over even in intact cells.

PHYLOGENY

To study the neural development of an organism is also to study a brief instant in the evolution of its species, since phylogeny is merely the summed history of all ontogenies. But what neural features have actually been modified to account for the evolution of new behavioral features between species? Since sets of homologous neurones are not recognizable, it is likely that the introduction of new classes of neurons has been associated with the evolution of new phyla (Shaw and Meinertzhagen, 1986). On the other hand, it appears that another pathway is needed to explain the evolution of behavioral

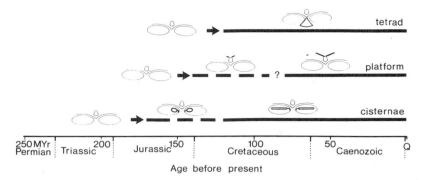

Fig. 6. Evolution of synaptic features at the photoreceptor tetrad synapse of the fly's lamina, represented by
schematic transverse sections of the synapse. In each panel the feature that has undergone modification
is darkened. Upper panel: Synaptic evolution can occur by single-step addition of postsynaptic
elements, such as the insertion about 120 million years ago of two elements derived from a single
amacrine cell process (darkened). Thereby, an ancestral dyad is transformed into the tetrad typical of
advanced Diptera. Middle and lower panels: Evolutionary changes can be more gradual, such as those
that have affected the ultrastructure of synaptic organelles. Middle panel: During phylogeny, the
presynaptic dense bar of the photoreceptor terminal has acquired a surmounting platform that appears to
have expanded during evolution. Lower panel: The large, flattened subsynaptic cisternae of L1 and L2
found in recent flies are not present in forms closest to ancestral Diptera, while they have a small,
tubular shape in intermediate species.

divergences within a phylum, such as have occurred amongst insects. For example, all the families of
Diptera (true flies) examined so far have shown a remarkable homogeneity of cell number, shape, and
position of their photoreceptors, and of the number and morphological classes of their lamina neurons
(Shaw and Meinertzhagen, 1986), even though they show a wide range of visual behavior. By reason
of their consistency, the cells are reasoned to be true evolutionary homologues in all species. What has
been modified during the course of evolution is the synaptic connectivity between the sets of these
previously existing neurons. The photoreceptor tetrad synapse, found amongst evolutionarily more
recent flies (such as *Musca*), seems to have derived from a dyad in forms closer to ancestral Diptera.
This dyad in those species is contributed by the processes of L1 and L2 only (Fig. 6), and the addition
of the two a processes at polar positions to generate the more recent tetrad appears to have occurred in a
single step about 120 million years ago. In addition to the recruitment of novel elements to existing
synapses, other classes of synapses seem to have disappeared. For example, in several species the
amacrine processes are also presynaptic to the photoreceptor terminals, constituting a feedback synapse.
This is, however, absent in *Musca*, implying that evolutionary loss of synaptic elements also occurs
(Shaw and Meinertzhagen, 1986).

Evolution also works at a much finer level, so that there is not only loss or addition of synaptic
classes, but also alterations in the fine structure of synapse-associated sub-cellular organelles (Shaw and
Meinertzhagen, 1986). The presynaptic ribbon of the photoreceptor terminal for instance, although
present throughout Diptera, acquired its surmounting platform only recently in phyletic history (Fig. 6).
Additionally, the postsynaptic cisternae of L1 and L2 at the tetrad synapse, although widely found in
recent Diptera, are smaller in less recent species and absent in those closest to the ancestral forms (Fig.
6).

The major branch points in the evolutionary modifications sustained by neurological features of the
eye and optic lobe correspond closely with the phyletic tree of Diptera established from classical
features, such as wing venation. This implies that neural features are good indicators of evolutionary
change. Indeed, the high selection pressure on neural organization through the adaptive power of its
product, animal behavior, and the large amount of the genome involved in establishing its organization
(John and Miklos, 1988), both suggest the possibility that neural changes may even offer indicators of

phyletic relationships that are more refined, genetically more broadly based, and thus superior to more accessible features of superficial morphology.

Which element was the most likely driving force in the evolution of the tetrad, the presynaptic or the postsynaptic element?

Since it is the postsynaptic elements that are added in the transition from a dyad to a tetrad, it seems more reasonable to assume that they acted as its driving force. A further clue comes from recent work in the visual system of mammals, which suggests that the ultrastructural differentiation of retinal ganglion cell axons, when these are re-routed, is largely regulated by the target cells of the ectopic environment (Campbell and Frost, 1987).

CONCLUSIONS

Analysis of the organization and development of the first optic neuropil of the fly's optic lobe leads to two apparently paradoxical conclusions. On the one hand, the development of the cartridge structure and synapse formation appear to obey very strict organizational rules. The organization of the cartridge is highly stereotypical and its development is very predictable; synaptic combinations and frequencies are almost invariant, and cell type, shape and position are all highly conserved. On the other hand, the developmental processes are highly interactive. Lamina development depends on receptor innervation, synaptogenesis is subject to modifications associated with visual experience and can be modified during the course of evolution; even the adult state may be one of dynamic equilibrium. Thus it may be much more appropriate to consider the organizational rigidity of the lamina as the stability of its dynamically regulated state, with the fine-tuning of the lamina at the synaptic level occurring in response to internal and environmental variables.

What is the functional significance, if any, of: 1) receptor tetrad formation during dipteran evolution, or 2) changes in L2 feedback synaptic frequency as a response to differential visual experience?

The lamina of the fly's optic lobe is concerned primarily with coding of visual temporal contrasts (Laughlin, 1981; Shaw, 1981). The temporal resolution of light contrasts and ultimately of visual behavior may be critical to the sophisticated aerial manoeuvres typical of the flight of advanced Diptera. Since the a processes of amacrine cells are also presynaptic to the photoreceptors in at least some recent Diptera (Shaw and Meinertzhagen, 1986), the addition of these same processes at the receptor afferent synapse may have led to the enhanced temporal resolution of transient visual stimuli through the feedback loop so provided.

The L2 feedback synapse also appears to participate in contrast enhancement by terminating photoreceptor signals that the postsynaptic cells have already seen (Shaw, 1984). If perturbations in L2 synaptic frequencies proportionally alter their synaptic output, then the increased synaptic frequency following dark-rearing may compensate for the low levels of contrasts to which the animal is exposed in the visually deprived environment, by enhancing its ability to detect contrasts. An interesting parallel is found in adult bees deprived of light of specific wavelengths. These bees had fewer synaptic profiles in the terminals of photoreceptors maximally sensitive to those wavelengths, but at their afferent sites (Hertel, 1983). The two sets of results are consonant if one considers that the opposite effects of relative visual deprivation in the bee and the fly act upon two synapses - afferent and feedback - that work in opposite directions to each other.

Given the high degree of cell determination during neurogenesis of the fly's lamina, is it fair to say that there are substantially more stereotypic developmental programs in insects than in mammals?

Not necessarily so. First, the proper development of the lamina is the product of a complex sequence of interactions, and not the execution of a simple, rigid program. In addition, developmental phenomena of cellular induction and regulation, cell death and competition, once thought unique to vertebrates, have been clearly demonstrated in invertebrates (Stent and Weisblat, 1985; Murphey, 1986). The only defining differences between invertebrate and vertebrate neuronal organization may then be cell size, shape and number (Bullock, 1978). The myth of the inflexible invertebrate (Murphey, 1986) was historically related to the influential concept of their identifiable neurons. Individual neurons of invertebrates such as insects can often be recognized invariably by such criteria as cell size, shape and position, as a consequence of which they were thought to arise from and remain part of a rigid program of determination. On the other hand, vertebrate neurons are apparently not recognizable beyond the broad level of cell class (e.g. pyramidal, stellate cells). However, diversification of cell classes is generally associated with increases in cell number and body mass that have occurred during phylogeny, specifically in higher vertebrates (Bullock, 1978) but not restrictively so. As techniques and studies on the identity of cells in the vertebrate CNS become more refined, neuronal classification may well extend correspondingly, as is becoming obvious now for the mammalian retina (Masland, 1988). Thus, the increased cellular redundancy in higher vertebrates may be somewhat offset by the diversification of cell classes, which we only now may begin to perceive.

REFERENCES

Bennett, M. R., and Pettigrew, A. G., 1975, The formation of neuromuscular synapses, *Cold Spring Harb. Symp. Quant. Biol.*, 40:409.

Brandstätter, J. H., Shaw, S. R., and Meinertzhagen, I. A., 1989, Synaptic disassembly after photo-degeneration of receptor terminals in the lamina of the fly's optic lobe, *Soc. Neurosci. Abstr.*, 15:1388.

Bullock, T. H., 1978, Identifiable and addressed neurons in the vertebrates, in: "Neurobiology of the Mauthner Cell," D. Faber and H. Korn, eds., Raven Press, New York, p. 1.

Burry, R. W., Kniss, D. A., and Scribner, L. R., 1984, Mechanisms of synapse formation and maturation, *Curr. Topics Neurosci. Res. Synapses*, 1:1.

Campbell, G., and Frost, D. O., 1987, Target-controlled differentiation of axon terminals and synaptic organization, *Proc. Natl. Acad. Sci. USA*, 84:6929.

Constantine-Paton, M., and Norden, J. J., 1986, Synapse regulation in the developing visual system, in: "Development of Order in the Visual System," S. R. Hilfer, and J. B. Sheffield, eds., Springer-Verlag, New York, p. 1.

Cotman, C. W., and Nieto-Sampedro, M., 1984, Cell biology of synaptic plasticity, *Science*, 225:1287.

Dowling, J. E., and Boycott, B. B., 1966, Organization of the primate retina: Electron microscopy, *Proc. R. Soc. Lond. [Biol.]*, 166:80.

Easter, S. S., Purves, D., Rakic, P., and Spitzer, N. C., 1985, The changing view of neural specificity, *Science*, 230:507.

Ferrús, A., and Garcia-Bellido, A., 1976, Morphogenetic mutants detected in mitotic recombination clones, *Nature*, 260:425.

Fröhlich, A., and Meinertzhagen, I. A., 1983, Quantitative features of synapse formation in the fly's visual system. I. The presynaptic photoreceptor terminal, *J. Neurosci.*, 3:2336.

Fröhlich, A., and Meinertzhagen, I. A., 1987, Regulation of synaptic frequency: Comparison of the effects of hypoinnervation with those of hyperinnervation in the fly's compound eye, *J. Neurobiol.*, 18:343.

Hertel, H., 1982, The effect of spectral light deprivation on the spectral sensitivity of the honeybee, *J. Comp. Physiol. (A)*, 147:365.

Hertel, H., 1983, Change of synapse frequency in certain photoreceptors of the honey bee after chromatic deprivation, *J. Comp. Physiol. (A)*, 151:477.

John, B., and Miklos, G., 1988, "The Eukaryote Genome in Development and Evolution," Allen and Unwin, London.

Kral, K., and Meinertzhagen, I. A., 1989, Anatomical plasticity of synapses in the lamina of the optic lobe of the fly, *Phil. Trans. R. Soc. Lond. [Biol.]*, 323:155.

Laughlin, S., 1981, Neural principles in the peripheral visual systems of invertebrates, in: "Handbook of Sensory Physiology," Vol. VII/6B, Comparative Physiology and Evolution of Vision in Invertebrates, H. Autrum, ed., Springer-Verlag, New York.

Macagno, E. R., 1984, Formation of ordered connections in the visual system of *Daphnia magna*, *Bioscience*, 34:308.

Masland, R. H., 1988, Amacrine cells, *Trends Neurosci.*, 11:405.

Meinertzhagen, I. A., 1973, Development of the compound eye and optic lobe of insects, in: "Developmental Neurobiology of Arthropods," D. Young, ed., Cambridge University Press, Cambridge, p. 51.

Meinertzhagen, I. A., 1984, The rules of synaptic assembly in the developing insect lamina, in: "Photoreception and Vision in Invertebrates," M. A. Ali, ed., NATO ASI Series A, Vol. 74, Plenum Press, New York, p. 635.

Meinertzhagen, I. A., 1989, Fly photoreceptor synapses: Their development, evolution, and plasticity, *J. Neurobiol.*, 20:276.

Meinertzhagen, I. A., and Fröhlich, A., 1983, The regulation of synapse formation in the fly's visual system, *Trends Neurosci.*, 6:223.

Meyerowitz, E. M., and Kankel, D.R., 1978, A genetic analysis of visual system development in *Drosophila melanogaster*, *Dev. Biol.*, 62:112.

Mimura, K., 1986, Development of visual pattern discrimination in the fly depends on light experience, *Science*, 232: 83.

Mimura, K., 1987, Persistence and extinction of the effect of visual pattern deprivation in the fly, *Exp. Biol.*, 46:155.

Murphey, R. K., 1986, The myth of the inflexible invertebrate: Competition and synaptic remodelling in the development of invertebrate nervous systems, *J. Neurobiol.*, 17:585.

Nicol, D., and Meinertzhagen, I. A., 1982a, An analysis of the number and composition of the synaptic populations formed by photoreceptors of the fly, *J. Comp. Neurol.*, 207:29.

Nicol, D., and Meinertzhagen, I. A., 1982b, Regulation in the number of fly photoreceptor synapses: The effects of alterations in the number of presynaptic cells, *J. Comp. Neurol.*, 207:45.

Rauschecker, J. P., and Marler, P., 1987, "Imprinting and Cortical Plasticity: Comparative Aspects of Sensitive Periods," Wiley, New York.

Shaw, S. R., 1981, Anatomy and physiology of identified non-spiking cells in the photoreceptor-lamina complex of the compound eye of insects, especially Diptera, in: "Neurones without Impulses," A. Roberts, and B. M. H. Bush, eds., Society Exptl. Biol. Seminar Series, Vol. 6, Cambridge University Press, Cambridge, UK, p. 61.

Shaw, S. R., 1984, Early visual processing in insects, *J. Exp. Biol.*, 112:225.

Shaw, S. R., and Meinertzhagen, I. A., 1986, Evolutionary progression at synaptic connections made by identified homologous neurones, *Proc. Natl. Acad. Sci. USA*, 83:7961.

Stent, G. S., and Weisblat, D. A., 1985, Cell lineage in the development of invertebrate nervous systems, *Annu. Rev. Neurosci.*, 8:45.

Stevens, C. F., 1989, Strengthening the synapses, *Nature*, 338:460.

Strausfeld, N. J., and Campos-Ortega, J. A., 1977, Vision in insects: Pathways possibly underlying neural adaptation and lateral inhibition, *Science*, 195:894.

Strausfeld, N. J., and Nässel, D. R., 1981, Neuroarchitectures serving compound eyes of Crustacea and insects, in: "Handbook of Sensory Physiology," Vol. VII/6B, "Comparative Physiology and Evolution of Vision in Invertebrates," H. Autrum, ed., Springer-Verlag, New York, p. 1.

Trujillo-Cenóz, O., 1965, Some aspects of the structural organization of the intermediate etina of dipterans, *J. Ultrastruct. Res.*, 13:1.

Trujillo-Cenóz, O., and Melamed, J., 1973, The development of the retina-lamina complex in muscoid flies, *J. Ultrastruct. Res.,* 42:554.

Watson, A. H. D., and Burrows, M., 1982, The ultrastructure of identified locust motor neurone and their synaptic relationships, *J. Comp. Neurol.,* 205:383.

POSTNATAL DEVELOPMENT OF THE CAT'S VISUAL PATHWAYS *

Larry R. Stanford (scribe)   ₁ S. Murry Sherman (lecturer)

Department of Comparative Biosciences and   Department of Neurobiology and
The Waisman Center on Mental Retardation   Behavior
and Human Development   State University of New York
University of Wisconsin   Stony Brook, New York, USA
Madison, Wisconsin, USA

INTRODUCTION

During postnatal life, there is a tremendous increase in both the weight and the volume of the brain. This increase cannot be attributed to the addition of new neurons, since mitosis of neurons is essentially completed by birth. Instead, this is due to the conjoint proliferation and elaboration of dendritic arbors and synaptic connections between neurons; this leads to enormous growth of the synaptic neuropil. The question that will be addressed here is the extent to which the development of these connections can be modified by the environment or, conversely, the extent to which these connections can develop normally in spite of experimental alterations to the normal sensory environment.

Using the visual system as a model, two fundamental questions related to this general problem in neural development are discussed. First, where in the developing visual system do the primary deficits induced by visual deprivation occur? For example, visual deprivation may cause cortical neurons to develop abnormal receptive field properties either because their inputs from the lateral geniculate nucleus develop abnormally, in which case the cortical deficits are secondary, or because these cortical neurons are the first cells in the visual pathways to be directly affected by the deprivation, in which case these deficits are primary. Second, if any of these primary sites can be defined, what are the mechanisms by which the environment affects the developmental processes?

HISTORICAL BACKGROUND

We can begin the discussion of these questions with the classical receptive field studies of neurons in the striate cortex (i.e., the primary visual cortex) by Hubel and Wiesel (1962). These authors found that most of these cortical neurons are binocular, since they could be driven by either eye, although, for any individual cell, the relative strength of the input from each of the two eyes might vary considerably. If the entire population of these cortical cells was considered, however, there was reasonable equivalence in the influence of the inputs from the contralateral and ipsilateral eyes.

Wiesel and Hubel (1963b) found that this balance could be disrupted if one eye was sutured closed soon after birth. In such monocularly deprived animals, nearly all of the neurons in the visual

---

* This chapter to be cited as: Stanford, L. R., and Sherman, S. M., 1990, Postnatal development of the cat's visual pathways, in: "Systems Approaches to Developmental Neurobiology," P. A. Raymond, S. S. Easter, Jr., and G. M. Innocenti, eds., Plenum Press, New York.

cortex could be driven only by input through the eye that had not been sutured closed (i.e., the nondeprived eye). One might then predict that binocular deprivation, or the suturing of both eyes soon after birth, would lead to twice the disruption of monocular deprivation, thereby leading to very few cortical neurons that could be influenced by visual stimuli. Surprisingly, however, rearing with binocular deprivation permitted such neurons to develop clear visual responses and a fairly balanced binocular input, although these neurons did display significant receptive field abnormalities (Wiesel and Hubel, 1965).

These findings led Hubel and Wiesel to the profound insight that deprivation *per se* was not the overriding factor in determining the extent of the abnormalities produced by these rearing conditions, but rather the balance of activity supported by the two eyes interacted in some competitive process to control the development of connections. Thus, as long as the balance of influence between the two eyes was preserved (as in binocular deprivation), many cortical cells could be influenced by both eyes. If, however, this balance was upset, with one eye receiving visual stimulation while the other was largely deprived of it, the result was much more devastating to the development of the visual system.

By examining the time course of the development of these abnormalities, Hubel and Wiesel (1970) also introduced the influential concept of a critical period for visual development. They found that normal development was disrupted only if monocular or binocular lid suture was performed during the first three months or so after birth. Deprivation during this time caused deficits that were permanent, and no amount of normal visual experience outside of the critical period could counteract the effects of visual deprivation during the critical period. Conversely, if the visual deprivation began after this critical period, no disruption of the visual pathways ensued.

In order to determine the location of the primary deficits caused by eyelid suture, Wiesel and Hubel (1963a) also studied the effects of this visual deprivation on neurons in the lateral geniculate nucleus of the thalamus and, to a limited extent, on retinal ganglion cells. They detected no abnormalities in these cells, leading them to conclude that the geniculocortical synapse represented the primary site of disruption caused by rearing with eyelid suture.

At the time Hubel and Wiesel produced the above mentioned seminal work in the early 1960s, the conventional wisdom viewed all retinal ganglion cells and geniculate neurons as divided into symmetrical on- and off- center moieties that were otherwise functionally homogeneous. Newer insights into the effects of visual deprivation were not made until new evidence appeared demonstrating that these cell populations were actually quite heterogeneous. Evidence built on these new insights indicates that, in fact, primary deficits due to early visual deprivation seem to develop at the level of the lateral geniculate nucleus. Therefore, two brief but necessary detours are taken to describe: 1) the organization of the cat's lateral geniculate nucleus; and 2) the concepts of parallel visual pathways that began with the discovery of X and Y cells in the retina by Enroth-Cugell and Robson (1966).

OVERVIEW OF THE CAT'S LATERAL GENICULATE NUCLEUS

Retinogeniculate axons are the axons of retinal ganglion cells that contribute to geniculocortical innervation. They travel through the optic nerve to terminate in the lateral geniculate nucleus, which is the principal visual nucleus of the thalamus. This nucleus is organized into a series of laminae that alternately receive input from one or the other eye. The most dorsal of these, Lamina A, is innervated by the retinogeniculate axons from the contralateral eye. Lamina A1, immediately ventral to Lamina A, receives retinogeniculate input from the ipsilateral eye. Below Lamina A1 lie the C-laminae, individually known as Laminae C, C1, C2, and C3. Lamina C is the most dorsal. Generally, the dorsal strip of lamina C contains relatively large neurons, while the rest of the C-laminae has smaller cells; this has led to the former being designated as the "magnocellular C lamina" and the latter, as the "parvocellular C laminae". Magnocellular C, like Lamina A, receives input from the contralateral eye. In addition to these laminated portions of the lateral geniculate nucleus, there are other regions, the geniculate wing and medial interlaminar nucleus, which are not well understood and need not concern us further in this account.

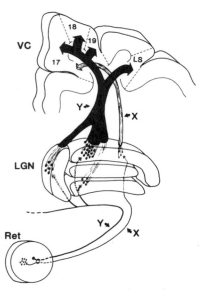

Fig. 1. Hypothetical schematic diagram of the retinogeniculocortical X and Y pathways. For clarity, only the projection pattern from one eye is illustrated. Each retinal Y cell axon diverges to innervate many cells in a number of different regions of the LGN, and each LGN Y cell innvervates a number of visual cortical cells in both the primary visual cortex (Area 17) and other visual cortical areas. Each retinal X cell provides input to relatively fewer LGN neurons in only the A laminae of the LGN. These LGN X cells then innervate cortical neurons in Area 17 only. By virtue of this difference in the divergence of the X and Y pathways, the relatively few Y cells in the retina come to dominate visual cortex. Ret, retina; LGN, lateral geniculate nucleus; VC, visual cortex. (Reprinted from Sherman, 1985a.)

PARALLEL X AND Y PATHWAYS

A number of functionally independent pathways are represented in the lateral geniculate nucleus, two of which, the X and Y pathways, are shown schematically in Figure 1 (for reviews, see Stone et al., 1979; Sherman and Spear, 1982; Sherman, 1985a). These pathways, as mentioned above, were first described as separable subpopulations of retinal ganglion cells by Enroth-Cugell and Robson (1966). More recent studies have convincingly demonstrated that retinal X and Y cells are actually the starting point of two functionally independent, parallel pathways that remain segregated through the lateral geniculate nucleus and through an as yet unspecified number of synaptic zones within the visual cortex. X cells and Y cells in both the retina and lateral geniculate nucleus can be recognized as separate populations on the basis of morphological and physiological criteria. Although it is beyond the scope of this lecture to treat these differences in detail, a brief summary of a few of the distinguishing functional characteristics follows. Most important to the premise under consideration is that X cells have smaller receptive fields than do Y cells. Thus X cells respond best to visual stimuli of high spatial frequency, which represent the fine detail in a visual scene. Y cells are much more responsive to low spatial frequencies and thus signal the basic forms in a visual scene. Also, X cells tend to have smaller somata and thinner axons than do Y cells, and as a consequence X axons conduct more slowly than do Y axons.

Each geniculate neuron is, typically, innervated by a single retinogeniculate axon. There is thus little convergence in retinogeniculate circuitry, which is one reason why the unique X and Y response properties established in retina are preserved among the postsynaptic geniculate neurons. There are, however, many more geniculate neurons than there are retinogeniculate axons, thus requiring considerable divergence in retinogeniculate circuitry.

Given the clear presence of X and Y (and other) parallel pathways involved in the processing of visual information, the key question becomes: What function is served by processing visual information in parallel? The hypothesis proposed here, based on evidence from anatomical, physiological, and behavioral experiments, is that the fundamental and primary visual processing is done by the Y pathway and that the X cell pathway functions secondarily to maximize spatial detail or acuity. Details of this hypothesis can be found in Sherman (1985a), and other hypotheses have also been advanced (Stone et al., 1979; Lennie, 1980). Some of the logic for the hypothesis of primacy of the Y pathway is provided below in consideration of the anatomical organization of the X and Y pathways and in behavioral tests of cats that can be interpreted in the context of these pathways.

Anatomical Organization

Anatomical studies of parallel processing in the cat's visual system require prior knowledge of which neurons to be studied anatomically are X and which are Y. This has usually been accomplished by recording from these neurons intracellularly with a micropipette filled with a marker, usually horseradish peroxidase (HRP), and then iontophoresing the marker into the physiologically defined neuron. This confers the considerable advantage that, for any given neuron, both physiological and morphological data are conjointly obtained.

However, other less direct correlations between structure and function have been made. For example, Wässle and his colleagues (Wässle et al.,1981a,b) were able to establish these relationships for retinal X and Y cells: morphologically, these two cell types are quite distinct, Y cells being associated with the anatomical class of α-cells and X cells, with β-cells. These relationships were confirmed with intracellular marking as described above (Stanford and Sherman, 1985; Stanford, 1987).

More important to the present discussion, however, the ability to equate a functional class of cell to its morphological counterpart provides an anatomical basis for defining the distributions of retinal ganglion cell classes within the retina. That is, with these correlations, it is possible to use the microscope rather than the oscilloscope to determine the actual distributions of cell types. The anatomical approach permits one, in theory, to account for every neuron in realizing the distributions, whereas recording alone is always plagued by problems of unknown electrode sampling errors (see Friedlander et al., 1981; Friedlander and Stanford, 1983). Thus Wässle and his colleagues were able to demonstrate with a reasonable degree of certainty that X cells outnumber Y cells in the retina by approximately 10:1, with this ratio increasing slightly with distance from the area centralis.

While the numerical superiority of retinal X cells would seem to contradict the contention that the Y cell system is the more important of the parallel pathways involved in visual processing, other experiments have shown that the relative strength of the Y pathway is greatly enhanced at successive levels as the visual cortex is reached. For instance, as mentioned above, there is considerable divergence in retinogeniculate connections, and Y axons seem to diverge much more than X axons, at both retinogeniculate and geniculocortical levels. Thus, when individual retinogeniculate axon arbors are labeled with HRP, the Y arbors occupy a much greater volume with many more synaptic boutons than is the case for X arbors. Also, each X axon innervates essentially only Lamina A or A1, while each Y axon typically innervates Lamina A or A1 and, if from the contralateral eye, the magnocellular C-laminae. Since the visual responses of thalamic neurons are dictated by their retinal input, these data suggest that the number of Y cells in the thalamus would be, proportionately, higher than the number in the retina, a conclusion supported by anatomical studies of geniculate X and Y cells.

This relationship between the structure and function of geniculate neurons is somewhat more complex than that described for retinal ganglion cells, primarily because of the morphological diversity of geniculate cells (Friedlander, et al., 1981; Stanford, et al., 1983). The Y cells are a fairly homogeneous group morphologically, and these cells correspond to the class 1 cell defined by Guillery (1966) from Golgi impregnations. The X cells are, anatomically, quite heterogeneous, involving a variety of cell types seen morphologically; they are mostly subsumed under the class 2 type described by Guillery (1966), although a minority (<5%) have the same class 1 morphology as do all Y cells. As noted below, this diversity of X cell morphology may have an interesting developmental basis.

Regardless of the explanation for the structure/function correlations, appreciation of the anatomical identity of geniculate X and Y cells permits the same sort of determination of their distributions as achieved by Wässle and colleagues (Wässle et al., 1981a,b) for retina. Unlike retina, where the X to Y ratio is roughly 10:1, this ratio for geniculate relay cells (i.e., those projecting to cortex) is probably less than 2:1. We estimate that, on average, each retinogeniculate X axon contacts roughly 5 geniculate relay cells while each retinal Y axon innervates 25 to 50 such cells. There has thus been a major relative increase in strength of the Y pathway at the level of the lateral geniculate nucleus, and we suggest that this is largely due to the much more extensive arbors of the retinogeniculate Y axons compared to those of the X axons (see Figure 1). Analogous studies of geniculocortical axon arbors indicate that these axons exhibit a similar relative expansion as seen among retinogeniculate axons: each geniculate Y cell innervates much more cortical territory, and thus presumably many more cortical cells, than does each X axon.

As a result of different extents of axonal arborizations between X and Y axons at both the retinogeniculate and geniculocortical levels, the minority of Y retinal ganglion cells come to dominate cortical processing. This might be explained as follows. The lower spatial frequencies are especially important to the cat for spatial vision, and the Y pathway carries this information to cortex. Thus, much cortex is devoted to its analysis, but a dense retinal grain is not needed to encode these lower frequencies, which explains the low density of Y cells in retina. Once primary spatial vision is handled on the basis of lower frequencies by the Y pathway, the X pathway can be used for specialized functions, such as maximizing spatial resolution based on higher spatial frequencies. The encoding of these higher frequencies does require a relatively dense retinal grain, but since this is of less importance to the cat's spatial vision, less cortex is devoted to its analysis. It must be emphasized that, while this may be a plausible explanation of the functional organization of the X and Y pathways, it is still nothing more than a hypothesis (for further discussion, see Sherman, 1985a).

Behavioral Studies

There is also behavioral evidence in support of this hypothesis. An interesting difference between the X and Y pathways in cats that serves as a background for the behavioral studies is the nature of geniculocortical projections: geniculate X cells innervate only striate cortex, while Y cells, as a population, directly innervate striate cortex plus many areas of extrastriate cortex (see Fig. 1). Thus complete bilateral destruction of striate cortex produces a cat with no cortical representation of the X pathway and some unspecified but significant proportion of the Y pathway still intact. Several investigators have reported that such destriate cats suffer remarkably minor losses of visual function, mostly limited to a mild acuity loss and sensitivity deficits limited to higher spatial frequencies (Berkeley and Sprague, 1979; Lehmkuhle et al., 1982). Thus, part of the Y pathway seems sufficient for fairly normal spatial vision, especially if visual stimuli do not involve fine details.

Although it is getting ahead of the story, early eyelid suture disrupts the development of geniculate Y cells, and it is interesting that such visually deprived cats respond very poorly on tests of visual function, behaving almost as if blind, and their sensitivity losses, as predicted, are considerable for lower spatial frequencies. This, too, is consistent with the relative importance suggested for the Y pathway. Of particular interest is the clear demonstration that normally reared cats with removal of striate cortex see much better than do cats reared with eyelid suture and no such cortical removal. This implies that, no matter how abnormally developed the striate cortex is as a result of early eyelid suture, there must be other primary sites of abnormal development to explain the poor vision suffered by these cats. A global failure of geniculate Y cells to develop is consistent with this logic, since, as shown by Figure 1, such a failure would indirectly affect all areas of visual cortex.

EFFECTS OF REARING WITH EYELID SUTURE

There is now considerable evidence that rearing with eyelid suture prevents the normal development of most, but not all, Y cells in the lateral geniculate nucleus (Sherman et al., 1972; reviewed in Sherman and Spear, 1982). Geniculate X cells develop relatively normally during eyelid suture, as do retinal X and Y cells. This raises two key questions. First, to what extent can abnormal development described in other visual structures be explained as secondary to this failure of Y cell development at the level of the lateral geniculate nucleus? Second, what are the developmental mechanisms that cause Y cells to be differentially affected by these deprivations?

Superior Colliculus

Data that address the first question have been obtained from a number of experiments. However, for the purposes of the present discussion, studies of the superior colliculus can serve to illustrate the effects of abnormally low geniculate Y cell numbers on other visual structures. The superior colliculus is an important subcortical visual structure located dorsally and anteriorly in the midbrain. It has 7 layers, but its dorsal three layers, which are purely visual and homologous to the optic tectum of nonmammalian vertebrates, are all that concern us here. Both retina and visual cortex provide innervation to the superior colliculus.

Hoffmann (1973) investigated the visual inputs to the superior colliculus in cats. He described two pathways from retinal Y cells. One is a direct retinocollicular pathway that mostly crosses in the optic chiasm to innervate the superior colliculus from the contralateral eye. The other is an indirect pathway involving a neuronal chain: a retinal Y cell innervates a geniculate Y cell that, in turn, innervates a corticocollicular cell; this indirect pathway provides fairly balanced, binocular input to the superior colliculus. There is no evidence of any involvement of the X pathway in collicular innervation. In an elegant series of experiments, Wickelgren and Sterling (1969a,b) worked out the effects on the response properties of collicular neurons after lesioning visual cortex and/or rearing cats with eyelid sutures. These authors found that, in normal cats, cells in the SC, much like the corticocollicular cells in the visual cortex, had binocular receptive fields, were most responsive to moving stimuli, and preferred stimuli moving in a particular direction. Removal of visual cortex and early binocular deprivation produced nearly the same changes in collicular neurons. The receptive fields of these cells were now dominated by input from the contralateral eye with no directional selectivity and generally poor responses that showed no preference for moving stimuli. Whatever the explanation for these changes in responses, it is interesting that removal of cortex mimics the effects on the superior colliculus of early binocular deprivation, as if the direct retinocollicular pathway, which would not be directly affected by cortical removal in normally reared cats, develops fairly normally during binocular deprivation.

A similar conclusion is reached from Wickelgren and Sterling's studies of monocular deprivation, although the analysis is more complicated. Such deprivation produces collicular cells that respond essentially only to activation of the nondeprived eye, and they do so fairly normally, regardless of whether the nondeprived eye is ipsilateral or contralateral to the colliculus in question. This mimics the responses of the corticocollicular cells of these cats. However, if the visual cortex is removed in these cats, then the collicular responses are indistinguishable from those seen in normally reared cats with cortex removed (and, as noted, are also the same as that found in binocularly deprived cats). This effect of decortication is most dramatic for the colliculus contralateral to the deprived eye. Here, before the cortical removal, responses are normal, but only to the nondeprived eye, as if the deprived eye had no influence whatsoever over these neurons; after decortication, the deprived eye dominates cellular responses of collicular cells, although direction selectivity and the preference for moving targets is now lost. Whatever the explanation for this dramatic change, one conclusion is clear: removal of cortex eliminates any differences in collicular responses caused by early monocular deprivation. Thus the direct retinocollicular pathway must develop fairly normally in these visually deprived cats, and the abnormalities seen in colliculus are imposed by an abnormal corticocollicular input.

Later experiments by Hoffmann and Sherman (1974, 1975) extended these conclusions. These authors used electrical stimulation to determine the inputs to the superior colliculus in visually deprived cats. They found that the direct retinocollicular pathways developed normally after visual deprivation, but that the indirect pathway involving corticocollicular innervation was interrupted somewhere between the deprived eye and colliculus. Because electrical activation of the corticocollicular pathway produced fairly normal responses in visually deprived cats, Hoffmann and Sherman concluded that the indirect pathway to colliculus was disrupted subcortically. These authors went further to suggest (Hoffmann and Sherman, 1974,1975) that all of the data from these experiments are consistent with the notion that a single primary deficit, occurring among geniculate Y cells, can account for the entire spectrum of deficits shown by Wickelgren and Sterling in the superior colliculus. The abnormalities seen among SC cells are thus secondary to a disruption of the normal Y cell pathway ascending through the lateral geniculate nucleus to the visual cortex.

Retinogeniculate Connections

The mechanisms that cause development of the Y cell pathway to be selectively affected by lid suture have yet to be securely defined. However, anatomical studies of geniculate cells and their retinal afferents in visually deprived cats, using the aforementioned techniques of marking physiologically defined neurons, have provided a number of important insights.

Lateral geniculate nucleus. Some factors that contribute to the Y cell dysfunction following early visual deprivation were suggested by anatomical studies of geniculate neurons (Friedlander et al., 1982). As expected from earlier microelectrode sampling studies, these authors recorded a significant number of cells in the lateral geniculate nucleus of monocularly deprived cats that were quite abnormal, responding poorly, or not at all, to visual stimuli. However, the conduction velocity of the retinal inputs to many of these neurons suggested that they were innervated by Y cell axons. Morphologically, these neurons were unlike any geniculate cells previously described in normal cats, having very small somata and extensive but tortuous and beaded dendritic arbors. More surprisingly, a significant number of geniculate neurons were found that had the morphological features typical of normal Y cells (i.e., class 1) but were driven by input from retinal X cells. As noted above, such class 1 X cells were relatively rare in normal cats (<5%), but 1/3 of geniculate X cells innervated by the deprived eye had such class 1 morphology. Recent evidence indicates that binocular deprivation causes similar abnormalities in structure/function relationships among geniculate neurons (Raczkowski et al., 1982).

Retinogeniculate Axons

These effects of visual deprivation on geniculate neuronal morphology support the notion that the developmental deficits resulting from such deprivation reflect a disruption in the normal retinogeniculate connections. More direct evidence for this notion is provided by intracellular labeling of retinogeniculate arbors in visually deprived cats (Sur et al., 1982). As described above, normal retinogeniculate X axons support terminal arbors that are restricted to the geniculate A-laminae; those of Y axons ramify extensively in the geniculate A-laminae and, if from the contralateral eye, the magnocellular C lamina.

Monocular or binocular deprivation had relatively little effect on the morphology of retinogeniculate X axons, although there was some slight increase in the volume of their terminal arbors. Retinogeniculate Y arbors, on the other hand, were drastically affected by these forms of visual deprivation. The terminal arbors of most Y axons were quite abnormally small in the A-laminae, both in volume and in the number of synaptic terminals. Some of these Y axons, in fact, had no terminal arbor at all in the A-laminae. Curiously, the contralaterally projecting arbors of the deprived Y axons in the magnocellular C-lamina seemed entirely normal, even when no other arbor was present in Lamina A. The observation that deprived Y arbors fail to develop normally where X arbors exist (the A-laminae) but do so where X arbors do not extend (the C-laminae) suggests a developmental mechanism of competitive interactions between these two classes of retinogeniculate arbor, and this is considered more fully below.

Thus the failure of geniculate Y cells to develop normally during eyelid suture can readily be explained on the basis of these morphological abnormalities among retinogeniculate axon arbors. The inability of many Y axons to innervate the A-laminae explains why few Y cells develop, and many poorly responsive cells with abnormal morphology may receive insufficient retinal input to develop normally. Also, the large number of geniculate X cells with class 1 morphology, given the normal association of this morphology with Y inputs, suggests that many geniculate cells that normally would have accepted Y inputs instead receive X inputs, and this is consistent with the abnormally large retinogeniculate X arbors after visual deprivation.

While experiments that compare the structure/function relationships of neurons in the X and Y cell pathways in normal and deprived animals can describe the outcome of disrupting normal visual input, they provide no evidence concerning the reasons why the Y cell pathway is more susceptible to alterations in the normal visual environment. Since it is well documented that these disruptions only occur if lid suture is performed during the critical period, it seems reasonable that some insight into this question might be gained by examining the development of the parallel X and Y pathways.

NORMAL DEVELOPMENT OF RETINOGENICULATE ARBORS

Prenatal Development

The most thorough study of prenatal development of retinogeniculate axons has recently been described by Shatz (1983). By injecting different anatomical tracers in the two eyes of embryonic kittens, Shatz found that the first retinal axons reach the lateral geniculate nucleus at about embryonic day 32 (E32). These first axons to reach the lateral geniculate nucleus emanate exclusively from the contralateral eye. About three days later, axons from the ipsilateral eye invade the lateral geniculate nucleus and, initially, there is considerable overlap in the territory occupied by the axons from the two eyes. Then begins a gradual segregation of the inputs from the two eyes until, at birth, the afferent input to the nucleus is essentially adult-like in terms of its laminar segregation pattern.

By making very small injections of tracer into the optic tract, Sretavan and Shatz (1984) labeled single retinogeniculate axons in prenatal kittens. At first (E43), the ingrowing retinal axons exhibit short, fine side branches along their entire length within the lateral geniculate nucleus. During the next few prenatal weeks, these side branches eventually disappear as a mature arbor forms that is strictly limited to its appropriate laminar pattern. Unfortunately, it has not yet proved technically feasible to determine whether the axons studied by Shatz and her co-workers prenatally arose from retinogeniculate X axons, Y axons, or both. Therefore, studies of prenatal development cannot directly address the question of whether differences in the embryonic development of retinogeniculate X and Y axons contribute to the more damaging effects of early visual deprivation on the Y pathway. However, studies of postnatal development can and do.

Postnatal Development

The morphological features of retinogeniculate arbors in kittens at various postnatal ages have been recently described, and at the postnatal ages tested, it has been possible to identify X and Y axons (Sur et al., 1984; Friedlander et al., 1985). Retinogeniculate X axons develop much earlier than Y axons. The X axons already form large arbors in the A-laminae by three weeks postnatal (the earliest age tested), and there is a slight, but significant, decrease in their terminal arbor sizes until twelve weeks after birth, by which time the adult pattern is attained. In contrast at three weeks of age few Y axons have yet even reached the A-laminae, although many from the contralateral eye already have begun to form their arbors in the C- laminae. During the succeeding weeks, there is a monotonic increase in the size of these Y arbors in the A-laminae until, like the X axons, they attain their adult form at approximately 12 weeks of age. This suggests that retinogeniculate X axons develop and mature much earlier than do Y axons, and this conclusion is consistent with other studies of development of retinal ganglion cells and optic tract axons (Walsh et al., 1983; Ramoa et al., 1988).

The following hypothesis is suggested to account both for this pattern of postnatal retinogeniculate development as well as the effects of visual deprivation on this development (reviewed in Sherman, 1985b). Retinogeniculate X axons innervate the lateral geniculate nucleus first, and, as the only retinal innervation in the A-laminae, they are able to innervate geniculate cells fairly indiscriminately. They thus have large arbors by 3 weeks postnatal. As the later developing Y axons enter the A-laminae, they must compete with the already present X arbors for control of geniculate cells, and they compete successfully only for synaptic space on morphological class 1 neurons. Thus, under normal conditions, the vast majority of class 1 cells are Y, and X axons innervate all the remaining geniculate cells. Visual deprivation somehow disrupts this process by placing the later developing retinogeniculate Y axons at a competitive disadvantage; it is interesting in this regard that the elaboration of these retinogeniculate Y arbors in the A-laminae occurs nearly entirely during the critical period as defined by Hubel and Wiesel (1970; see above). Although the rules that govern this presumed competition are far from clear, the fact that retinogeniculate Y axons are able, during visual deprivation, to establish normal terminal arbors in the C-laminae, which is the only major site in the lateral geniculate nucleus that retinal X cells normally do not innervate, strongly suggests that competitive interactions do, in fact, underlie this developmental process.

Data from an analogous series of experiments in which one eye was removed in kittens at various ages also lend support to this notion that the developmental time course of retinogeniculate X and Y axons is important in the regulation of their competitive interactions.

Postnatal Enucleation

In one set of studies, the projections of retinogeniculate axons were examined in cats that had one eye removed soon after birth (Guillery, 1972; Hickey, 1975). Retinogeniculate axons from the remaining eye "sprouted"to innervate geniculate laminae that normally received retinal input from the enucleated eye (i.e., lamina A if the remaining eye was ipsilateral, and lamina A1, if contralateral). Such sprouting only occurred if the enucleation was performed within the first 10 postnatal days. Garraghty et al. (1986b) later demonstrated that all of this sprouting was due to retinogeniculate Y axons: every X axon from the remaining eye innervated only the proper lamina, and every Y axon extended part of its arbor across the interlaminar zone into the inappropriate lamina.

Several explanations were proposed for this clear difference between retinogeniculate X and Y axons. One was the possibility that, due to the rapid later growth of these Y axons, they enjoyed a competitive advantage in the ability to occupy the denervated geniculate zones. To test this, Garraghty et al. (1986a) tried to place the developing Y axons at a disadvantage by suturing closed the remaining eye when the other was,removed. In such cats, the retinogeniculate X arbors were still strictly limited to their appropriate laminae. That the retinogeniculate Y axons were indeed at a disadvantage during this rearing condition seems evident, because very little of their arbors formed in the appropriate laminae where X axons already had a foothold; instead, most of these Y arbors were devoted to the inappropriate laminae, while only a small part of these arbors invaded inappropriate laminae when the remaining eye was left open. Thus even when given an advantage, X axons do not sprout.

Prenatal Enucleation

If competitive advantage does not explain why Y but not X axons can sprout, then perhaps it has to do with the age of enucleation. It might be that the later maturing Y axons still possess the capacity to sprout for a week or so after birth, at which time their advanced maturity precludes such plasticity, and the earlier maturing X axons have already passed this maturation stage by birth. Garraghty et al. (1988) tested this possibility by investigating retinogeniculate development in cats that had been monocularly enucleated at E44. At this early age, even X axons should still be sufficiently immature to sprout unless such ability is never conferred to them. Although the prenatal enucleations so obscured geniculate lamination patterns that clear interpretation of the data is difficult, the innervation patterns of these cats are nonetheless strikingly similar to those obtained in postnatally enucleated cats: retinogeniculate X arbors are confined to a zone in the A-laminae that seems appropriate for their eye of origin, while many of the Y arbors span the entire A-laminae.

This inability of retinal X cell axons to sprout, therefore, seems not to be due to their earlier development. While the mechanisms governing sprouting are unknown, these data suggest that fundamentally different rules might apply to the X and Y pathways in terms of retinogeniculate development. Perhaps the X pathway, being the first to innervate the lateral geniculate nucleus, is somehow constrained to terminate only in laminae appropriate to the eye of origin. This might be necessary, for instance, to insure that the normal lamination pattern is formed during the early stages of geniculate development. Later arriving pathways, such as the Y pathway, might then be shaped more by competitive interactions, following rules that are less rigid than those defining the development of the X axons that establish lamination in the geniculate.

CONCLUSIONS

Some of the most important conclusions from the experiments described above are as follows. First, if the processes underlying the development of the visual pathways are to be understood, an appreciation of the heterogeneity in the pathway from the retina through the lateral geniculate nucleus to the visual cortex is essential. There is now ample evidence that the development of the X and Y pathways are governed by very different mechanisms. Second, the hypothesis that all primary sites of abnormalities due to early visual deprivation are cortical seems untenable in light of the data that have become available since the early studies of Hubel and Wiesel (1962, 1963, 1965, see above). A major primary abnormality is induced by visual deprivation in the retinogeniculate connections of the Y pathway. Finally, although the reasons for the relative susceptibility of the Y pathway to perturbations of the developing visual environment have not yet been defined, the experiments described here do suggest that the late development of the retinogeniculate Y axons' and the fact that they must compete during the critical period with the already established X axons' contributes to the severity of the deficits seen in the Y pathway of visually deprived cats.

What criteria were used to define X and Y cell responses?

A number of different response properties were used to distinguish between X cells and Y cells. First, it should be mentioned that X and Y cells, in both the retina and the lateral geniculate nucleus, have an antagonistic center/surround receptive field organization. For both of these classes of cells, also, the elements that contribute to the center and surround sum stimuli fairly linearly. That is, for an "on" center cell, the output of the cell will be the sum of the illumination of the "on" center and the antagonistic "off" surround. Y cells, however, have an additional, non-linear component within their receptive fields. One commonly used test to distinguish Y cells involves using a stimulus that can evoke this nonlinear response; this is usually done by flashing a relatively high spatial frequency sine-wave grating on the receptive field and observing the nonlinear response. This typically appears as a "doubling" response, a response at twice the temporal rate of the stimulus. Unlike the linear component in a Y cell's receptive field, the doubling response is independent of the spatial phase, or position, of the grating within the receptive field. The presence of a nonlinear component, which produces this doubling, is thus one criterion used to distinguish X from Y cells in our experiments. Another characteristic that can separate these two groups of cells is receptive field center size; at any given retinal eccentricity, Y cells have receptive field centers that are approximately three times larger than those of X cells. Finally, axonal conduction velocity can also be used to distinguish X and Y cells. Y cells have axons that conduct action potentials at 30 to 40 meters per second while X cell axons conduct only at approximately one half that velocity.

You discussed data from studies that recorded from X cells and Y cells in kittens and in visually deprived cats. Which response properties can also be used to distinguish X and Y cells in these animals?

That actually presents somewhat of a problem. While we have well documented criteria for making this distinction in normal adult animals, some question always remains about how reliably the criteria used in the adult animal can distinguish cell groups in an immature system, or one that has been experimentally modified. We can only address this issue indirectly by citing some of the results of the experiments discussed here. In three to four week old kittens, for instance, which represent the earliest developmental age of the animals used in these experiments, there was a very good correlation among the responses normally associated with the two cell classes. Perhaps the strongest evidence, however, comes from those experiments in which retinal ganglion cell axons were identified in the optic tract and subsequently filled with horseradish peroxidase. When these experiments were performed in kittens, the retrogradely filled cell bodies demonstrated in the retina showed the same correlation between physiological and morphological cell class that had previously been demonstrated in adult cats. That is, the Y cells displayed alpha morphology, and the X cells, beta morphology.

Are there any abnormalities in visually deprived cats in the X cell pathway in either the lateral geniculate nucleus or the visual cortex?

There seems to be very little effect of these rearing paradigms on the X pathway. The only effect that has been documented at this time is a slight increase in receptive field center size among retinal and geniculate X cells. It should be emphasized, however, that there is some controversy concerning this increase in receptive field size among X cells; some laboratories have reported this effect while others have been unable to detect any change in the receptive fields of these neurons.

REFERENCES

Berkeley, M.A. and J.M. Sprague, 1979, Striate cortex and visual acuity functions in the cat, *J. Comp. Neurol.*, 187:679.

Enroth-Cugell, C. and J.G. Robson, 1966, The contrast sensitivity of retinal ganglion cells of the cat, *J. Physiol. (London)*, 187:517.

Friedlander, M.J., C. S. Lin, L.R. Stanford, and S. Murray Sherman, 1981, Morphology of functionally identified neurons in the lateral geniculate nucleus of the cat, *J. Neurophysiol.*, 46:80.

Friedlander, M.J., K.A.C. Martin, and C. Vahle-Hinz, 1985, The structure of the terminal arborizations of physiologically identified retinal ganglion cell Y axons in the kitten, *J. Physiol. (London)*, 359:293.

Friedlander, M.J. and L.R. Stanford, 1984, The effects of monocular deprivation on the distribution of cell types in the LGNd: A sampling study with fine-tipped micropipettes, *Exp. Brain Res.*, 53:451.

Friedlander, M.J., L.R. Stanford, and S. Murray Sherman, 1982, Effects of monocular deprivation on the structure/function relationship of individual neurons in the cat's lateral geniculate nucleus, *J. Neurosci.*, 2:321.

Garraghty, P.E., C.J. Shatz, D.W. Sretavan, and M. Sur, 1988, Axon arbors of X and Y retinal ganglion cells are differentially affected by prenatal disruption of binocular inputs, *Proc. Natl.. Acad. Sci. USA*, 85:7361.

Garraghty, P.E., M. Sur, and S.M. Sherman, 1986a, The role of competitive interactions in the postnatal development of X and Y retinogeniculate axons, *J. Comp. Neurol.*, 251:198.

Garraghty, P.E., M. Sur, R.E. Weller, and S.M. Sherman, 1986b, The morphology of retinogeniculate X and Y axon arbors in monocularly enucleated cats, *J. Comp. Neurol.*, 251:216.

Guillery, R.W., 1966, A study of Golgi preparations from the dorsal lateral geniculate nucleus of the adult cat, *J. Comp. Neurol.*, 128:21.

Guillery, R.W., 1972, Experiments to determine whether retinogeniculate axons can form translaminar collateral sprouts in the dorsal lateral geniculate nucleus of the cat, *J. Comp. Neurol.*, 146:407.

Hickey, T.L., 1975, Translaminar growth of axons in the kitten dorsal lateral geniculate nucleus following removal of one eye, *J. Comp.Neurol.*, 161:259.

Hoffman, K.-P., 1973, Conduction velocity in pathways from retina to superior colliculus in the cat: a correlation with receptive field properties, *J. Neurophysiol.*, 36:409.

Hoffman, K.-P., and S.M. Sherman, 1974, Effects of early monocular deprivation on visual input to cat superior colliculus, *J. Neurophysiol.*, 37:1267.

Hoffman, K.-P., and S.M. Sherman, 1975, Effect of early binocular deprivation on visual input to cat superior colliculus, *J. Neurophysiol.*, 38:1049.

Hubel, D.H., and T.N. Wiesel, 1962, Receptive fields, binocular interaction, and functional architecture in the cat's visual cortex, *J. Physiol. (London)*, 160:106.

Hubel, D.H. and T.N.Wiesel, 1970, The period of susceptibility to the physiological effects of unilateral eye closure in kittens, *J. Physiol. (London)*, 206:419.

Lehmkuhle, S., K.E. Kratz, and S.M. Sherman, 1982, Spatial and temporal sensitivity of normal and amblyopic cats, *J. Neurophysiol.*, 48:372.

Lennie, P., 1980, Parallel visual pathways, *Vision Res*, 20:561.

Raczkowski, D., L.R. Stanford, and S.M. Sherman, 1982, Binocular lid suture causes the development of abnormal structure/function relationships among lateral geniculate neurons of the cat, *Soc. Neurosci. Abst.*, 8:816.

Ramoa, A.S., G. Campbell, and C.J. Shatz, 1988, Dendritic growth and remodelling of cat retinal ganglion cells during fetal and postnatal development, *J. Neurosci.*, 8:4239.

Shatz, C. J., 1983, The prenatal development of the cat's retinogeniculate pathway, *J. Neurosci.*, 3:482.

Sherman, S.M., 1985a, Functional organization of the W-, X-, and Y-cell pathways: a review and hypothesis, in: "Progress in Psychobiology and Physiological Psychology," Vol. 11, Sprague, J.M., and Epstein, A.N., eds., Academic Press, New York, p. 233.

Sherman, S.M., 1985b, Development of retinal projections to the cat's lateral geniculate nucleus, *Trends Neurosci.*, 8:350.

Sherman, S.M., K.-P. Hoffmann, and J. Stone, 1972, Loss of a specific cell type from dorsal lateral geniculate nucleus in visually deprived cats, *J. Neurophysiol.*,35:532.

Sherman, S.M., and P.D. Spear, 1982, Organization of the visual pathways in normal and visually deprived cats, *Physiol. Rev.*, 62: 738.

Sretavan, D.W., and C.J. Shatz, 1984, Prenatal development of retinogeniculate axons during the period of segregation, *Nature*, 308:845.

Stanford, L.R., 1987, X-cells in the cat retina: Relationships between the morphology and physiology of a class of cat retinal ganglion cells, *J. Neurophysiol.*, 58:940.

Stanford, L. R., M.J. Friedlander, and S.M. Sherman, 1983, Morphological and physiological properties of geniculate W-cells of the cat: A comparison with X- and Y-cells, *J. Neurophysiol.*, 50:582.

Stanford, L.R. and S..M. Sherman, 1984, Structure/function relationships of retinal ganglion cells in the cat, *Brain Res.*, 297:381.

Stone, J., B. Dreher, and A. Leventhal, 1979, Hierarchical and parallel mechanisms in the organization of visual cortex, *Brain Res. Rev.*, 1: 345.

Sur, M., A.L. Humphrey, and S.M. Sherman, 1982, Monocular deprivation affects X- and Y-cell retinogeniculate terminations in cats, *Nature,* 300:183.

Sur, M., R.E. Weller, and S.M. Sherman, 1984, Development of X- and Y-cell retinogeniculate terminations in kittens, *Nature*, 310:246.

Walsh, C., E.H. Polley, T.L. Hickey, and R.W. Guillery, 1983, Generation of cat retinal ganglion cells in relation to central pathways, *Nature*, 302:611.

Wässle, H., B.B. Boycott, and R.B. Illing, 1981a, Morphology and mosaic of on- and off-beta cells in the cat retina and some functional considerations, *Proc. R. Soc. Lond. [Biol.]*, 212:177.

Wässle, H., L. Peichl, and B.B. Boycott, 1981b, Morphology and topography of on- and off-alpha cells in the cat retina, *Proc. R. Soc. Lond. [Biol.]*, 212: 157.

Wickelgren, B.G., and P. Sterling, 1969a, Influence of visual cortex on receptive fields in the superior colliculus of the cat, *J. Neurophysiol.*, 32:16.

Wickelgren, B.G., and P. Sterling, 1969b, Effects on the superior colliculus of cortical removal in visually deprived cats, *Nature*, 224:1032.

Wiesel, T.N. and D.H. Hubel, 1963a, Effects of visual deprivation on morphology and physiology of cells in the cat's lateral geniculate body, *J. Neurophysiol.*, 26, 978.

Wiesel, T.N., and D.H. Hubel, 1963a, Effects of visual deprivation on morphology and physiology of cells in the cat's lateral geniculate body, *J. Neurophysiol.*, 26:978.

Wiesel, T.N., and D.H. Hubel, 1963b, Single-cell responses in striate cortex of kittens deprived of vision in one eye, *J. Neurophysiol.*, 26: 1003.

Wiesel, T.N., and D.H. Hubel, 1965, Comparison of the effects of unilateral and bilateral eye closure on cortical unit responses in kittens, *J. Neurophysiol.*, 28:1029.

THEORETICAL APPROACHES AND CELLULAR ANALOGS OF FUNCTIONAL PLASTICITY IN THE DEVELOPING AND ADULT VERTEBRATE VISUAL CORTEX [*]

Daniel Shulz (scribe), Yves Frégnac (lecturer)

Laboratoire de Neurobiologie et
Neuropharmacologie du Développement
Université Paris-Sud,
91405 Orsay cedex, FRANCE

INTRODUCTION

Visual cortical neurons acquire their functional identity through a number of developmental events, particularly those occurring postnatally, when the animal starts to explore its outside environment. Once the integrative properties of neurons are expressed, do they process incoming signals in the same way throughout life, or can they be considered as adaptive devices capable of modifying their functional properties? This chapter will discuss the importance of activity dependent processes involved in functional plasticity, and the determination of the learning capacities of cells in the primary visual cortex of developing and adult mammals.

Three types of approaches will be presented in the study of visual cortical epigenesis. The first step is theoretical, and consists in defining rules of synaptic plasticity which could account for the rapid functional changes observed during a critical postnatal period in kitten visual cortex (area 17). The hypothesis is that co-activity, i.e., temporal correlation between pre- and post-synaptic activity or between activities in different afferent fibers, controls synaptic efficiency changes. A specific algorithm of synaptic plasticity ("covariance hypothesis"), which has been applied previously in cerebellum (Sejnowski, 1977) and in visual cortex (Bienenstock et al., 1982), has been used to simulate the functional reorganization due to manipulation of visual input during postnatal development, and the predictions that result will be discussed.

A second approach, based on electrophysiological recordings in vivo, is a biological implementation of the covariance algorithm, and demonstrates cellular analogs of visual cortical plasticity. Four protocols have been devised, where locally imposed patterns of activity in the cortex of anesthetized and paralyzed animals induce long-term functional changes during the time of recording of individual neurons. The common aspect of these protocols is the external control (by the experimenter) of the temporal contingency between given characteristics of the visual message and imposed levels of post-synaptic activity of the recorded cell.

Finally, the third approach addresses the synaptic nature of the functional modifications. Possible biophysical mechanisms, which could explain how changes in the co-activity level increase or decrease the efficiency of transmission of neocortical synapses, will be outlined.

---

[*] This chapter to be cited as: Shulz, D., and Frégnac, Y., 1990, Theoretical approaches and cellular analogs of functional plasticity in the developing and adult vertebrate visual cortex, in: "Systems Approaches to Developmental Neurobiology," P. A. Raymond, S. S. Easter, Jr., and G. M. Innocenti, eds., Plenum Press, New York.

STRATEGIES FOR THE STUDY OF CELLULAR PLASTICITY

Cellular plasticity is defined here as the intrinsic capacity of a neuron to change its reactive properties as a function of past activity. Although the function of sensory neurons is classically presented in almost perceptual terms, attempts in vertebrates to relate changes of cellular function with changes in perceptual performances or behavior are far less demonstrative than those made in invertebrates. For instance, Alkon and collaborators, studying the cellular basis of classical conditioning in the marine slug *Hermissenda*, could show that artificial pairing of an intracellular current with photic stimulation of a single photoreceptor of type B is a sufficient condition to induce a predicted behavioral change (such as foot contraction) indicative of the establishment of a conditioned response (Farley et al., 1983; Alkon, 1988). In this invertebrate semi-intact preparation, cellular changes are causally related to behavioral learning. This is not the case in vertebrates, where certain rearing procedures known to dramatically affect the representation of orientation preference in visual cortex do not relate to changes in the global perception of orientation by the organism. One should note, however, that traces of conditioning procedures suggesting cellular learning can be found in the visual and associative areas (Spinelli and Jensen, 1979), but the distributed nature of transmission of information in the central nervous system of vertebrates explains the relative failure to establish causal links between cellular learning and expressed changes in behavior.

Changes in the integrative properties of visual cortical cells are under the influence of spontaneous and evoked activity. In the developing kitten, before eye-opening, visual pathways receive a tonic influence from spontaneously active elements in the retina (dark discharge). This level of tonic activity is filtered along the retino-geniculo-cortical pathway, and it is not surprising that in the visual cortex, where the level of spontaneous activity is low and where most post-synaptic firing corresponds to activation from the visual environment, sensitivity to visual experience is maximal. Classically, three different roles have been attributed to visual activity in the first stages of development. The functional verification hypothesis introduced by Hubel and Wiesel (1963) implies that visual activity is simply validating some connections which are already present. Conversely, Pettigrew and co-workers (Pettigrew et al., 1973; Pettigrew and Garey, 1974) proposed in the seventies that oriented growth processes could be under the influence of evoked activity, and that consequently neuronal selectivity in visual cortex was the mirror of sensory experience. Finally, the selectionist point of view, developed by Changeux and collaborators (Changeux et al., 1973; Changeux and Danchin, 1976), considers that, after the initial establishment of a supernumerary envelope of connections under strict genetic constraints, activity will selectively stabilize certain synapses and lead to the loss of other contacts.

Functional epigenesis at the cortical level is generally thought to occur during a critical period of postnatal development (Hubel and Wiesel, 1970, Wiesel, 1982). Factors critically involved in the mechanisms of cellular plasticity should then be different in kittens and adults. Does this mean that adult neurons have lost the capacity to change their properties, or does their mature microenvironment no longer provide them the key to express functional changes? A first difference between a developing and an adult visual cortex is the level of inhibitory constraints. The removal of inhibition by bicuculline in adult visual cortex induces, in otherwise regular spiking cortical neurons (Artola and Singer, 1987), the same bursting behavior that is present in most neurons in the young animal (Kato et al., 1988), and makes them susceptible to undergo plastic changes. A second difference could be that glial environment changes with age, as was recently suggested in a preliminary study by Müller and collaborators (1988) who could restore sensitivity to visual experience outside the critical period by grafting glia from kitten into adult visual cortex. A third possibility is that all the machinery for cellular plasticity is still present in the adult, but that the proper extraretinal gating signals are no longer present. For instance, it has been reported that the laminar pattern of noradrenergic projections in visual cortex may vary with age. Thus, one of the main problems in understanding critical periods could be in determining the nature of gating factors controlling the transitions in the internal state of a neuron, from a passive relay mode to an adaptive mode.

IN SEARCH OF AN ALGORITHM OF SYNAPTIC PLASTICITY

The functional architecture of adult visual cortex reveals a built in tendency of the network to reinforce functional proximity and neighborhood relationships. Neurons in the same vertical column as well as in distant isofunctional columns tend to be co-active, as shown by cross-correlation studies which reveal coherence or phase-locked activity at distant points in the cortex sharing the same functional specificity (Gray and Singer, 1989). The regularity seen in the visual cortical assembly, which expresses specific co-activity states, could be the result of intrinsic temporal correlations within the visual pathway which are found in neighboring cells of the same functional type in the retina (Mastronarde, 1983). Co-activity is probably implicated in the process by which connections are reinforced or weakened.

The idea that co-activity controls the coupling between neurons was already present in the principle of association proposed by William James in 1890. This founder of psychophysiology stated that "when two elementary brain processes are active together or in immediate succession, one of them, on re-occurring, tends to propagate its excitement into the other". This general rule was restated more precisely by Donald Hebb in 1949, who proposed that maintained temporal correlation between pre- and post-synaptic activity leads to increase in the efficiency of synaptic transmission. In order to avoid saturation of the synaptic efficiencies due to spontaneously occurring coincidences in activity, different normalization rules were added to Hebb's principle (Marr, 1969; von der Malsburg, 1973; Stent, 1973), most of which result in spatial competition between converging afferents onto the same target cell.

The integrative function of a neuron, i.e. the way a cell integrates incoming signals in the different afferent fibers, can be defined by assuming that the post-synaptic activity is the sum of inputs amplified by the corresponding synaptic efficiencies minus a certain threshold activity. This formal neuron, considered to be a simple transmitting device, can be made adaptive by allowing synaptic efficiencies to vary as a function of pre- and post-synaptic signals and as a function of time. In order to describe changes in synaptic efficiency, Sejnowski in 1977 and Bienenstock and collaborators in 1982 introduced a refined version of Hebb's postulate, which uses covariance between pre- and post-synaptic activities, and which bears its own normative property. In this algorithm, the instantaneous pre- and post-synaptic terms are compared with the mean pre- and post-synaptic activities respectively, and the product of their differences (covariance) gives the sign and amplitude of the predicted synaptic changes.

WHY DO VISUAL CORTICAL CELLS NEED AN EXTRARETINAL "TEACHER?"

Functional properties of visual cortical cells are very stable in the anesthetized and paralyzed preparation. Attempts to induce modifications of the integrative power of a single neuron by repetitive visual stimulation have shown the difficulty in inducing long-lasting and reliable changes in orientation selectivity and ocular dominance under those conditions (Pettigrew et al., 1973; Imbert and Buisseret, 1975; Frégnac and Bienenstock, 1981; review in Frégnac and Imbert, 1984). Several types of experimental approaches (Kasamatsu and Pettigrew, 1978; Buisseret et al., 1978; Freeman and Bonds, 1979; Geiger and Singer, 1986) indicate that extraretinal activation is a necessary requisite to induce functional modifications, and that perhaps a certain threshold in the activity of the post-synaptic site must be reached in order to induce such changes (von der Malsburg, 1973). This requirement is probably fulfilled in the alert animal having a normal visuo-motor experience, including extraretinal signals and attentional processes, which should gate cortical plasticity.

There are two kinds of extraretinal gating signals which could be of importance for expressing plasticity. First, Kasamatsu and collaborators provided appealing but controversial evidence (review in Kasmatsu, 1983 and Frégnac, 1987) suggesting that the ascending noradrenergic system might be involved in maintaining the sensitivity of the visual cortex to monocular deprivation during the critical period. Second, eye movements and mainly extraocular proprioceptive signals running through the ophthalmic branch of the trigeminal nerve appear to be crucial in gating visual cortical plasticity. For instance, restoration of orientation specificity in dark-reared kittens following a brief flash of visual experience depends on ocular motility (Buisseret et al., 1978) and on extraocular muscle proprioception (Trotter et al., 1981; 1983). Trotter, Frégnac and collaborators described—both in normally reared and visually deprived kittens—critical periods for the unilateral (Trotter et al., 1987; Graves et al., 1987) and bilateral (Graves et al., 1987) section of the ophthalmic branch of the trigeminal nerve, which fall within the temporal limits of the classical critical period of sensitivity to monocular deprivation (Hubel and Wiesel, 1970). Consequently extraocular proprioceptive inflow appears to play a role in the maturation and plasticity of visual cortical receptive properties (reviewed in Frégnac, 1987).

One of the few experimental paradigms in which changes in ocular dominance or orientation preference could be obtained in the anesthetized and paralyzed preparation was the pairing of visual stimulation with passive eye movements (Freeman and Bonds, 1979; Frégnac and Bienenstock, 1981). However, this associative procedure concerns the whole cortex, and all neurons were probably conditioned at the same time. Another type of approach used in order to change functional properties of individual visual cortical cells during the time of recording, was to locally mimic the gating action of extraretinal signals, which are lacking in the anesthetized and paralyzed animal, by modulating at the site of recording the temporal correlation between the afferent visual activity and the post-synaptic activity of the recorded cell.

CELLULAR ANALOGS OF VISUAL CORTICAL PLASTICITY *IN VIVO*.

In order to test predictions of the covariance algorithm, we developed, in collaboration with Elie Bienenstock, an electrophysiological paradigm that allowed us to produce, during the time of recording of one cell, functional changes analogous to those classically described during visual cortical development (Frégnac et al., 1988; Frégnac and Shulz, 1989; Frégnac et al., 1989). The control of the temporal correlation between the afferent visual message and the post-synaptic activity was obtained by the association of a iontophoretic current (less than +/- 10 nA) through the juxtacellular recording electrode (2-20 MOhm, 3M KCl) with the presentation of a given stimulus within the receptive field of the cell. Four different properties intrinsic to visual cortical organization were tested: ocular dominance (Fig. 1), orientation selectivity (Fig. 2), interocular orientation disparity (Fig. 3) and the spatial sensitivity profile of the receptive field (Fig. 4).

Plasticity in Ocular Dominance

In normally reared and dark-reared kittens, most cells are binocularly activated (Imbert and Buisseret, 1975; Frégnac and Imbert, 1978). However, ocular dominance can be dramatically affected by closing one eye during a critical period of postnatal life (Wiesel and Hubel, 1963; Hubel and Wiesel, 1970). For example, if only a few hours of monocular visual experience is given to a dark-reared animal of 6 weeks of age, most cells are found to be as orientation selective as in normally reared kittens of the same age, and respond exclusively to the open eye (Fig. 1; Trotter et al., 1983).

In order to induce such fast changes in ocular dominance during the time of recording of a single neuron, we artificially helped the cell to respond to the presentation of the stimulus to the preferred stimulus to one eye and blocked the cell's firing while presenting the same stimulus to the other eye. We could demonstrate, by using this differential pairing procedure, the induction of significant long lasting changes in ocular dominance in about 30% of cells recorded in visual cortex of kittens and adult cats (see Fig. 1). The great majority of these changes were in favor of the positively reinforced eye, as predicted from the covariance hypothesis.

Plasticity in Orientation Selectivity

A second property of visual cortical cells which has been shown to depend on visual experience is orientation selectivity (reviewed in Frégnac and Imbert, 1984). Cells in visual cortex not only integrate information from both eyes but also respond to slits of light correctly oriented within the receptive field. Before 18 days of age, the kinetics of development of orientation selectivity seem to be the same in normally-reared and dark-reared animals (Frégnac, 1979a). However, this intrinsic process of maturation afterwards becomes dependent on visual experience. For instance, if an animal is totally deprived of vision from birth until 6 weeks of age, most cells are found to be unoriented. At that age, 6 hours of normal visual experience seem to undergo a maturation process which has been masked by the absence of vision (Imbert and Buisseret, 1975; Frégnac, 1979b).

This explains the success of the protocols using restricted visual exposure carried out in the 70s (Hirsch and Spinelli, 1970; Blakemore and Cooper, 1970). Animals, usually kept in darkness, were

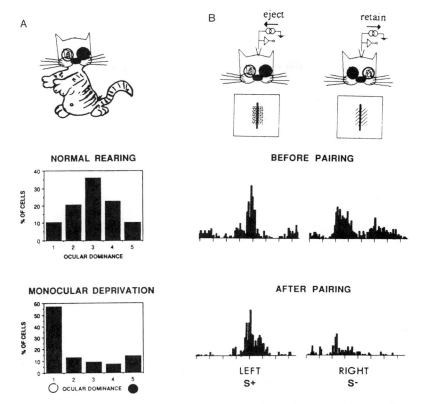

Fig. 1. **A)** **Population analysis:** comparison of ocular dominance histograms in normally reared and monocularly exposed kittens (data adapted from Trotter et al., 1983 and 1987). In 6 week old kittens, most cells are binocularly activated under normal rearing conditions (classes 2 to 4 in NR histogram), whereas monocular vision imposed for a few hours at that age results in most cells being dominated by the open eye (classes 1 and 2 in MD histogram).

B) **Single cell analysis:** modification of the ocular dominance of a single cell in visual cortex of an anesthetized and paralyzed animal. This cell, recorded in an adult cat, responds before pairing equally through both eyes. During pairing (not shown) the left eye stimulation was associated with an increase in activity imposed by a positive current passed through the KCl recording electrode (S+), and right eye stimulation was associated with a decrease in the cell's response induced by a negative current (S-). After pairing, the cell shifted its preference towards the eye which had been positively reinforced (S+).

exposed during a few hours every day to striped environments (Fig. 2), and comparison of orientation preference of cortical cells before and after the visual experience showed that most neurons were tuned to the orientation to which they had been exposed. Two different interpretations concerning the processes involved in these effects were proposed, selective versus instructive mechanisms. In view of the inherent limitations of analysis based on the comparison of populations of neurons recorded in different animals, no definitive answer could be given.

In order to address this question more directly, we applied the same protocol of associative conditioning to the orientation selectivity of single cortical cells. The response of the recorded cell was artificially reinforced during the presentation of a given orientation (S+) and suppressed while presenting the orthogonal orientation (S-) through the same eye (see Fig. 2). About 40% of the

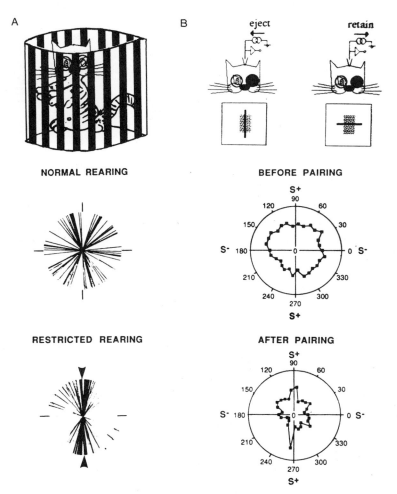

A

NORMAL REARING

RESTRICTED REARING

B

eject

retain

BEFORE PAIRING

S+
90
120   60
150   30
S⁻ 180   0 S⁻
210   330
240   300
270
S+

AFTER PAIRING

S+
90
120   60
150   30
S⁻ 180   0 S⁻
210   330
240   300
270
S+

Fig. 2. **A) Population analysis:** comparison of the distribution of preferred orientations in visual cortex of normally reared kittens and kittens reared in a vertically striped environment. Under normal rearing conditions, all orientations are equally represented in area 17 (each line corresponds to the preferred orientation for one given cell). After the restricted rearing, most cells recorded in primary visual cortex show a preferred orientation near the one imposed by the rearing (data adapted from Blakemore and Cooper, 1970).

B) Single cell analysis: modification of the orientation tuning curve of a single cell in visual cortex of an anesthetized and paralyzed animal. The polar tuning curves indicate the level of firing to the presentation of a bar of light as a function of its orientation (expressed on a 360 degree scale, since for a given orientation the bar can be moved in two opposite directions). This cell, recorded in a 12 week old kitten, responded before pairing to every orientation. During pairing (not shown) the alternate presentations of a vertical (90°) and an horizontal (0°) orientation were associated respectively with a high level of activity (S⁺), and a low level of response (S⁻). After pairing, the cell became tuned to the vertical orientation (S⁺), and the response to the horizontal orientation (S⁻) was markedly reduced. The increase in responsiveness for the reinforced orientation affected both directions of movement of the oriented bar (90° and 270°).

conditioned cells showed a significant change in their relative preference between the two orientations, and in more than 90% of these cases the shift was in favor of the orientation associated with a high level of response during conditioning.

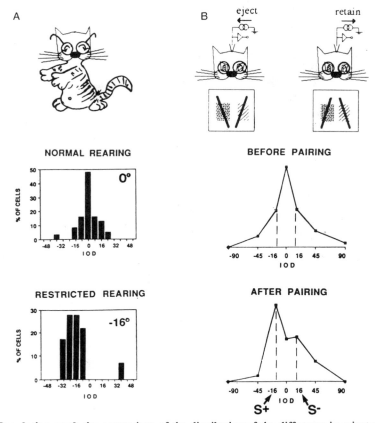

Fig. 3. **A) Population analysis:** comparison of the distribution of the difference in orientation preferences seen through each eye, in normal kittens (IOD=0°) and in kittens reared with prisms imposing an optical rotation between each visual field (IOD=-16°). Under normal rearing conditions (or rearing with neutral goggles: 0°) most cells in primary visual cortex show an IOD centered around 0°. Conversely, if the animal experiences binocular vision though prisms imposing a -16° disparity, most cells in cortex show a preferred IOD centered on the imposed disparity (data adapted from Shinkman and Bruce, 1977).

B) Single cell analysis: modification of the preferred interocular orientation disparity of a single cell recorded in primary visual cortex of a 10 week old kitten. Before pairing, the cell was tuned to the 0° disparity, and showed equal levels of response to -16° and +16° disparities. During pairing (not shown), the -16° and +16° disparities were associated respectively with high (S$^+$) and low (S$^-$) levels of activity. After pairing, the cell became tuned to the reinforced disparity (i.e.,-16°).

The orientation preference paradigm allowed us to study the generalization of the effects to stimuli other than those used during the conditioning (Fig. 2). In most cases, responsiveness was also increased for orientations close to the S$^+$ stimulus and was decreased for orientations close to the S$^-$ orientation. The induced orientation shift was related to the initial selectivity of the neuron: the probability of observing large orientation shifts was significantly higher in initially unoriented neurons than in already selective ones.

Plasticity in Interocular Orientation Disparity

Inspection of specific functional properties of visual cortical neurons through each eye shows that the two receptive fields are very similarly organized (Hubel and Wiesel, 1962). However, a certain number of differences are found between the receptive fields of the two eyes, for instance, in retinal positional disparity and in orientation preference disparity.

Disparities in the preferred orientation for each eye have been observed in the primary visual cortex of cats and kittens (Blakemore et al., 1972; Nelson et al., 1977) and have been proposed as a possible cue for stereopsis (Blakemore et al., 1972). The matching between the preferred orientations for each eye shows a very high level of plasticity: in order to create an artificial interocular orientation disparity (IOD), Shinkman and collaborators (Shinkman and Bruce, 1977; review in Shinkman et al., 1983) exposed dark-reared kittens to a normal visual environment through prisms which optically rotated the visual field of each eye in opposite directions. The electrophysiological analysis of the part of visual cortex subserving central vision (where IOD imposed by prisms was not accompanied by positional disparity) showed that most cortical cells would remain binocularly activated for disparity values less than 20 degrees. In this latter case, the difference in the orientation preference seen by each eye reflected, on average, the value imposed by the prism (compare situations 0 and -16 degrees in Figure 3).

A third protocol of associative cellular conditioning was developed in order to study plasticity of the selectivity of binocular integration to IOD. Activity of the recorded cell activity was artificially increased during the presentation of a given orientation disparity configuration (i.e., simultaneous presentation of different orientations for each eye) and decreased or even blocked during the presentation of a different orientation disparity (Fig. 3). In order to compare the temporal evolution of binocular and monocular responses, orientation tuning curves were established during control periods (no current applied) for dichoptic stimulation and for independent stimulation of each eye.

We could observe selective changes in the preferred IOD in about 40 % of paired neurons (Fig. 3). A finding which pleads for the associative nature of these functional modifications is the observation that binocular responses were affected to a much larger extent than monocular ones. In half of the modified cells the changes were expressed or retained only in the binocular viewing condition, during which control of activity had been imposed.

Plasticity in the Spatial Sensitivity Profile of Receptive Fields

The three paradigms discussed above mimic at the cellular level rearing situations known to profoundly affect visual cortical functions. However, there is a lack of quantitative evidence demonstrating that the spatial organization of the receptive field itself can be shaped by visual experience (but see Pettigrew and Freeman, 1973 and Singer and Tretter, 1976). The fourth protocol more directly addresses this issue (Frégnac et al., 1989), and could help us to understand how modifications in the responses of cortical cells assessed with moving stimuli may be related to discrete changes in the spatial organization of their receptive field. Moreover, independent manipulations of the level of responses to the presentation (ON) and extinction (OFF) of a static stimulus in a fixed position of the receptive field are thought to lead to a better separation of inputs (in term of activated synapses), since it is known (at least in the ferret) that ON and OFF pathways remain segregated to a significant extent up to the cortical level. During the differential pairing procedure the response of the recorded cell was increased during presentation of a static, optimally oriented, bar of light (ON response in Fig. 4) and decreased during the extinction of the same stimulus (OFF response in Fig. 4). We could induce significant modifications in the relative level of ON and OFF responses in a given position of the receptive field in about 30 % of cells (see Fig. 4). Significant changes could be also obtained in the adult cortex, indicating that although two distinct stable states in receptive field organization are classically observed, namely Simple and Complex receptive fields, it is possible by certain artificial procedures to reveal masked responses in subzones of the receptive field and make Complex a Simple cell.

PUTATIVE MECHANISMS OF SYNAPTIC PLASTICITY

A first general conclusion, drawn from the phenomenology of the observed changes, is that imposed temporal correlation between post-synaptic activity and given characteristics of the visual message induces functional modifications in receptive field properties which are analogous to those observed during epigenetic development. A second conclusion, more unexpected, is that visual

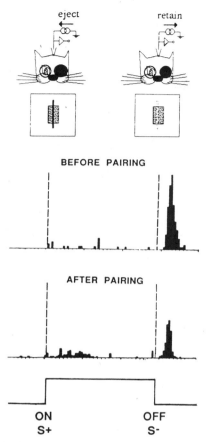

Fig. 4. **Single cell analysis:** modification of the relative levels of ON and OFF responses of a Simple cell recorded in visual cortex of a 27 week old cat. Before pairing, a static bar of light was presented repetitively within a given position of the receptive field (RF). During pairing (not shown), presentation of the visual stimulus (ON) was associated with an increase in the cell's activity, and extinction of the same stimulus (OFF) in the same position of the RF was associated with a decrease of the response. After this pairing procedure, the cell showed an increased ON response and a decreased OFF response. Note that this differential modification in RF type, from Simple to Complex-like, cannot be explained by a global change in the excitability level of the cell.

cortical neurons - under such artificial conditions - are able to undergo activity-dependent changes even at the adult age.

Interpretation of our electrophysiological recordings in terms of synaptic changes is supported by recent results obtained in motor (Baranyi and Féher, 1978; Baranyi and Szente, 1987), frontal (Sutor and Hablitz, 1989), visual (Artola and Singer, 1987) and associative (Bindman et al., 1988) cortices and hippocampus (Kelso et al., 1986; Wigström et al., 1986) of the adult cat and rat. In these central structures, pairing of afferent stimulation (single pulse or weak tetanization) with depolarization of the target neuron - a situation equivalent to the S+ condition of our protocol - produces long-lasting enhancement of excitatory post-synaptic potentials. Membrane depolarization is thought to relieve the magnesium block of the ionophore coupled with the post-synaptic NMDA receptor. Calcium entry through this unmasked channel could then trigger second messenger processes leading to long-term increase in synaptic efficiency.

Much less evidence is available concerning the effects of pairing afferent stimulation with hyperpolarization of the target cell, which could constitute a situation equivalent to the S- condition in our protocol. Reiter and Stryker (1988) provided evidence that suppression of post-synaptic activity by intracortical perfusion of muscimol (a GABA agonist) during monocular deprivation in the middle of the critical period leads afterwards to most cells being dominated by the closed eye. This somehow paradoxical result is in line with our own working hypothesis according to which a maintained period of failure in synaptic transmission induces a selective weakening of the efficiency of the active synapses.

Although it is classically thought that there is a unique membrane potential threshold above which a neuron switches from a relay mode to an adaptive state, and that inhibition blocks cellular plasticity (Malinow and Miller, 1986; Baranyi and Szente, 1987), these data open the suggestion of two different thresholds above and below which, respectively, increases and decreases in synaptic efficiency will be observed.

The covariance algorithm successfully simulated the specification process of functional characteristics of visual cortical cells during development, such as orientation selectivity and ocular dominance. Does it predict any age dependency in plasticity which could explain the end of the critical period?

The decrease in functional plasticity with postnatal age observed in normally reared kittens appears to be correlated with the progressive development of visual cortical cell's properties such as orientation selectivity. The end of the critical period could be a logical consequence of the specification process of the neocortical network, where available competition between different functional inputs on a given target neuron becomes restricted and inhibitory influences from already specified neighboring neurons increase the stability of the network. In contrast, it has been demonstrated that the end of the critical period can be delayed following an initial period of visual deprivation which maintains the visual cortical network in a non selective stage (see discusion in Frégnac, 1985). In the covariance model, Bienenstock, et al. (1982) have introduced a floating threshold of synaptic plasticity (linked to the mean activity of the cell), which predicts a higher susceptibility to environmental manipulation in neurons which are initially poorly responsive compared to cells which are already specialized and show a high level of postsynaptic activity.

The hypothesis of a "teacher" seems similar to that of global validation signals allowing the expression of specific cellular changes. How are these signals generated and what is their functional nature?

The visual cortex can be considered as a self-organizing assembly. Cells within this assembly become adaptive under certain physiological conditions during which "print now" signals are generated internally by the central nervous system and appear to be linked to the motivation and attention states, the motor act or behavior that has helped to sample the visual information.

ACKNOWLEDGEMENTS

Part of this work has been done in collaboration with Elie Bienenstock, Simon Thorpe and Dominique Debanne. Current research is supported by grants from MRES (87C0187), CEE (ST2J0416C), NEDO and FRM. We wish to thank Michèle Gautier for her technical assistance and Kirsty Grant for help with the English.

REFERENCES

Alkon, D. , 1988, "Memory Traces in the Brain," Cambridge University Press.

Artola, A., and Singer, W., 1987, Long-term potentiation and NMDA receptors in rat visual cortex. *Nature,* 330: 649.

Baranyi, A., and Féher, O., 1978, Conditioned changes of synaptic transmission in the motor cortex of the cat, *Exp. Brain Res.,* 33:283.

Baranyi, A., and Szente, M.B., 1987, Long-lasting potentiation of synaptic transmission requires postsynaptic modifications in the neocortex, *Brain Res.,* 423: 378.

Bienenstock, E., Cooper, L.N., and Munro, P., 1982, Theory for the development of neuron selectivity: orientation specificity and binocular interaction in visual cortex. *J. Neurosci.,* 2: 23.

Bindman, L. J., Murphy, K. P. S. J., and Pockett, S., 1988, Postsynaptic control of the induction of long-term changes in efficacy of transmission at neocortical synapses in slices of rat brain, *J. Neurophysiol.,* 60:1053.

Blakemore, C., and Cooper, G. F., 1970, Development of the brain depends on the visual environment, *Nature,* 228:477.

Blakemore, C., Fiorentini, A., and Maffei, L., 1972, A second neural mechanism of binocular depth discrimination, *J. Physiol.,* 226:727.

Buisseret, P., Gary-Bobo, E., and Imbert, M., 1978, Ocular motility and recovery of orientational properties of visual cortical neurones in dark-reared kittens, *Nature,* 272:816.

Changeux, J. P., and Danchin, A., 1976, Selective stabilization of developing synapses as a mechanism for the specification of neuronal networks, *Nature,* 264:705.

Changeux, J. P., Courrège, P., and Danchin, A., 1973, A theory of the epigenesis of neuronal networks by selective stabilization of synapses, *Proc. Natl. Acad. Sci. USA,* 70: 2974.

Farley, J., Richards, W. G., Ling, L. J., Liman, E., and Alkon, D. L., 1983, Membrane changes in a single photoreceptor cause associative learning in *Hermissenda, Science,* 221:1201.

Freeman, R. D., and Bonds, A. B., 1979, Cortical plasticity in monocularly deprived immobilized kittens depends on eye movement, *Science,* 206:1093.

Frégnac, Y., 1979a, Development of orientation selectivity in the primary visual cortex of normally and dark reared kittens. I. Kinetics, *Biol. Cybern.,* 34:187.

Frégnac, Y., 1979b, Development of orientation selectivity in the primary visual cortex of normally and dark reared kittens. II. Models, *Biol. Cybern.,* 34:195.

Frégnac, Y., 1985, Functional multicompartment models: a kinetic study of the development of orientation selectivity, in: "Models of the Visual Cortex," D. Rose and V. G. Dobson, eds., J. Wiley and Sons, New York, p. 172.

Frégnac, Y., 1987, Cellular mechanisms of epigenesis in cat visual cortex, in: "Imprinting and cortical plasticity," J. Rauschecker and P. Marler, eds., J. Wiley and Sons, New York, p. 221.

Frégnac, Y., and Bienenstock, E., 1981, Specific functional modification of individual cortical neurons triggered by vision and passive eye movement in immobilized kittens, in: "Pathophysiology of the Visual System," Documenta Opthalmol. Proc. Ser., vol. 30, L. Maffei, ed., W. Junk, The Hague, p. 100.

Frégnac, Y., and Imbert, M., 1978, Early development of visual cortical cells in normal and dark reared kittens: relationship between orientation selectivity and ocular dominance, *J. Physiol.,* 278:27.

Frégnac, Y., and Imbert, M., 1984, Development of neuronal selectivity in the primary visual cortex of the cat, *Physiol. Rev.,* 64: 325.

Frégnac, Y., and Shulz, D., 1989, Hebbian synapses in visual cortex, in: "Seeing Contour and Color," K. Kulikowski, ed., Pergamon Press, Elmsford, NY, p. 711.

Frégnac, Y., Shulz, D., Thorpe, S., and Bienenstock, E., 1988, A cellular analog of visual cortical plasticity, *Nature,* 333: 367.

Frégnac, Y., Shulz, D., and Debanne, D., 1989, The role of co-activity in shaping visual cortical receptive fields, *Biomed. Res.,* 10(S2):11.

Geiger, H., and Singer, W., 1986, A possible role of Ca++ currents in developmental plasticity, *Exp. Brain Res.,* 14:256.

Graves,A., Trotter,Y., and Frégnac,Y., 1987, Role of extraocular muscle proprioception in the development of depth perception in cats, *J. Neurophysiol.,* 58: 816.

Gray, C. M., and Singer, W., 1989, Stimulus-specific neuronal oscillations in orientation columns of cat visual cortex, *Proc. Natl. Acad. Sci. USA,* 86:1698.

Hebb, D. O., 1949, "The Organization of Behavior," J. Wiley and Sons, New York.

Hirsch, H. V. B., and Spinelli, D. N., 1970, Visual experience modifies distribution of horizontally and vertically oriented receptive fields in cats, *Science,* 168:869.

Hubel, D. H., and Wiesel, T.N., 1962, Receptive fields, binocular interaction and functional architecture in the cat's visual cortex, *J. Physiol.,* 160:106.

Hubel, D. H., and Wiesel, T.N., 1963, Receptive field of cells in striate cortex of very young, visually inexperienced kittens, *J. Neurophysiol.,* 26:994.

Hubel, D. H., and Wiesel, T.N., 1970, The period of susceptibility to the physiological effects of unilateral eye closure in kittens, *J. Physiol.,* 206:419.

Imbert, M., and Buisseret, P., 1975, Receptive field characteristics and plastic properties of visual cortical cells in kittens reared with or without visual experience, *Exp. Brain Res.,* 22:25.

Kasamatsu, T., 1983, Neuronal plasticity maintained by the central norepinephrine system in the cat visual cortex, in: "Progress in Psychobiology and Physiological Psychology, vol. 10," J. M. Sprague and A. M. Epstein, eds., Academic Press, London, p. 1.

Kato, N., Artola, A., and Singer, W., 1988, Susceptibility of visual cortical neurones to undergo long-term potentiation decreases with age, *Proc. Eur. Neurosci. Assoc.,* 11: A311.

Kelso, S. R., Ganong, A.H., and Brown, T.J.,1986, Hebbian synapses in hippocampus. *Proc. Natl. Acad. Sci. USA.* , 83:5326.

Malinow, R., and Miller, J. P., 1986, Postsynaptic hyperpolarization during conditioning reversibly blocks induction of long-term potentiation, *Nature,* 320:529.

Marr , D., 1969, A theory of cerebellar cortex, *J. Physiol.,* 202:437.

Mastronarde, D. N., 1983, Interactions between ganglion cells in cat retina, *J. Neurophysiol.,* 49:350.

Müller, C.M., Engel, A.K. and Singer, W., 1988, Development of astrocytes in the cat visual cortex, *Soc. Neurosci. Abstr.,* 14: 745.

Nelson, J. I., Kato, H., and Bishop, P. O., 1977, Discrimination of orientation and position disparities by binocularly activated neurons in cat striate cortex, *J Neurophysiol.,* 40:260.

Pettigrew, J. D., and Garey, L. J., 1974, Selective modification of single neuron properties in the visual cortex of kittens, *Brain Res.,* 66:160.

Pettigrew, J. D., and Freeman, R. D., 1973, Visual experience without lines: effect on developing cortical neurons, *Science,* 182:599.

Pettigrew, J. D., and Kasamatsu, T., 1978, Local perfusion of noradrenaline maintains visual cortical plasticity, *Nature,* 271:761.

Pettigrew, J. D., Olson, C., and Barlow, H. B., 1973, Kitten visual cortex: short-term, stimulus induced changes in connectivity, *Science,* 180:1202.

Reiter, H.O., and Stryker, M.P.,1988, Neural plasticity without postsynaptic action potentials: less-active inputs become dominant when kitten visual cortical cells are pharmacologically inhibited, *Proc. Natl. Acad. Sci. USA,* 85:3623.

Sejnowski, J., 1977, Storing covariance with non-linearly interacting neurons, *J. Math. Biol.,* 4: 303.

Shinkman, P.G., and Bruce, C.J., 1977, Binocular differences in cortical receptive fields of kittens after rotationally disparate binocular experience, *Science,* 197: 285.

Shinkman, P.G., Isley, M. R., and Rogers, D. G., 1983, Prolonged dark rearing and development of interocular orientation disparity in the visual cortex, *J. Neurophysiol.,* 49:717.

Singer, W., and Tretter, F., 1976, Unusually large receptive fields in cats with restricted visual experience, *Exp. Brain Res.,* 26:171.

Spinelli, D. N., and Jensen, F. E., 1979, Plasticity: The mirror of experience, *Science,* 203: 75.

Stanton, P.K., and Sejnowski, T.J., 1989, Associative long-term depression in the hippocampus induced by hebbian covariance, *Nature,* 339:215.

Stent, G., 1973, A physiological mechanism for Hebb's postulate of learning, *Proc. Natl. Acad. Sci. USA,* 70: 997.

Sutor, B., and Hablitz, J. J., 1989, Long-term potentiation in frontal cortex: role of NMDA-modulated polysynaptic excitatory pathways, *Neurosci. Lett.,* 97:111.

Trotter, Y., Gary-Bobo, E., and Buisseret, P., 1981, Recovery of orientation selectivity in kitten primary visual cortex is slowed down by bilateral section of ophthalmic trigeminal afferents, *Dev. Brain Res.,* 1:450.

Trotter, Y., Frégnac,Y., and Buisseret, P., 1983, Synergie de la vision et de la proprioception extraoculaire dans les mécanismes de plasticité fonctionnelle du cortex visuel primaire du Chaton, *C. R. Acad. Soc. Paris,* 296:665.

Trotter, Y., Frégnac,Y., and Buisseret, P., 1987, The period of susceptibility of visual cortical binocularity to unilateral proprioceptive deafferentation of extraocular muscles, *J. Neurophysiol.,* 58:795.

Von der Malsburg, C.,1973, Self-organization of orientation sensitive cells in the striate cortex, *Kybernetik,* 14: 85.

Wiesel, T. N., and Hubel, D. H., 1963, Single-cell responses in striate cortex of kitten deprived of vision in one eye, *J. Neurophysiol.,* 26:1003.

Wiesel, T.N., 1982, Postnatal development of the visual cortex and the influence of environment (Nobel lecture), *Nature,* 299: 583.

Wigström, H., Gustafsson, B., Huang, Y. Y., and Abraham, W. C., 1986, Hippocampal long-term potentiation is induced by pairing single afferent volleys with intracellularly injected depolarizing current pulses, *Acta Physiol. Scand.,* 126:317.

ABSTRACTS

DEVELOPMENT OF THE CORPUS CALLOSUM IN CATS. A QUANTITATIVE AND QUALITATIVE STUDY

P. Berbel[1], G.M. Innocenti[2], J.J. Prieto[1] and R. Kraftsik[2]
1) Dpto. Histologia, Univ. Alicante, 03690-Alicante, SPAIN and
2) Inst. d'Anatomie, Rue due Bugnon 9, 1005-Lausanne, SWITZERLAND

Changes in the anatomy of the corpus callosum (CC), and in the number, size and structure of callosal axons (ca) between embryonic day 38 (E38) and postnatal day 150 (P150) were studied light- and electromicroscopically in 25 kittens[1]. The development of microtubules (T) and neurofilaments (F) of ca in 11 kittens from E58 and P150 was studied in "standard" (st) axons, i.e., transversally cut, free of artifacts that may alter quantification, and without organelles or other elements that may displace Ts and Fs.

The development of CC was divided in three phases: i) Embryonic development (E36, 53, 58): Characterized by an increase in the number of axons (from 48.05 million at E53 to 57.56 million at E58), peaking at birth. Mean axon diameter were 0.26 μm at E53 and 0.27 at E58. ii) Early postnatal development (P39, 57, 92, 107, 150): The number of axons still decreased (48.77 million at P39 and 35.43 million at P150). Nevertheless, the CC grew dramatically in length and thickness; the latter especially in the genu. The growth was probably due to increases in the proportion of myelinated axons (1.6% at P26 and 32.3% at P150) and in the mean axon diameter (0.35 μm at P39 and 0.46 μm at P150).

The number of Ts (nT) and Fs (nF) were proportional to axon's cross sectional area (A). Both increased more rapidly in small (≤ 0.23 μm^2) than in large axons (> 0.23 μm^2), but the rate of increase changed more markedly for nT than for nF. Density of Ts increased with age (93.8 Ts per μm^2 at E53 and 125.9 at P150); density of Fs increased as well (40.0 Fs per μm^2 at E53 and 55.0 at P150). The mean distance between Ts (DT) decreased (0.081 μm at E53 to 0.076 μm at P150). In contrast, the distance between Fs (DF) increased slightly (0.075 μm at E53 to 0.1 μm at P26); afterwards, it remained constant (0.093 μm at P150). 95% of axons at P150 showed a DT between 0.028 and 0.11 μm, and a DF between 0.025 μm and 0.18 μm. The ratio nF/(Nf+nT) decreased from 0.48 at E53 to 0.35 at P150. During this period, the overlap of both Ts and Fs domains increased, although, the mean distance between the geometric centers of the domains remained almost the same (0.081 μm at E53 and 0.084 μm at P150).

Reference:
1) P. Berbel and G.M. Innocenti, 1988, *J. Comp. Neurol.*, 276:132-156.

MUTATIONS AT THE *fused rhabdomeres* (*fur*) LOCUS AFFECT RHABDOMERE MORPHOLOGY AND PHOTORECEPTOR FUNCTION IN *DROSOPHILIA MELANOGASTER*

Ann Blake, Laurel B. Bernstein, Peter M. O'Day, Matthew Lonergan, T.R. Venkatesh
Institutes of Neuroscience and Molecular Biology, University of Oregon
Eugene, OR 97403, USA

The *Drosophila* compound eye is a precise modular and reiterated structure comprised of some 800 simple units, the ommatidia. Each ommatidium is a discrete cluster of cells, including eight photoreceptor cells of three subtypes, defined by their characteristic position, spectral sensitivity, and connectivity to the optic ganglia. The plasma membrane of each photoreceptor cell is elaborately infolded to form the structures known as the rhabdomeres. These extend the length of the cell, and are studded with the primary photopigments, the rhodopsins. We are interested in the development of the rhabdomeres and their role in the proper function of the retina.

Drosophila genetics permits the analysis of developing pattern and function in the compound eye. A great number of mutations have been characterized that affect various aspects of phototransduction and retinal development.

We have characterized a new mutation generated by hybrid dysgenesis which has marked effects on both rhabdomere morphology and photoreceptor function. The *fused rhabdomeres* (*fur*) locus has been localized to the proximal region of the X chromosome by classic recombination and deficiency mapping. Mutations at the *fur* locus cause fusion of the rhabdomeres of neighboring photoreceptor cells within an ommatidium. An apparent longitudinal compaction of the rhabdomere structure is also seen. The degree of rhabdomere fusion is variable within a given eye, but the longitudinal compaction is consistent across the entire retina.

The *fur* mutation also produced several distinct physiological abnormalities. The retinas of *fur* flies have a one order of magnitude decrease in sensitivity to light relative to wild-type retinas. This loss of sensitivity is wavelength-independent, indicating a generalized deficit rather than a loss of a wavelength-specific class of primary photopigment. The second detectable functional deficit is the absence, in white-eyed *fur*, of a prolonged depolarizing afterpotential (PDA) characteristic of wild-type white-eyed flies.

It has been possible to generate partial and complete revertants of *fur*, thus providing genetic evidence that the mutant phenotype is the result of a P element insertion. Complete revertants show complete resortation of both structural and functional deficits.

To examine further the role of the *fur* gene product in rhabdomere morphology and the relation of morphological deficits to functional abnormalities, we are pursuing the molecular cloning of *fur* utilizing the inserted P element tag.

OPTIC FLOW REQUIREMENTS FOR THE DEVELOPMENT OF VISUALLY GUIDED BEHAVIOUR IN KITTENS

Eli Brenner and Frans W. Cornelissen
Neuro-ethology group, University of Utrecht
Padualaan 8, 3584 CH Utrecht, THE NETHERLANDS

Twenty years ago, Held, Hein, Diamond and Gower showed that kittens only learn to use vision to guide their behaviour if they are free to walk around in an environment containing visible contours. Moving them around passively was not sufficient. When a kitten moves around, the image of the environment shifts on its retina and is subjected to systematic deformations. During development, these shifts and deformations (the optic flow) are presumably associatd with the movements that cause them. The present study aims to determine which aspects of the optic flow are essential for the development of visually guided behaviour. This is done by limiting the environment in a manner that confines the aspects of optic flow that the kitten encounters without restricting their movements. The visual environments consist of scattered dots or streaks of light.

Kittens were raised in the dark, and each spent several hours a day in one of the specially designed visual environments. Controls were subjected to the same environment in complete darkness or illuminated at either a scotopic or photopic level. The exposure conditions were selected in a manner that enables us to distinguish between environments with and without aspects of optic flow such as "motion parallax", "global expansion" and "specific deformation" (which could be used to determine relative distance, ego-locomotion and orientation of surfaces, respectively). Kittens were exposed to the limited visual environments for a total of 49 hours, after which various forms of visually guided behaviour were examined: ocular pursuit of a moving target, visually guided extension and reaching, visual orientation in a known environment, depth perception and finding a target. Improvement or acquisition of these behaviours was examined after consecutive 4 hour periods of exposure to normal light.

The results show substantial differences between cats raised in different environments. The most striking difference is that the development of visually guided orientation requires the presence of oriented contours. It is also influenced by the level of illumination and the presence of more complex visual information (e.g. texture), and is clearly independent of the tangibility of visual contours. Apparently the optic flow must arise from self-induced motion; it is not enough to be able to confirm visual experience with information from another modality. The development of depth perception requires photopic stimulation, whereas some behaviour only requires that the level of illumination during testing is similar to that during exposure (i.e. scotopic).

In the cat primary visual cortex, each cell only responds to contours of a specific orientation. The development of this orientational selectivity is guided by experience. Similarly, we find that kittens need oriented contours and the displacements and deformations they undergo during egomotion to learn to use vision to guide their behaviour. The lateral suprasylvian visual cortex is presumably specialized in evaluating ego-motion. Its cells have properties one would expect in an area that extracts the expansion component from the optic flow: selectivity for direction of motion, rather than contour orientation, and an over-representation of motion away from the area centralis. We have recently shown that this specialization can develop without the experience with expanding flow fields that kittens normally get during forward locomotion (Brenner and Rauschecker, submitted). This too is in good agreement with the present study: expansion and motion parallax are not crucial for behavioural development. This does not necessarily mean that these aspects of optic flow are less important for visually guided behaviour, but they are not the aspects of visual experience that guide development.

RETINAL DEVELOPMENT IN THE ZEBRAFISH: TOWARD A GENETIC APPROACH TO DEVELOPMENT OF THE VERTEBRATE VISUAL SYSTEM

C. Fulwiler, E. Schmidt, J.E. Dowling and W. Gilbert
Program in Neuroscience, Harvard Medical School and The Biological Laboratories, Harvard University
16 Divinity Avenue, Cambridge, MA 02138, USA

We are studying development of the zebrafish visual system in two ways: behavioral assays of visual function in young larvae, and anatomical studies of the embryonic and larval retina. These studies are intended to provide the necessary background for attempts to find mutants affecting the retina using genetic methods.

Larvae have been studied behaviorally from the time of hatching at 3 days. We find that larvae show a positive phototaxis which is maximal at 7 days. Interestingly, in the second week of larval life the response reverses and by two weeks the animals are negatively phototactic. There appears to be a strong genetic component to this behavior as clonal lines of zebrafish are significantly more uniform in the response than wild type. We also find, as described by others (Clark, Ph.D. thesis, U. Oregon, 1981), that optokinetic nystagmus is quite reliable and easy to detect in 4 day larvae. These two assays should prove useful in large-scale screening for visual mutants in young larvae.

We are also studying normal development in the retina using light and electron microscopy in combinatoin with immunohistochemistry. We have used monoclonal antibodies (made by K. Larrison, Masters thesis, U Oregon) as markers for the developing cellular and synaptic layers, and a series of antibodies against neurotransmitters and their synthetic enzymes to follow the development of individual neuronal cell types and their pathways. The earliest time we detect transmitter expression is about 2 days. Electron mircoscopy is also being used to examine synapse formation in the plexiform layers.

Finally, we have pursued alternative mutagenesis strategies based on insertion of DNA into the germline. For example, we are able to remove immature oocytes prior to germinal vesicle breakdown for microinjection into the nucleus, and culture them to maturity in vitro. DNA constructs containing the lacZ gene under the control of different promoters are being used to assay for transformation.

DIFFERENTIAL BEHAVIOUR OF *XENOPUS* RETINAL FIBRES ON VARIOUS SUBSTRATES IN VITRO

Douglas Gooday
MRC Neural Development and Regeneration Group, King's Building
West Mains Road, Edinburgh, EH9 3JT, SCOTLAND

The behaviour of nerve fibres from different parts of the retina has been studied in vitro, on various substrates, in an attempt to examine whether intrinsic differences in behaviour of fibres from the different retinal quadrants could play a role in segregating the fibres during development of the retino-tectal projection.

On a laminin substrate explants of nasal and temporal retina give rise to identical patterns of outgrowth; 200-300 fine fascicles are produced by each explant, which grow up to 1500um in 4 days.

Glial cell monolayers were prepared from cell suspensions of the diencephalon and tectum of stage 54 tadpoles; the neuronal cells were removed and the glial cells were grown to confluence. Anti-GFAP staining (clone G-A-5) showed that the monolayers were pure populations of astrocytic cells.

On monolayers of diencephalic glial cells a similar pattern of outgrowth is produced to that on laminin. There are, however, fewer fascicles; 100-200 per explant, and the average length is around 1000um. Nasal and temporal explants produce identical outgrowth patterns.

On tectal glial monolayers nasal and temporal explants produce different patterns of fibre growth. Nasal explants produce a similar pattern to that of both types of explant on diencephalic glia. On tectal glia which have been grown to a high density (1000+ cells/mm^2) the fascicles are slightly shorter, 800-1000um, and thicker, but the overall pattern of growth remains the same.

Temporal explants produce a restricted outgrowth on tectal glia. On monolayers which are just confluent (700-1000 cells/mm^2) fibres are bundled into fascicles of up to 10um diameter, there are far fewer fascicles per explant, and they are shorter, rarely exceeding 700um. On densely packed tectal glia, the growth is even more restricted with usually fewer than 5 very short fat fascicles per explant.

In addition to culturing retinal explants on glia, the behaviour of retinal fibres growing on other retinal fibres has been studied to assess whether there is any evidence for selective fasciculation in certain fibre populations. Using the experimental protocol devised by Bonhoeffer and Huf (1985) nasal and temporal fibres have been confronted with a choice of growing on either other nasal or temporal fibres. Out of 8 nasal cases all showed no preference and grew equally on nasal and temporal fibres, whereas in 17 out of 22 temporal cases the fibres showed a perference for growing along other temporal fibres.

These findings are indicative of three phenomena: 1. there are cell surface differences between tectal and diencephalic glial cells, 2. these differences are recognized by temporal fibres and to a lesser extent by nasal fibres, 3. there are cell surface differences between nasal and temporal growth cones.

Reference:
Bonhoeffer, F. and Huf, J., 1985, Position-dependent properties of retinal axons and their growth cones, *Nature*, 315:409-410.

GENETIC SCREEN FOR MUTANTS AFFECTING NEURONAL CONNECTIVITY IN THE VISUAL SYSTEM OF *DROSOPHILA MELANOGASTER*

Megan E. Grether and Hermann Steller
Department of Biology and Department of Brain and Cognitive Sciences, MIT,
Cambridge, MA 02139, USA

The overall objective of our research is to understand how genes control the assembly of a functional nervous system during embryonic development. In particular, we are interested in how genes specify the unique cellular identity of individual neurons and how these neurons find and recognize their correct synaptic partners to form a precisely wired network of cells.

To address these issues we use a simple model system, the larval visual system of *Drosophila melanogaster*. The larval visual system forms a well described neuronal circuit. It consists of 12 photoreceptor cells whose axons form the larval optic nerve, and their synaptic preparations of embryos or larvae by staining with a photoreceptor cell specific monoclonal antibody. This makes possible the identification and analysis of mutants with abnormal axonal projections of the larval optic nerve.

The gene *disconnected* (*disco*) is required for the establishment of stable connections between the larval photoreceptor neurons and their synaptic partners during embryonic development. We have systematically screened for additional mutations that affect the development of the larval visual system. We have examined a large fraction of the *Drosophila* genome for such loci by analysing the projection of the larval optic nerve in embryos homozygous for deletions.

From these studies it is evident that a relatively small number of deletions affect the formaiton of specific neuronal connections in the larval visual system. Furthermore, ectopic position of the target cells due to defects in morphogenetic movements does not necessarily prevent "normal" connectivity between the larval optic nerve and these targets. We have also observed axonal outgrowth from the larval photoreceptor cells in the absence of the target cells (or the entire brain hemispheres, e.g., in *tailless* embryos).

Two of the deficiency stocks, Df(2R)L+48 and Df(3L)w4, ru h e ca/TM6B contain phenotypes of particular interest to us. In each case, the larval optic nerve projects to an ectopic position in the brain of what otherwise appears to be a basically normal embryo. We are currently trying to identify the loci responsible for these phenotypes by genetic mapping.

AXONAL GUIDANCE IN THE MAMMALIAN RETINOTECTAL SYSTEM: A MODEL FROM PATHWAY TO TARGET

Mark H. Hankin and Raymond D. Lund
Department of Neurobiology, Anatomy and Cell Sciences
University of Pittsburgh, Pittsburgh, PA, USA

Several years ago we examined the possibility of transplanting embryonic neural tissue to the neonatal rodent brain in the hope of providing an *in vivo* preparation which might complement ongoing *in vitro* studies of axonal guidance. The goal of these studies was to confront growing optic axons in an experimental preparation with the complex microenvironment of the developing rodent brain, and subsequently to analyze their detailed outgrowth patterns and abilities with respect to normal or abnormal substrates, pathways and target fields.

Our attention has focused on the processes responsible for development of the mammalian retinotectal projection. As a result of these investigations, we have begun to define the nature of the cues which guide retinal axons along the optic tract, and which direct them to terminate in their principal nucleus in the dorsal midbrain, the superior colliculus (SC).

Here we summarize a number of studies wihch have contributed to this overall goal. Examination of the earliest axons from retinal transplants shows that optic axons prefer to grow along the subpial margin ("pathway") of the brainstem, remain within about 20 um of the glia limitans, and show directed outgrowth towards the superior colliculus. Transplant-derived optic axons growing within the midbrain neuropil show oriented outgrowth as if responding to a diffusible chemotropic signal emanating from the SC. Work in the *ocular retardation* mutant mouse, which is anophthalmic by birth and whose superior colliculus does not receive retinal input, suggests that tectal cells can only exert a neurotropic influence once they have received an initial optic innervation. While perhaps able to use glia and their processes as substrates for outgrowth within the SC, retinal axons do not appear to receive directional cues from the geometric alignment of these elements.

We have recently begun to explore the molecular cues responsible for outgrowth along the subpial pathway by attempting to perturb selectively retinal axon outgrowth in this region. To do this we have preincubated mouse retinae with a mouse-specific antibody to the neuronal cell-surface glycoprotein M6 prior to transplantation in the rat brainstem. In culture, anti-M6 blocks neurite outgrowth from cerebellar neurons[1]. The resulting optic axon outgrowth, rather than being inhibited as in culture, was directed into the depth of the midbrain. Therefore, these studies indicate that specific cell surface components may be critical in enabling optic axons to recognize subpial pathway guidance cues.

Finally, a study of the molecules present along the subpial margin of the brainstem demonstrate that NCAM and L1 (NgCAM) are present along the subpial pathway. However, L1 is positioned to play a selective role in the outgrowth along the optic tract (but not the SC) since it is to localized to the subpial margin.

In normal circumstances, it may be suggested, growing optic axons follow substrate cues close to the brainstem surface and, directly by polar cues towards to dorsolateral midbrain, thereby reach the tectum. Once there, they quickly form the first synapses, and this process may stimulate neurons or associated glia in the tectum to produce a neurotropic factor. This may serve several purposes. It could divert axons from the surface substrate; it could improve the efficiency of tectopetal growth by late growing axons; it could serve to change the growth process from one of extension to one of terminal ramification.

It would appear therefore that the quite artificial circumstances presented by intracerebral transplantation may have dissociated biological processes that would, otherwise, be hard to recognize by studying normal development.

Reference:
1) Lagenaur, L.F., Fushiki, S. and Schachner, M., 1984, *Soc. Neurosci. Abstr.*, 10:759.

DENDRITIC GROWTH OF DAPI-ACCUMULATING AMACRINE CELLS IN THE RETINA OF THE GOLDFISH

Peter F. Hitchcock and Ronald N. Brown, Jr.
Departments of Ophthalmology and Anatomy and Cell Biology
The University of Michigan, Ann Arbor, MI 48109, USA

The retina of the goldfish grows throughout the animal's life, in part, by expansion (Johns and Easter, 1977, J. Comp. Neurol., 17:33). With this expansion, there is continual formation of new synapses by amacrine cells in central retina (Fisher and Easter, 1979, J. Comp. Neurol., 185:373), without cell addition. To determine the growth related structural changes of amacrine cells, those that accumulated intraocularly injected 4,6=diamidino-2-pheynlindole (DAPI) were compared in wholemounted retinas from small, young fish (6.5-9.3 cm body length; 2.8-3.0 mm lens dia.) and large old ones (16.5-18.0 cm body lengh; 4.2-4.3 mm lens dia.). The dendritic arbors of DAPI-labelled neurons were stained by intracellular injections of lucifer yellow under visual control. Dendritic field areas and the number of dendritic terminals were quantitatively compared between cells in small (S) and large (L) retina.

Based upon dendritic morphology, two types of amacrine cells were seen: starburst and fusiform. For both cell types the dendritic fields were significantly larger in the larger retinas (starburst, $S=0.1um^2$, n=18 vs. $L=0.2um^2$, n=12; fusiform, $S=0.09um^2$, n=16 vs. $L=0.3um^2$, n=12). For starburst cells the number of terminal dendrites remained constant (S=25.4 vs. L=26.5), whereas the fusiform cells in the large retinas had significantly more dendritic terminals than those in the small retinas (S=30.4 vs. L=41.5). This latter result was due to new, small dendritic processes being added to existing dendrites, primarily near the soma.

These data show that with retinal expansion, the growth of amacrine cells is cell-type specific; their dendritic arbors can grow interstitially only, or by a combination of interstitial growth and the formation of new dendritic processes. Assuming that the cells described here participate in the continuing synaptogenesis, these data also suggest that amacrine cells can insert new pre-synaptic elements into the membrane of existing dendrites and/or grow new pre-synaptic processes.

PERTURBATION OF AXON GROWTH AND GUIDANCE IN THE GRASSHOPPER LIMB BUD BY CHROMOPHORE ASSISTED LASER INACTIVATION

Daniel G. Jay[1] and Haig Keshishian[2]
1) Department of Neurobiology, Harvard Medical School, Boston, MA
2) Department of Biology, Yale University, New Haven, CT, USA

This is a progress report on the application of chromophore assisted laser inactivation (CALI) to study the axonal growth and guidance of the T1 pioneer neurons in the grasshopper limb bud. This procedure inactivates single protein functions in an embryo by injection of the embryo with a dye-labeled antibody and subjecting it to intense laser light of a wavelength absorbed by the dye but not by cellular components. The dye is effective in targeting the laser energy to the bound proteins which denatures them while other proteins in the system are not likely to be affected. Previously this procedure has been tested with enzymes in solution and on the surfaces of red blood cells.

For this study dye-labeled anti-horseradish peroxidase (which binds specifically to a subset of neuronal membrane proteins in insects) was injected into 31% grasshopper embryos that were subjected to laser irradiation. The progress of axonal growth was visualized by immunocytochemistry after 24 hours of further incubation. Preliminary data show a perturbation of the progress of axonal growth and guidance from the limb bud by laser irradiation for dye labeled anti-horseradish peroxidase treated embryos in a majority of the cases observed. Embryos injected with anti-horseradish peroxidase without dye were not perturbed by laser light. Embryos injected with dye-labeled bovine serum albumin showed some effects in a small number of cases. These experiments suggest a role for one or more of the anti-horseradish peroxidase cross reactive antigens in axon growth and guidance. In addition, the experiments demonstrate the applicability of CALI to studying molecular events in neurodevelopment.

THE ROLE OF NORMAL VISUAL INPUT IN THE SYNAPTIC DEVELOPMENT OF THALAMIC RECIPIENT NEURONS OF MONKEY VISUAL CORTEX

J.S. Lund, S.M. Holbach and W.-W. Chung
Center for Neuroscience and Department of Psychiatry
University of Pittsburgh, Pittsburgh, PA 15261, USA

We have examined the development of spine-bearing stellate neurons as seen in Golgi Rapid impregnations in two important thalamic input layers (laminae 4Ca and 4CB) of primary visual cortex of *Macaca nemestrina* monkeys. The dendritic spines on these neurons are the primary sites of thalamic inputs for the visual cortex; the neurons of 4CB receive input from the parvocellular layer of the lateral geniculate nucleus (LGN) and this input is driven primarily by color and fine detail in the visual input. The neurons of 4Ca receive input from the magnocellular layers of the LGN and are driven primarily by pathways which are very sensitive to luminance contrast and motion.

In previous studies we found the visual cortex spine bearing neurons of the normal animal to go through a period of rapid formation then loss of spines in the first few postnatal months. We have now examined this phenomenon in more detail comparing proximal, intermediate and distal regions of the dendrites for timing of the production and loss of spines for different ages of normal animals and animals reared under conditions of visual deprivation.

For normal 4Ca neurons peak spine coverage occurs as a wave moving in time down the dendrites from distal to proximal over the period from 2-4 months of postnatal age. For the 4CB neurons peak spine populations occur at 2-3 months of age on the intermediate and distal segments, but nearer 6 months on the proximal segments. Peak spine coverage on all dendritic segments is markedly increased above the normal in 4CB neurons (but not in 4Ca) when animals are reared with bilateral eyelid suture to 3 months of age; however, animals reared to 5 years of age with bilateral closure have neurons with normal adult spine coverage. Rearing in the dark to 3 and 6 months of age causes marked retardation in both spine acquisition and loss on all segments, and an overall reduction in peak spine coverage on both a and B neurons. Monocular rearing retards spine loss on the distal dendrite segments of a and B neurons.

These investigations reveal a complex set of maturational events in synapse formation occurring during the first few postnatal months of life. The time of these events is in part innate and in part determined by the quality of the stimuli driving activity of the visual pathways.

CYTOPROTECTIVE EFFECT OF ILOPROST ON CORTICAL BRAIN TISSUE GRAFTS IN RATS

S. Palaoglu[1], A. Erbengi[1], A. Sav[2], S. Kaya[3], T. Erbengi[3], R.K. Turker[4]
1) Department of Neurosurgery, Medical Faculty of Hacettepe University, Ankara
2) Department of Pathology, State Hospital of Numune, Ankara
3) Department of Histology and Embryology, Medical Faculty of Istanbul University
4) Department of Pharmacology, Medical Faculty of Ankara University
TURKEY

The cytoprotective effect of iloprost was studied on isolated embryonic cortical brain tissue grafts of rats, using light and transmission electron microscopy. The brain tissue pieces were stored either in saline or 50 ng/ml iloprost solution for 30 minutes, 3, 6, 24 hours at $+4^{\circ}C$. It was demonstrated that iloprost significantly protected the neuronal integration of the tissue pieces compared with saline preserved pieces. Tissues preserved in iloprost showed only minimal dissolution of the tissue with minimal extracellular edema only in the later stages of preservation. Afterwards, the cytoprotective effect of iloprost on the viability and survival of embryonic cortical brian tissue grafts were examined ultrastructurally under light and electron microscopy 4 weeks after a transplantation surgery. It was shown that neural grafts awaited in iloprost solution (50 ng/ml) for 3 hours were more or less in a normal cytoarchitecture compared to saline preserved grafts. Moreover, it was demonstrated that 4 weeks after transplantation, graft tissues stored in iloprost solution for 3 hours before implantation maintained a successful survival. Thus, a higher cellular population with new vascularizaton areas, preservation of myelin formation were accepted as a desirable integration of the graft tissue into the host brain tissue.

References:
1) Demirel, E., Turker, R.K., 1989, Possible calcium channel modulating activity of iloprost in rabbit isolated vascular segments, *Gen. Pharmacol.* (in press).
2) Finger, S., Dunnett, S.B., 1989, Nimodipine enhances growth and vascularization of neural grafts, *Exp. Neurol.*, 104:1-9.
3) Houle, J.D., Das, G.D., 1980, Freezing and transplantation of brain tissue in rats, *Experientia*, 1114-1115.
4) Korfali, E., Doygun, M., Ulus IH, Rakunt C, Aksoy K, 1988, Effects of neuronotrophic factors on adrenal medulla grafts implanted into adult rat brains, *Neurosurg.*, 22:994-998.
5) Langkopf, B., Rebmann, U., Schabel J, Pauer HD, Heymann H, Forster W, 1986, Improvement in preservation of ischemically imparied renal transplants of pigs by iloprost (ZK 36374), *Prost. Leuk Md.*, 21:23-29.
6) Palaoglu, S., Benli, K., Pamir, N., Erbengi, T., Erbengi, A., 1988, Examination of autologous and embryonic cortical brain tissue transplantation to adult brain cortex in rats, *Surg. Neurol.*, 29:183-190.
7) Renkawek, K., Herbaczynska-Cedro, K., Mossakowshi, J.M., 1986, The effect of porstacyclin on the morphological and enzymatic properties of CNS cultures exposed to anoxia, *Acta. Neurol. Scand.*, 73:11-21.
8) Turker, R.K., Demirel, E., Ercan, Z.S., 1988, Iloprost preserves kidney function against anoxia, *Prostaglandins Leukotrienes and Essential Fatty Acids,* 31:45-52.

VEIN-SPECIFIC EXTRACELLULAR ANTIGENS IN THE WING OF *DROSOPHILA MELANOGASTER*

P.B. Snyder, M.A. Murray and J. Palka
Department of Zoology, University of Washington
Seattle, WA 98115, USA

Prompted by an interest in the mechanisms of axon navigation employed by pioneer mechanosensory axons in the *Drososphila* wing, we have been using monoclonal antibodies (MAbs) generated against prepupal wings (2-6 hr after pupariation [AP] as probes to investigate the molecular landscape of the wing epithelium. We have isolated two MAbs which, in the wing blade, bind preferentially to the longitudinal veins (most strongly to L3, L4 and L5). Studies of the temporal development of the spatial patterning of the two antigens reveal that, though their patterns are similar after about 4 hr AP, they have very different distributions prior to this point. Prior to the flattening of the wing blade, 6G7 is uniformly distributed throughout the lumen of the wing; it becomes vein-limited only later. 2G2, by contrast, is initially present in a diffuse pattern with concentrations along the wing margin. However, by 2 hr SP (prior to morphological differentiation of the veins), it is already associated with presumptive vein precursors.

Both antigens show altered distributions in wings derived from flies in which vein formation has been genetically suppressed. Neither antigen is limited in expression to the wing. Staining is also seen in other imaginal disc derivatives and in basement membrane associated with gut, CNS and body wall muscle. The pattern of staining exhibited by the two MAbs in other tissues is not identical. Examination of tissue sections reveals that the antigens are extracellular and associated with the basal surface of the wing epithelium.

The highly patterned distribution of 2G2 and 6G7 seen in the wing is in marked contrast to other extracellular matrix proteins, such as laminin and fibronection, which have very uniform distribution in the wing. While it is not likely that these antigens are directly involved in axonal navigation, they may mediate cell-cell adhesion and/or tissue morphogenesis.

DEVELOPMENT OF *XENOPUS LAEVIS* TROCHLEAR MOTONEURONS

Ronald Sonntag and Bernd Fritzsch
University of Bielefeld, Faculty of Biology
4800 Bielefeld, FRG

Throughout vertebrate evolution, the trochlear nucleus innervates a single eye muscle, the superior oblique (SOM)[1,2]. Because of this fact and its distinct anatomical features[3] - the trochlear nerve (N.IV) is the only motor nerve which crosses dorsally at the caudal midbrain - the trochlear system is ideally suited for comparative developmental studies in a homologous system that has conserved its basic function, eye rotation.

During ontogeny of bird trochlear motoneurons and of limb innervating spinal motoneurons, an early phase of proliferation results in more than twice the adult numbers of motoneurons. A phase of motoneuron death establishes the adult motoneuron number. In amniotes it is suggested that motoneuron death is regulated by a process of numerical mathing with primary myotubes[4], whereas recent data of frog lumbar motoneurons do not support a numerical matching[5].

In amphibians both processes, motoneuron death and proliferation, occur simultaneously after the first motoneurons reached the SOM[6,7]. ^{3}H-thymidine injections at different developmental stages followed by HRP-filling of trochlear motoneurons 4-6 weeks later[7] showed that the proliferation ends later than the decrease in numbers. The full establishment of adult motoneuron numbers is reached at metamorphosis (Figure). We found no primary motoneurons as defined by established criteria such as birth date and morphology[8]. However the high ratio of innervation until

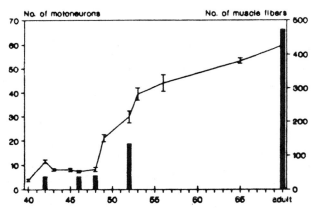

Fig: In *Xenopys laevis* the number of trochlear motoneurons decreases during st. 42-46 from a mean of 11.6 to 7.5. After st. 48 the number increases until st. 65 to a mean of 52 motoneurons. Mean +/- sem are shown. Bars indicate the mean number of muscle fibers. Although the muscle fiber number increases after st. 48 the motoneuron:muscle fiber ratio remains at about 1:4.5 until st. 52. In contrast, the adult ratio is 1:8. The x-axis indicates developmental stages.

premetamorphic st.52 probably reflects physiological properties of the larval oculomotor system, which may be different from the adult (Figure).

To investigate a possible pioneering role of the earliest born and most caudal situated trochlear motorneurons[7], we severed the N.IV axons during their contralateral decussation in the velum medullare. Surgery of N.IV axons in embryonic *Xenopus* (st. 34-36) resulted in small numbers of trochlear motoneurons innervating the SOM at st.56. This small population included the most caudal motorneurons as well as ipsilateral motoneurons, which are not present at any stage in normal animals. Axonal surgery at st. 40-48 resulted in fibers of the oculomotor nerve (N.III) innervating the SOM, while in numerous animals no regeneration of N.IV was observed[9]. These results confirm recent data on regeneration of N.III and N.IV[10] and extend them by showing differences in the regenerative capability depending on the age of the animal.

In conclusion the trochlear system in *Xenopus* laevis which is functional throughout development is subject to continuous changes with regard to insertion of new muscle fibers and motoneurons and shows complex responses to trochlear axon surgery during ontogeny. *Supported by the DFG (SFB 223).*

References:
1) Fritzsch & Sonntag, 1988, *Cell Tiss. Res.*, 252:223-229.
2) Fritzsch & Sonntag, 1989, in: "Dynamics and Plasticity of Neuronal Systems," Elsner& Singer, eds., Stuttgart, Thieme, p337.
3) Fritzsch & Sonntag, 1987, *Anat. Embryol.*, 177:105-114.
4) Tanaka & Landmesser, 1986, *J. Neurosci.*, 6:2889-99.
5) Lamb et al., 1988, in: "Developmental neurobiology of the frog," Pollack & Bibb, eds., A.R. Liss, New York, pp. 53-76.
6) Sonntag & Fritzsch, 1987, *Neurosci. Lett.*, 77:143-148
7) Sonntag & Fritzsch, 1989, *Progr. Zool.*, 37 (in press).
8) Metcalfe & Westerfield, this volume.
9) Sonntag & Fritzsch, 1989, *Soc. Neurosci. Abstr.*
10) Scherer, 1986, *J. Neurosci.*, 6:764-773.

NEURONAL MATURATION AND AXON GUIDANCE IN THE MOUSE TRIGEMINAL SYSTEM: AN IMMUNOHISTOCHEMICAL STUDY

D.Y.R. Stainier and W. Gilbert
Biological Laboratories, Harvard University
Cambridge, MA 02138, USA

We are investigating the outgrowth and pathfinding characteristics of the trigeminal sensory neurons in the embryonic mouse.

Wholemount preparations and cryostat sections of E9 and E12 mouse embryos are being processed immunohistochemically with several MAb's, each with a different specificity. MAb B30 (Stainer, D. and W. Gilbert, *J. Neurosci.*, 9:2468) stains the surface of mesencephalic trigeminal neurons (mesV) in the CNS as well as other sensory neurons in the cranial ganglia (including the trigeminal ganglion) and dorsal root ganglia. MAb E1.9 labels growing axons and cell bodies of various sensory neurons in the CNS and PNS as well as some motor neurons. E1.9 immunoreactivity exhibits a precise temporal and spatial regulation, appearing first in the CNS at late E8 and disappearing by E12.

By early E9, sparsely distributed E1.9 immunoreactive neurons in the presumptive trigeminal ganglion send out short axons. The first outgrowth defines the ophthalmic projection and axons grow out as individual fibers, each growth cone growing independently in a common direction. Shortly after, other neurons send out axons that form the maxillary and mandibular projections. By late E9, B30 immunoreactivity defines mesV neurons as they project axons from their midbrain location to the brainstem where they exit the CNS at the pontine region. These central axons mix with B30 immunoreactive neurons and axons of the trigeminal ganglion and join one of the three projections. At this stage B30 reveals the true bipolarity of the trigeminal ganglion neurons; they send short processes dorsally that enter the CNS at the pontine region while their peripheral processes are already quite long. By early E10, the ophthalmic projection has already reached past the eye cup where axons are sending short collaterals. While leading axons still behave as pioneer axons, later ones seem to join nerve bundles.

By late E10, early E11, the leading axons seem to have reached the vicinity fo their targets and more axons can be seen joining the nerve bundles as they leave the ganglion. Indeed, B30 immunoreactivity clearly shows at this stage three distinct axon bundles leaving the ganglion. This separation originates inside the ganglion as trigeminal neurons, by now pseudounipolar, seem to distribute themselves according to their general target area. Shortly after that, E1.9 immunoreactivity disappears while the B30 antigens are detectable throughout synaptogenesis and until about two weeks after birth.

INVESTIGATIONS OF THE FORMATION OF ORDERED RETINOTECTAL PROJECTIONS TO ROTATED TECTA

Jeremy S.H. Taylor and R.V. Stirling
Department of Human Anatomy, University of Oxford, Oxford OX1 3QX, UK and
Eye Research Institute, Boston, MA, USA

The results of experiments in which the tectal precursor tissue of *Xenopus* was rotated, suggested that the polarity of the retinotectal projection did not always conform with the rostrocaudally reversed structure of the tectum[1]. This implied that the cues orienting the topography of the retinotectal projection are not specifically related to the polarity of the tectum. This suggestion has long been in need of substantiation using more modern methods of analysis.

We rotated the embryonic dorsal midbrain precursor and allowed animals to survive to post-metamorphoic juvenile frogs. HRP was used to label selected populations of retinal ganglion cell axons, allowing the route of the optic tract and both the topography and orientation of the retinotectal projection, to be determined. In some cases electrophysiological recording of the retinotectal projection was made prior to HRP labelling.

In all cases where retinal axons projected to a rotated tectum (as determined by its rostrocaudally reversed structure), the pattern of innervation was correspondingly reversed. Fibres from temporal retina terminated caudally and those from nasal retina more rostrally. Interestingly, the polarity of the projection across the mediolateral axis of the tectum was normal. Where the embryonic operation results in a splitting of the tectum, the orientation of the projection was normal to the unrotated part-tectum and reversed over the rotated part-tectum. With the exception of a few single fibres, the direction of innervation was always reversed from caudal to rostral, and arose from an abnormally caudal optic tract. The internal order of the projections appeared to be less precise than normal, but was retinotopic. Of 112 projections we have analysed we have not found evidence for a separate polarity of the projection when compared with that of the tectum.

These results shed doubt on the idea of modifiable tectal labels and of a "diencephalic organizer". Our results support the idea that retinal axons recognize rostrocaudal tectal polarity[2], and that they progressively shift their terminations with the growth of the tectum.

References:
1) Chung, S-H and Cooke, J., 1978, *Proc. R. Soc. Lond. [Biol]*, 201:335.
2) Walter, J. Kern-Veits, B., Huf, J., Stolz, B. and Bonhoeffer, F., 1987, *Development*, 101:685.

THE FORMATION OF THE RETINOTOPIC MAP IN THE MAMMALIAN GENICULO-CORTICAL PROJECTION

Andrew J. Trevelyan and Ian D. Thompson
University Laboratory of Physiology
Parks Road, Oxford OX1 3 PT, UK

We are using a double-label protocol to study the precision of the geniculo-cortical projection. Our aim is to determine how the projection develops prior to the eyes opening, and to what extent the adult pattern is moulded by early visual experience. The protocol, using latex microspheres conjugated to two different fluorochromes, is being evaluated in adult hamsters. Separate injections of the fluorescent tracers are made in area 17 and the pattern of labelling in the dorsal lateral geniculate nucleus (dLGN) is analysed under an epifluorescence microscope. By varying the distance between injection sites, the precision of the map can be determined from the degree of overlap of the two populations of fluorescently labelled cells in the dLGN, whilst the proportion of double-labelled cells indicates whether any imprecision is due to the size of arborization or the scatter of axons. After completing a description of the development in normal animals, we hope to study the effects of albinism and monocular enucleation.

DEVELOPMENT OF TECTAL NEURONS IN THE PERCIFORM TELEOST *HAPLOCHROMIS BURTONI*: A GOLGI STUDY

Claudia Wilm and Bernd Fritzsch
Faculty of Biology, University of Bielefeld
P.O. Box 8640, D-4800 Bielefeld 1, FRG

The differentiation of tectum mesencephali of *Haplochromis burtoni* (Teleostei, Cichlidae) was studied using a modified Golgi rapid impregnation[1]. The tectum serves orientation and movement of the eyes and the body, essential for food location. We wanted to know, whether the need for early function of the teleostean brain as compared to birds and mammals, is reflected in the mode of tectal development. The tectum of teleosts serves integation of several modaliites, the afferents of which are stratified in four distinct tectal layers[2]. The main feature of tectal neurons is the ramification of their dendrites also in specific tectal layers. Therefore the pattern of lamination of the tectum is reflected both in the dendritic stratification of tectal neurons and the projection of fibers from various sources. Our analysis concentrated on the gradient of differentiation of four neuronal types, type I, IIIu, VI and XII[2] in 15-day-old larvae. The essential results of the developmental study are as follows[3]:

1. The tectum of 10- to 18-day-old larvae exhibits a gradient in maturation with the most differentiated cells at the rostral pole and the undifferentiated ones at the caudal U-shaped margin of the tectum. The gradient of maturation corresponds to the mode of tectal growth[4].

2. Morphogenesis and growth are largely independent developmental events. Tectal neurons first develop their typical dendritic morphology. The characteristic tectal lamination, as indicated by the spatial relationships of the dendrites of tectal neurons, is acquired already in 15-day-old larvae as a miniature of the adult pattern. In a second step, the dendritic field of tectal neurons more than doubles in size in radial and horizontal direction without changing the characteristic morphology and position relative to other types of tectal neurons. Intersegments of dendrites elongate considerably. Dendritic and axonal reorganization and/or intersegmental growth may take place. No study on other brain areas in vertebrates shows a comparable developmental mode. This developmental mode may reflect the need for early functioning of the developing tectum of teleost larvae.

3. The tectal cell types I and VI show variable positions of their perikaryon in 15-day-old larvae, but not in adults. It is suggested that they translocate their perikaryon inside their stem dendrite, while their dendrites are already well developed. *Supported by the DFG (Fr 572).*

References:
1) Wilm, C. and Fritzsch, B., 1985, *Mikroskopie*, 42:252-258.
2) Meek, J., 1983, *Brain Res. Rev.*, 6:247-297.
3) Wilm, C. and Fritzsch, B., 1989, *Dev. Brain Res.*, 47:35-52.
4) Raymond, P.A., 1986, *J. Neurosci.*, 6: 2479-2488.

INDUCTION OF AN IPSILATERAL RETINOFUGAL PROJECTION IN THE BONY FISH, *HAPLOCHROMIS BURTONI* (CICHLIDAE)

Claudia Wilm and Bernd Fritzsch
Faculty of Biology, University of Bielefeld
P.O. Box 8640, D-4800 Bielefeld 1, FRG

Most teleosts possess only a small ipsilateral retinotectal projection or none at all. In contrast, regenerating optic projections show transient errors, such as increased numbers of ipsilaterally coursing fibers, which are subsequently largely eliminated[1]. We studied the conditions for the development and maintenance, as well as the specificity of one of these aberrant projections, the enhanced ipsilateral retinofugal projections (EIRPs) in early juveniles and adults of *Haplochromis burtoni* (Cichlidae). Retinal projections were labelled in three different ways: a) with HRP, b) bilaterally labelled with fluorescent dextran-amines, or c) with the lipophilic fluorescent dye diI in aldehyde fixed animals.

After unilateral nerve crush (NCuni) an EIRP develops initially (seven days postcrush)[2]. Persisting EIRPs (four months and longer postoperatively) exist in only 10% (5 out of 50) of the enucleated animals (EN), in none of the animals with an unilaterally crushed optic nerve (NCuni), in 79% of the animals with bilaterally crushed optic nerves (NCbi), and in all of the animals which were unilaterally enucleated and which received the remaining optic nerve additionally crushed (EN + NC). This indicates that nerve crush leads to ipsilaterally growing fibers, most likely because of the disturbed fiber order in the regenerating nerve and tract. We believe that in the five animals with an EIRP after unilateral enucleation the remaining optic nerve was disturbed by the operation. The long term maintenance of an ipsilateral projection requires either a disturbed (NCbi) or an eliminated contralateral projection (EN + NC). This may lead to alternating stripes of retinofugal fibers of each eye on the tectum of animals with bilaterally crushed (NCbi) optic nerves. Ipsilateral fibers of the EIRP recross at the rostral diencephalon, which is unusual in normal projections. It is in this area of the monocular fiber-crossing[3], where the rearrangement of retinal fibers from the optic nerve into the optic tract configuration takes place, that regenerating fibers are misguided to the ipsilateral brain side. Therefore, not fiber-fiber interactions between the fibers of the two eyes but the fiber-substrate interaction leads to ipsilateral projections when the ingrowing fibers are disordered.

The EIRP is specific for all optic areas. In long term denervated animals, unilaterally enucleated with 6.5 days or 26 days of age and which received a crush of the remaining optic nerve at 1 to 1.5 years later, the probability of reinnervation is reduced for some ipsilateral diencephalic areas. However, the ability to develop an EIRP is independent of the age of the animal, independent of the time lapse between enucleation and nerve lesion and independent of persisting debris. In juveniles the size of the EIRP is independent of the time lapse between enucleation and nerve lesion. But in long term enucleated animals, which developed without an optic projection of the ipsilateral side, the size of the EIRP and its tectal extent is reduced compared to animals with an intact optic projection until the operation. *Supported by the DFG (FR 572).*

References:
1) Springer, A.D., 1980, *Brain Res.*, 199:214-218.
2) Wilm, C. and Fritzsch, B., 1989, in: "Dynamics and Plasticity in Neuronal Systems," N. Elsner and W. Singer, eds., Thieme, Stuttgart, New York, p. 44.
3) Maggs, A.and Scholes, J., 1986, *J. Neurosci.*, 6:424-438.

THE PATHWAYS FOLLOWED BY REGENERATING FIBRES AT THE OPTIC CHIASMA IN *XENOPUS*

M.A. Wilson and R.M. Gaze
MRC Neural Development & Regeneration Group, Department of Zoology
University of Edinburgh, King's Buildings
West Mains Road, Edinburgh, EH9 3JT, SCOTLAND

In a midlarval *Xenopus* the older optic nerve fibres (myelinated and unmyelinated) cross deep in the chiasma and then pass up the deeper part of the optic tract, whereas the younger fibres cross superficially and run up the optic tract at the diencephalic margin. When an optic nerve is crushed and allowed to regenerate, many of the fibres reach the chiasma within 10 days. In contrast to the distribution of normal fibres, regenerating fibres usually all pass up the outer edge of the diencephalon. It is possible that this behaviour is the result of regeneration fibres following residual undegenerated fibres of the original projection.

If an eye is removed, 5 days later a substantial number of apparently intact fibres can be seen in the degenerating nerve close to the chiasma. These fibres label well when HRP is applied to the re-severed stump of the nerve, and they can be followed into the optic tract.

Ten days after eye removal a few persistent unmyelinated fibres are still present in the nerve close to the chiasma. They are always at the periphery of the nerve and stain poorly with uranyl acetate and lead citrate. They can occasionally be labelled with HRP via the residual nerve and followed into the diencephalon bridge.

In normal tadpoles, older optic fibres (unmyelinated and myelinated) make a herring-bone pattern as they cross deep in the chiasma. Ten days after eye removal, degenerating fibres are found in this deep position, usually unaccompanied by unmyelinated fibres oriented in the same direction. In this region all, or most, unmyelinated fibres appear to run in one direction only, and to come from the other eye.

It would seem that the residual unmyelinated fibres present in the optic nerve at the time newly regenerating fibres reach the diencephalon, comprise some of the smallest (and youngest) optic fibres; and it is possible that they lead regenerating fibres into the ventral parts of the chiasma and thus into the peripheral part of the optic tract.

CHANGES IN MORPHOLOGY OF UNCROSSED RETINAL GANGLION CELLS IN HAMSTERS AFTER REMOVAL OF ONE EYE AT BIRTH

Richard J.T. Wingate
University Laboratory of Physiology
Parks Road, Oxford OX1 3 PT, UK

I have used an *in vitro* technique to compare the detailed morphology of populations of retinal ganglion cells with different axonal targets. In the normal adult retina the majority of cells outside the temporal crescent project to the contralateral side of the brain, while the majority of the ipsilateral projection is from the temporal crescent. However, a small population of developmentally aberrant cells projects ipsilaterally from the nasal retina. By making a unilateral injection of rhodamine-latex microspheres into the terminal nuclei, these different populations are retrogradely labelled. Filled cell bodies are located in an *in vitro* retina preparation using a fixed stage compound microscope equipped with epifluorescence and Nomarski optics and then selectively impaled with a low resistance, glass microelectrode. Detailed morphology is revealed by the intracellular injection of lucifer yellow. Aberrant retinal ganglion cells are found to have abnormal dendritic arbors and an incomplete coverage. By removing one eye at birth, developmental cell death in aberrant cells is reduced. Cells from this increased population are found to have an apparently normal morphology.

LESION INDUCED MHC EXPRESSION IN THE DEVELOPING BRAIN

Kathleen T. Yee, Ava M. Smetanka, Kanchan Rao, Raymond D. Lund
Department of Neurobiology, Anatomy and Cell Science
University of Pittsburgh, Pittsburgh, PA, USA

In most tissues, cells express major histocompatibility complex (MHC) antigens. These molecules located on the cell surface serve to present foreign antigens to lymphocytes and thus initiate an immune rejection response. Cells of the mature central nervous system do not normally express MHC antigens and, accordingly, tissue can frequently survive transplantation to the central nervous system even though donor and host may be incompatible. It is clear, however, that not all transplants survive without rejection, and one factor is the age of the host at the time of transplantation. Thus, embryonic mouse retina transplanted into rat brain during the first postnatal week usually survives for many months. However, mouse retina transplanted into older hosts undergoes rapid rejection. Grafts placed in the dorsal midbrain of neonates which had become incorporated into host tissue can be induced to reject at later times by removing the host eye and causing degeneration in the vicinity of the graft. We have found that eye removal, alone, in mature animals, induces expression fo MHC antigens. Class I MHC antigens are mainly expressed in non-myelinated terminal areas and in the optic tract, while class II MHC antigen expression is found in areas of myelinated optic terminal degeneration.

Why, therefore, do grafts not reject when placed in neonatal brains? Why does the massive optic axon death that occurs in the first postnatal week not provoke rejection of grafts? And why does eye removal performed on young animals also not cause graft rejection? Two possible explanations are that the host immune response is immature at birth, and that MHC expression is regulated differently in young animals. To test the latter, we have used antibodies, OX-18 (against class I MHC antigens) and OX-6 (against class II MHC antigens) to examine expression patterns in normal young rats, and rats in which one eye had been removed. As in adults, normal young rats do not express class II MHC antigens, but in contrast, large areas of brain contain cells which express the class I antigen. After eye removal at birth, a focus of class I expression is seen in the superior colliculus and in the optic tract by postnatal day (PND) 5. In contrast, the first evidence of class II expression is seen in the optic tract after eye removal on PND 12, and in the superior colliculus after enucleation on PND 15.

It is suggested, since class II expression in adults is concentrated in areas of myelin degeneration and since it is first detected at the time of onset of myelination, that induction of class II expression is caused by a product of myelin degeneration. Thus, in the absence of myelin, the cell death that occurs in the developing brain is protected from immune surveillance by T helper lymphocyte mediated events. The appearance of class I MHC antigens in young brains suggests a somewhat different pattern of regulation than that causing expression of MHC class II antigens.

PARTICIPANTS

Mr. Frederic Assal
Institut d'anatomie
Université de Lausanne
CH1005 Lausanne
SWITZERLAND

Dr. Jonathan Bacon
School of Biological Sciences
University of Sussex
Falmer, Brighton BN19QG
UNITED KINGDOM

Dr. Peré Berbel
University of Alicante
Department of Histology
Alicante
SPAIN

Ms. Ann Blake
Institute of Neuroscience
University of Oregon
Eugene, OR 97403
USA

Dr. Friedrich Bonhoeffer
MPI für Entwicklungsbiologie
Spemannstr. 35
D7400 Tubingen
W. GERMANY

Ms. Janet Braisted
Department of Anatomy
  and Cell Biology
University of Michigan Medical School
4610 Med. Sci. II Bldg.
Ann Arbor, MI 48109
USA

Dr. Eli Brenner
Bollenhofsestraat 10
3572 VN Utrecht
THE NETHERLANDS

Dr. J. A. Campos-Ortega
Institut für Entwicklungsphysiologie
University of Cologne
Gyrhofstrasse 17
5000 Cologne 41
W. GERMANY

Dr. C. Dambly-Chaudiere
Laboratoire de Génétique
Université Libre de Bruxelles
Rue des Chevaux 67
1640 Rhode St. Genese
BELGIUM

Dr. Stephen Easter
Department of Biology
University of Michigan
2109 Nat. Sci. Bldg.
Ann Arbor, MI 48109
USA

Dr. Yves Frégnac
Neurobiology Research Center
University of Alabama at Birmingham
Birmingham, AL 35294
USA

Dr. Carl Fulwiler
Department of Cell and Molecular Biology
Harvard University
Cambridge, MA 02138
USA

Dr. Patricia Gaspar
INSERM U-106
Histologie normale et pathologique
  du systeme nerveux
Hopital de la Salpetriere
47, Boulevard de l'Hopital
75651 Paris Cedex 13
FRANCE

Dr. R. M. Gaze
MRC Neural Unit
Department of Zoology
University of Edinburgh
W. Mains Rd.
Edinburgh 3H9 3JT
UNITED KINGDOM

Dr. Alain Ghysen
Laboratoire de Génétique
Université Libre de Bruxelles
Rue des Chevaux 67
1640 Rhode St. Genese
BELGIUM

Douglas Gooday
Zoology Department
University of Edinburgh
W. Mains Rd.
Edinburgh 3H9 3JT
UNITED KINGDOM

Ms. Megan Grether
Department of Biology
MIT E25-442
Cambridge, MA 02139
USA

Dr. Mark Hankin
Department of Neurobiology, Anatomy,
   and Cell Science
818A Scaife Hall
University of Pittsburgh School of
   Medicine
3550 Terrace St.
Pittsburgh, PA 15261
USA

Dr. Peter Hitchcock
W. K. Kellog Eye Center
1000 Wall St.
Ann Arbor, MI 48105
USA

Dr. Giorgio Innocenti
Institut d'anatomie
Rue du Bugnon 9
CH1005 Lausanne
SWITZERLAND

Dr. Daniel Jay
Department of Neurobiology
Harvard Medical School
Boston, MA 02138
USA

Dr. Fernando Jiménez
Centro de Biologia Molecular
Facultad de Ciencias
Canto Blanco
Madrid 28049
SPAIN

Dr. Peter Kind
Department of Psychology
Dalhousie University
Halifax NS B3H 4J1
CANADA

Dr. Anthony LaMantia
Department of Anatomy and Neurobiology
Washington University
Box 8108
660 S. Euclid Ave.
St. Louis, MO 63110
USA

Dr. Jennifer Lund
Western Psychiatric Institute and Clinic
University of Pittsburgh
3811 O'Hara St.
Pittsburgh, PA 15213-2593
USA

Dr. Raymond Lund
Department of Neurobiology, Anatomy
   and Cell Science
University of Pittsburgh Medical School
3550 Terrace St.
Pittsburgh, PA 15261
USA

Ms. Riva Marcus
Department of Biology
Univertsity of.Michigan
Ann Arbor, MI 48109-1048
USA

Mr. René Marois
c/o Prof. T. Carew
Department of Psychology
Yale University
11A Yale Station
New Haven, CT 06520
USA

Dr. Ian Meinertzhagen
Department of Psychology
Dalhousie University
Halifax, NS B3H 4J1
CANADA

Ms. Clare Meissirel
INSERM U 94
Lyon (Bron)
FRANCE

Dr. Walter Metcalfe
Department of Biology
Institute of Neuroscience
University of Oregon
Eugene, OR 97403
USA

Dr. Zoltan Molnar
Department of Physiology
Oxford University
Oxford, OX1 3PT
UNITED KINGDOM

Dr. Selcuk Palaoglu
PK 760 Kizilay
06425 Ankara
TURKEY

Dr. Rolf D. Potthoff
Universitat Lubeck
Inst. f. Med. Psychology
Lubeck
GERMANY

Dr. Jorge J. Prieto
Department of Histology
University of Alicante
03690 Alicante
SPAIN

Dr. Dale Purves
Department of Anatomy and Neurobiology
Washington University Medical School
660 S. Euclid Ave.
St. Louis, MO 63110
USA

Dr. Pamela Raymond
Department of Anatomy and Cell Biology
University of Michigan Medical School
Ann Arbor, MI 48109-0616
USA

Dr. Linda Ross
Department of Biology
2109 Nat. Sci. Bldg.
Univeristy of Michigan
Ann Arbor, MI 48109-1048
USA

Dr. Mar Ruiz-Gómez
Laboratoire de Génétique
Faculté des sciences
Université Libre de Bruxelles
Rue des Chevaux 67
1640 Rhode St. Genese
BELGIUM

Dr. S. Murray Sherman
Department of Neurobiology
  and Behavior
SUNY
Graduate Biology Building
Stony Brook, NY 11794
USA

Dr. Daniel Shulz
Neurobiology Laboratory
Université de Paris Sud
Batiment 440
F 91405 Orsay Cedex
FRANCE

Dr. Peter Snyder
Department of Zoology NJ-15
University of Washington
Seattle, WA 98195
USA

Ronald Sonntag
University of Bielefeld
Faculty of Biology
P.O.B. 8640
D-4800 Bielefeld 1
WEST GERMANY

Dr. Constantino Sotelo
Laboratoire de Neuromorphologie
INSERM U 106
Hopital de la Salpetriere
F 75651 Paris Cedex 13
FRANCE

Didier Stainier
Department of Cellular and
  Developmental Biology
The Biological Laboratories
16 Divinity Ave
Harvard University
Cambridge, MA 02138
USA

Dr. Larry Stanford
Department of Structural
  and Functional Science
University of Wisconsin
School of Veterinary Medicine
2015 Linden Drive, W.
Madison, WI 53706
USA

Dr. Jeremy S. H. Taylor
Department of Human Anatomy
University of Oxford
South Parks Rd.
Oxford OX13QX
UNITED KINGDOM

Mr. Andrew Trevelyan
Department of Physiology
Oxford University
Oxford OX1 3PT
UNITED KINGDOM

Jacques Van Helden
Laboratoire de Genetique
Université Libre de Bruxelles
Rue des Chevaux
1640 Rhode St. Genese
BELGIUM

Dr. Monte Westerfield
Institute of Neuroscience
University of Oregon
Eugene, OR 97403
USA

Ms. Claudia Wilm
c/o Bernd Fritzsch
University of Bielefeld
Faculty of Biology
P O B 8690
48 Bielefeld 1
WEST GERMANY

Ms. Margaret Wilson
Department of Zoology
University of Edinburgh
Edinburgh 3H9 3JT
UNITED KINGDOM

Mr. Richard Wingate
Department of Physiology
Oxford University
Oxford OX1 3PT
UNITED KINGDOM

Ms. Kathleen Yee
Department of Neurobiology, Anatomy,
   and Cell Science
818 B Scaife Hall
University of Pittsburgh Medical School
Pittsburgh, PA 15261
USA

INDEX

Acetylcholine receptor, 44-45
Acetylcholinesterase histochemistry, 55
Acheta domesticus (cricket), 5-6
  giant interneuron, 5-6
  sensory system, cercal, 5-6
  X-neuron arborization, 6
Achaete-scute (gene) complex, 12-13, 23
  and DNA, 12, 13
Animal size
  and neuron morphology, 99-105
Antigen Thy-1, 82
Ambystoma tigrinum, 50, 55
Arborization
  axonal, 86-87, 148
  dendritic, 102
  neuronal, 6
  retinogeniculate, 148
Association principle neuronal, 154
Astrocyte, 82, 121
Axon
  arborization, 86-87, 148
  assay, 63-64
  blueprint hypothesis, 53-54
  callosal, 167
  in cat, 114-118
  and cobalt, 49
  fasciculation, 4, 62; *see also* Fascilin
  and fibronectin, 45
  and ganglion, retinal,63-65, 71
  and glycoprotein, 4
  growth, 42, 43, 54, 59-60,173
    cone, 81
  guidance of, 59-68, 81-89,171-173, 177
    tropic, 81
  and laminin, 45
  maintenance, trophic, 81
  mechanosensory, 175
  in monkey, 117
  navigation of, 175
  in nervous system, central (CNS), 16-18
  optical, 49, 50, 54, 56
  outgrowth, 84-86
  pathfinding of, 4, 81
  pathway of, 16-18
  pioneer -, 54, 75
  position-dependent, 43

Axon (*cont.*)
  preganglionic, 100, 102
  regeneration of, 54
  retinal, 60-67, 77, 178
  retinogeniculate, 142, 147-149
  staining of, 55
  survival in cortex, cerebral 119-121
  and target, role of, 18
  temporal, 64
  tracing methods for, 50
  of tract, optic, 73
  transient, 121
  transplantation of, 49
  of wing vein of *Drosophila*
    melanogaster, 175
  in zebrafish, 56

Bee, 136
Bicuculline, 154
Blastoderm, 3
Blastomere precursor cell, 42
Bouton, Synaptic, 106
Brachydanio rerio, see Zebrafish
Brain, vertebrate, 49-58, 82, 141
  formation, early, 49-58, 82
  in frog, 49-58
  in zebrafish, 55-57
  increase in
    volume, 141
    weight, 141
  postnatal, 141
Bulb, olfactory, murine, 108

α-Bungarotoxin, 44

Calbindin immunostaining, 92, 93
6-Carboxyfluorescein, 105
Cat, 114-120, 145-146, 153-165, 168-169
  behavior, 145
    visually guided, 168-169
  colliculus, superior, 146
  cortex, visual, 169
  deformation of image, 168-169
  depth perception, 169
  eyelid suture technique, 145
  flow, optic, requirements for, 168-169

Xenopus laevis (frog) *(cont.)*
  pathway, optic, in early brain, 49-53
  pioneer axon, 54, 75
  precursor tissue, tectal, rotated, 177-178
  projection
    retinofugal, 50-54
    retinotectal, 69, 85, 177-178
  retina, 33, 69, 170
  retinofugal system, 50-54
  retinotectal system, 69, 85, 177-178
  tadpole brain, 82
  tectum, 177-178
  tract, optic, 71
  visual system, 69079
    development of, 69-79
X-neuron, 6
X-pathway, 143, 145, 147

Y-cell, 150

Y-pathway, 145, 147

Zebrafish,
  axon, optical, 56
  brain formation, early 55-57
  development of, 42
    analysis, genetic, 42
  and gamma-rays, 42
  larva, 169
    phototaxis, 169
  motoneuron, primary, 41-47
  mutation, 42, 45
    spadetail, 45
  nystagmus, optokinetic, 169
  retina, 169
    development of, 169
  tracts, early, 55, 56
  and ultraviolet radiation, 42
  visual system, 169